D1709542

Drug Development

2nd Edition

Editor

Charles E. Hamner, D.V.M., Ph.D.
President
North Carolina Biotechnology Center
Research Triangle Park, North Carolina

CRC Press
Boca Raton   Ann Arbor   Boston

Library of Congress Cataloging-in-Publication Data

Drug development / editor, Charles E. Hamner.— 2nd ed.
    p.   cm.
   Includes bibliographical references.
   ISBN 0-8493-6319-5
   1. Pharmaceutical technology. 2. Pharmaceutical industry — United
States. I. Hamner, Charles E.
   [DNLM: 1. Drug Industry — United States. 2. Technology,
Pharmaceutical — United States.   QV 736 D7929]
   RS192.D77   1990
615′.19—dc20
DNLM/DLC
for Library of Congress

90-1500
CIP

This book represents information obtained from authentic and highly regarded sources. Reprinted material is quoted with permission, and sources are indicated. A wide variety of references are listed. Every reasonable effort has been made to give reliable data and information, but the author and the publisher cannot assume responsibility for the validity of all materials or for the consequences of their use.

All rights reserved. This book, or any parts thereof, may not be reproduced in any form without written consent from the publisher.

Direct all inquiries to CRC Press, Inc., 2000 Corporate Blvd., N.W., Boca Raton, Florida, 33431.

© 1990 by CRC Press, Inc.

International Standard Book Number 0-8493-6319-5

Library of Congress Card Number 90-1500
Printed in the United States

PREFACE

Hamner's new edition of *Drug Development* builds and improves upon his splendid first edition by modernizing the topics as well as adding areas which were previously ignored. The most notable addition is the two excellent chapters on biotechnology.

Overall the volume stands as a relatively comprehensive but not exhaustive summation of the complex process of drug development. It should serve as a useful tool for those charged with guiding development efforts as well as an educational tool for nontechnical managers who may be unaware of the nature and extent of the field's immense challenges.

Unless they have been close to drug development projects over a long period of time, few people understand what the tortuous pathway from discovery to market entails. It requires the carefully orchestrated coordination of divergent but interdependent technical functions — a challenge under any circumstances, but especially so when the coordination must be maintained for a decade or more. Even after this, many more years of nurturing and monitoring may be required.

It also requires the services and cooperation of people in what may be society's most sophisticated professions: chemists, biologists, engineers, physicists, computer experts, medical doctors, nurses, mathematicians, information specialists, statisticians, epidemiologists, patent lawyers, economists, accountants, marketers, planners, etc. Precisely because of its dependence on this broad range of professionals, drug development cannot be managed in the traditional sense. The "managers" must rather be strong leaders, accomplished and respected scientists themselves, who must exhibit broad vision, long-term perspective, trust in other professionals, and the ability to inspire others. Only in this way can they direct the activities of development without threatening the scientific creativity and freedom of the professionals carrying out the multitude of tasks. In this sense, the process of development is similar to the process of discovery. Both are best achieved by professionals in an atmosphere of freedom, respect, and flexibility. Managers quickly learn that reliance on conventional management practices applicable in other businesses or functions will create major problems in this unique industry.

In addition, drug development is one of the most highly regulated activities in our society. The federal agencies involved are often used as scapegoats for problems actually created by companies themselves. Although it may sound heretical for an executive from industry R & D to defend regulatory controls, they are, in fact, important and necessary. We have seen many cases of well-intentioned but poorly conceived science or enthusiastic but premature conclusions from poorly controlled clinical trials, to say nothing about "accidents" or even deliberate abuses or distortions by charlatans. The public and the ethical industry are best served by decisions based on good science, adherence to high standards, and independent, expert review of results, such as that performed by the FDA. If the industry starts with high-quality science, effective analyses and honest, responsive presentations, its regulatory problems will be few.

In this context, it is understandable that Hamner's work, while laudable, could not cover *all* aspects of drug development in satisfactory depth. Among the areas inadequately covered, and which are essential to the proper conduct of drug development in contemporary times, are (1) emphasis on certain underlying current technologies in science which are changing the basic approaches of discovery research from screening to rational processes (e.g., the "New Biology", molecular genetics, gene regulation, computer graphics, receptor advances, etc.); (2) the changing focus of discovery research from the easy diseases (infectious diseases and other acute conditions) to the more difficult chronic disorders, especially those associated with aging; (3) the growth of structural and biophysical approaches in the chemical design of new molecules; (4) the transition of toxicology to mechanistic and *in vitro* approaches, which will dominate and transform the future of this discipline (and make it an integral component of discovery research, rather than a function that just services regulatory demands); (5) the pivotal nature of drug metabolism, especially in preclinical phases, as a legitimate function inseparable from other scientific disciplines in rational drug discovery (rather than the traditional "service" role); (6) the extremely difficult, challenging, and essential role of chemistry in discovering new, simpler synthetic methods and adapting these to the practical scale-up needs of production (a *bona fide* and unique branch of chemistry); (7) the need of scientists to maintain a constant eye on the products once they are marketed, including conducting experiments for developing new indications, for just learning more, or for marketing support, as well as to monitor for unexpected adverse events which may take years to discover (and the new, legitimate discipline of pharmacoepidemiology); and (8) the emerging alliances between industrial and university laboratories.

On the whole, however, this book certainly reflects the overall flavor of drug development, as well as depicting in some depth several of the major activities involved in this lengthy and complicated process. It is a welcome addition to the bookshelves of those who work in the industry and those who wish to understand more about it.

Pedro Cuatrecasas, M.D.

EDITOR

Charles E. Hamner, Jr., D.V.M., Ph.D., is president of the North Carolina Biotechnology Center and Research Professor of Obstetrics and Gynecology at the University of North Carolina at Chapel Hill.

Dr. Hamner, 54, was Associate Vice President for Health Affairs at the University of Virginia Medical Center in Charlottesville, Virginia, where he was responsible for overseeing planning, development, and day-to-day operations at the medical center and was also a Professor of Obstetrics and Gynecology.

Dr. Hamner, a native of Schuyler, Virginia, held several administrative and research positions during his 23 years at the University of Virginia. He joined the UVA Medical Center in 1964 as an Assistant Professor of Surgery and became the director of the Division of Reproductive Biology in 1967. In 1977 he was appointed Assistant Vice President for Health Services at the medical school. Two years later he was appointed Associate Vice President for Health Affairs.

From 1974 to 1977, Dr. Hamner was also Director of Program Coordination for Research and Development at the A.H. Robbins Company in Richmond, Virginia. He coordinated an R&D budget of $14 million and the work of 284 scientists and technicians.

Dr. Hamner has a Bachelor's degree in Animal Husbandry from Virginia Polytechnic Institute and a Doctor of Veterinary Medicine Degree, a Master's Degree in Chemistry, and a Doctorate in Biochemistry, all from the University of Georgia. His specialties are the management of research and development of pharmaceuticals and the biochemistry of reproduction. He is licensed to practice veterinary medicine and surgery in Virginia and Georgia. He has served on Advisory Committees to the Rockefeller Foundation, World Health Organization, National Institutes of Health, and other state and federal agencies.

Dr. Hamner has authored more than 50 papers and is editor or co-author of 12 books on the biochemistry of reproductive biology and pharmaceutical product development. He is a member of the American Physiological Society, Society for the Study of Fertility, Society for the Study of Reproduction, Society for Experimental Biology and Medicine, and American Association for the Advancement of Science. He has been recipient of the "Sigma Xi Research Award" and a Research Cancer Development Award from the National Institutes of Health.

At the Biotechnology Center, Dr. Hamner oversees 36 full-time employees. The Center is a nonprofit corporation funded largely by the General Assembly. Its mission is to assure that North Carolina benefits economically from biotechnology. To carry out its mission, the Center promotes biotechnology research, industrial growth, and public awareness.

CONTRIBUTORS

Carlos R. Ayers, M.D.
Professor
Department of Internal Medicine
University of Virginia
Health Science Center
Charlottesville, Virginia

Alfred Burger, Ph.D.
Professor Emeritis
Department of Chemistry
University of Virginia
Charlottesville, Virginia

G. Steven Burrill, B.B.A.
National Director
High Technology Industry Services
Ernst & Young
San Francisco, California

Richard L. Chamberlain, M.S., Ph.D.
President
Medical Development Systems, Inc.
Deerfield, Illinois

Walter B. Cummings, Ph.D.
Director
Clinical Data Processing and Statistics
Burroughs Wellcome Company
Research Triangle Park, North Carolina

Mark D. Dibner, M.B.A., Ph.D.
Director
Biotechnology Information Division
North Carolina Biotechnology Center
Research Triangle Park, North Carolina

Richard E. Faust, Ph.D.
President
American Foundation for Pharmaceutical
  Education
North Plainfield, New Jersey

Ralph Fogleman, D.V.M.
Consultant to Toxicology and
  Regulatory Affairs
R. W. Fogleman & Associates
Upper Black Eddy, Pennsylvania

Gerald B. Hajian, M.S., Ph.D.
Head
Department of Statistical Services
Burroughs Wellcome Company
Research Triangle Park, North Carolina

Charles E. Hamner, D.V.M., Ph.D.
President
North Carolina Biotechnology Center
Research Triangle Park, North Carolina

David E. Jones, M.S.
Vice President
Special Products Division
A.H. Robbins Company
Richmond, Virginia

Winston Liao, M.P.H., Ph.D.
Associate Program Director
Center for Epidemiologic and
  Medical Studies
Research Triangle Institute
Research Triangle Park, North Carolina

John A. Owen, Jr., M.D.
Professor
Department of Internal Medicine
University of Virginia School of Medicine
Charlottesville, Virginia

Robert A. Paarlberg, M.S.
Manager, Washington Regulatory Liaison
U.S. Pharmaceutical Regulatory Affairs
The Upjohn Company
Kalamazoo, Michigan

William G. Pappas, J.D.
Partner
Parker, Poe, Adams & Bernstein
Raleigh, North Carolina

James W. Parker, Ph.D.
Senior Project Manager
The Upjohn Company
Kalamazoo, Michigan

Allen J. Polon, B.S.
Consultant in Pharmaceutical Marketing
Redington Beach, Florida

Kenneth D. Sibley, M.A.
Associate
Bell, Setzler, Park & Gibson
Raleigh, North Carolina

J. David Tucker, M.B.A.
Director
Logistics and Fine Chemical
  Manufacturing
Upjohn International
Kalamazoo, Michigan

Joyce Williams, M.B.A.
Vice President
Regulatory and Clinical Affairs
Telios Pharmaceuticals, Inc.
San Diego, California

Michael Williams, Ph.D., D.Sc.
Area Head
Neuroscience, D-464
Abbott Laboratories
Abbott Park, Illinois

John H. Wood, Ph.D.
Professor Emeritus
Department of Pharmacy and
  Pharmaceutics
Virginia Commonwealth University
Richmond, Virginia

ACKNOWLEDGMENTS

The compilation, review, and synthesis of these works come from a diverse group of knowledgeable authors. To form a logical and useful dissertation required a dedicated office staff and several trusted friends who have a wide range of experience in the pharmaceutical industry.

It is with great appreciation that I acknowledge Flora Moorman for her excellence in coordination and communications with the authors and consultants and filing and management of secretarial work; Barry Teater for his outstanding editorial reviews; and La Keta Elek, John Pace, and Tammy Hogan for their technical assistance. Finally, I am grateful to Dr. Pedro Cuatrecasas for the excellent preface and to each chapter author who followed the writing instructions and met the deadlines which allowed the manuscript to be delivered on schedule.

TABLE OF CONTENTS

Chapter 1

INTRODUCTION

Charles E. Hamner

Drug development continues to be a most exciting and complex business. It requires intuitiveness, entrepreneurship, attention to details, a good grasp of scientific information, and the ability to correlate basic laboratory tests and results with the clinical utilization. Although the Food and Drug Administration (FDA) has recently streamlined and clarified its new drug approval process, the bottom line remains the same: approvals are best obtained by having scientific results, both basic and clinical, that demonstrate the merits, uniqueness, and obvious advantages of a new entity in curing a disease.

A number of important scientific advances have occurred since the first edition of this book. These advances cover diverse areas from management information systems, biochemical and molecular biology/genetic engineering techniques, and bioprocessing systems to drug delivery methods. Many of the latter advancements have occurred in what is now termed the "biotechnology" industry. Therefore, several new chapters have been added and old chapters revised to reflect the changes occurring in the regulatory approach, new-product ideas, start-up of small biotechnology companies, and the extension of diagnostic and therapeutic markets. These changes will be very important to the growth of the pharmaceutical industry in the coming decade.

During preparation of the first edition three specific challenges faced the industry: how to improve productivity in research and development (R & D), how to develop better working relations with universities for transfer of biotechnology, and how to cope with inflation. The inflation problem has subsided. A number of excellent university/industrial affiliations have developed. Management of the R & D process has improved, but old problems of time lapse for FDA approval and management of information integration and accessibility remain. New challenges have emerged to include protection of intellectual properties, the patent approval process, and competition from abroad, especially Japan. These new challenges are focused in the biotechnology areas.

The amount of help the corporation derives from R & D investment is open to question because the minimum expected rate of return from investment in pharmaceutical R & D (after taxes) has been less than that of most industries; the industry, however, is reluctant to reduce R & D expenditures because of (1) the payoff potential of creating new products, (2) the hope of a major breakthrough, (3) the high profits experienced from previously marketed drugs, and (4) the recent promise of a reduction in the restrictiveness of the FDA in approving new drug applications (NDA). All of these factors would aid in developing new products and coping with competition.[1]

One of the major objectives of this book is to help solve the time and effort problems. The ultimate goal for a new-product development should be to carry out every activity correctly on the first attempt. Making this work for entire projects requires the most effective management, planning, coordination, monitoring, and control imaginable, plus considerable luck.[2] In an effort to provide insight into the problems of developing a drug and to identify practical approaches to solving these problems, practicing experts in each major area of drug development have prepared a chapter on their specific area. Their charge was to cover the key points of concern for a specified functional portion of the drug development scheme without going into great depth on scientific techniques that could be found in basic textbooks.

A number of books published in the past 20 years have taken different approaches to the discovery and development of drugs. Arnow[3] wrote a series of accounts about the discovery and development of early drugs. He pointed out that the odds for success in the search for new drugs are unbelievably small. Since the passage of the 1962 Drug Industry Act Amendments, the average number of new drugs marketed annually and the new entities in particular have appreciably diminished.

One publication has focused specifically on the development of contraceptives.[4] Many of the basic concepts leading to the discovery of original contraceptive methods were developed in the university or government laboratories. However, industry has been even more productive, since it possesses sufficient financial resources together with diversified, skilled manpower. Industry has been able to carry out the many development activities necessary throughout the various stages of chemical synthesis and analysis — pharmacology, toxicology, and clinical evaluation.

In the mid 1960s and the 1970s, there was deep concern over the reduced number of new drug approvals and the so-called "drug lag". The fact that many drugs routinely available in other countries could not be used in the U.S. spawned a plethora of meetings and publications. Wardell and Lasagna[5] examined the Drug Industry Act of 1962 (the so-called Kefauver-Harris Amendment to the Food, Drug and Cosmetic Act of 1938) to determine whether or not it constituted a turning point in the evolution of controls over the American pharmaceutical industry. They further addressed what influence the act had on the development, availability, and use of therapeutic drugs in this country, and what lessons could be derived.

Legislative and regulatory control over drugs have evolved parallel to, although somewhat behind, developments in medical and pharmaceutical sciences and biotechnology over the past century. Controls have steadily crept from purity to safety and, more recently, to concern for the efficacy of drugs and to their manner of use. The controls frequently utilized have impacted the following: (1) labeling, (2) advertising, (3) drug shipments in interstate commerce, (4) investigational plans — good clinical practices, and (5) approved drug usage. Further, certain regulations, such as those addressing good manufacturing practices and good laboratory practices, have helped eliminate unscrupulous manufacturers and developers. This book also discusses the interaction between scientific and governmental regulation and provides international comparisons in drug development with the therapeutic consequences.

A meeting held in 1975 on drug development and marketing helped to dispel the notion that drug manufacturing firms typically show relatively high rates of return on advertising and R & D.[6] Rubin[7] edited a multiauthored monograph in 1978, covering the promising therapeutic areas for drug discovery and evaluation from the vantage point of the industrial researcher. Mathieu and Murphy[8] in 1987 carefully reviewed the new regulatory environment. Williams and Malick[9] discussed the concepts of drug development and gave in-depth theoretical consideration to modern techniques for compound discovery and development of therapeutic entities. Beyer[2] published a book which addressed various teaching concepts and practices in drug discovery, as well as the need to bring new therapeutic agents to patients. The Beyer text is a fine blend of history, the scientific approach, and a variety of intangibles such as the environment, creativity, spontaneous discovery, and good fortune, which are important to overall success in drug discovery. Spilker[10] recently reviewed issues in drug discovery and the role of multinational drug companies.

REFERENCES

1. **Schwartzman, D.,** Pharmaceutical R & D expenditures and rates of return, in *Drug Development and Marketing,* Helms, R. B. Ed., American Enterprises Institute for Publishing Policy Research, Washington, D.C., 1975, 63.

2. **Beyer, K. H., Jr.,** Discover, *Development and Delivery of New Drugs,* S.P. Medical and Scientific Books, New York, 1978, 1.
3. **Arnow, L. E.,** *Health in a Bottle — Searching for the Drugs that Help,* Lippincott, Philadelphia, 1970, 9.
4. **Bennett, J. P.,** *Chemical Contraceptions,* Columbia University Press, New York, 1974, 1.
5. **Wardell, W. M. and Lasagna, L.,** *Regulation and Drug Development,* American Enterprises Institute for Publishing Policy Research, Washington, D.C., 1975, 1.
6. **Helms, R. B.,** *Drug Development and Marketing,* American Enterprises Institute for Publishing Policy Research, Washington, D.C., 1975, 3.
7. **Rubin, A. A.,** *New Drugs — Discovery and Development,* Marcel Dekker, New York, 1978, 1.
8. **Mathieu, M. P. and Murphy, W. J., III,** *New Drug Development: A Regulatory Overview,* Parexel International Corporation, Cambridge, MA, OMEC International, Washington, D.C., 1987, 1.
9. **Williams, M. and Malick, J. B.,** *Drug Discovery and Development,* Humana Press, Inc., Clifton, NJ, 1987, 1.
10. **Spilker, B.,** *Multinational Drug Companies, Issues in Drug Discovery and Development,* Raven Press, New York, 1989, 1.

Chapter 2

PROGRAM COORDINATION AND MANAGEMENT

Charles E. Hamner

TABLE OF CONTENTS

I. INTRODUCTION

During the late 1970s and 1980s, considerable progress has been made in managing the research and development (R & D) process. Managers have learned to cope with the complexity of large organizations and extensive federal regulations with the help of program management techniques utilizing computers and telecommunication systems, but the pressure on management to manage the production of new products has not lessened. However, the etiology of the pressure has shifted from problems of low output and inflation in the economy to competition in the marketplace. The competition is "biotechnology" based through the innovative use of molecular biology, genetic engineering and fermentation/cell culture techniques and processes. The pharmaceutical industry is shifting from a general chemical-based product approach to a biologically based product approach. This shift in approach to providing therapeutic entities will accelerate during the 1990s. It is hoped that in the long run simple organic chemicals will be found that can cause the same result as the complex biologics that are now under intense study.

The new technologies are requiring more collaboration than ever before of many organizations because of the mix of skills required, lack of trained technologists, and the enormity of associated costs to develop a therapeutic product. Therefore, the increased coordination requirements for R & D add to the demand that each project be carefully planned and managed. Yet, within each project, there needs to be a high order of responsible autonomy and an opportunity to be innovative. The managerial "trick" is to focus a wide array of intellectual and managerial commitments on a specific project, and to control the project without destroying the motivation and innovation of its participants along the way. To manage the complex activities involved in drug development, a number of techniques developed in other fields, such as industrial engineering, operations management, computer science, and business administration, have been applied.[3-6] The philosophy and methods involved in bringing together these management techniques for use in the pharmaceutical industry will now be discussed.

II. PLANNING A COURSE OF ACTION

Pharmaceutical R & D has a wide spectrum of activities ranging from exploratory research for finding new products to utilizing applied technology in developing new or improved products. There must be a long- and short-term considerations, balanced between freedom for innovation and creativity, and the control procedures for giving efficient and effective operations. Further, a clear understanding of corporate objectives is necessary along with resource availability and regulatory requirements, to provide a steady output of new products. A research plan is (1) keyed to the corporate business objectives and (2) developed to assure the proper selection and implementation of a project to fit the plans or activities of the manufacturing/ marketing divisions.

A. THE PROGRAM PROJECT PLAN

There are no simple and immediate answers for successful drug development. Managers are concerned with making policies, risking decisions, and directing activities. To accomplish these responsibilities they must understand the problem, determine and plan the solution, and correctly implement the program. Regardless of what organizational approach is taken, the program or functional plan should contain the following information: (1) goals, (2) objectives, (3) strategies (based on a resource statement of personnel, equipment, and facilities required), and (4) program evaluation.

1. Goals

Goals are long-term, broad, general statements setting forth the purpose and the results to be reached by a particular program. They specify "why" a program is being undertaken and provide direction to the manager in understanding the problem. The goal for the R & D division is based on the corporate objectives which have been developed by top-level management in consultation with various division heads (R & D, marketing, operations, finance, etc.) to reflect the perceived needs of the organization. These needs are usually based on: (1) lack of something considered requisite or useful because of a known opportunity and (2) a condition requiring relief or want in order not to miss on opportunity (usually in the area of advanced technology). Occasionally, there will be a situation, inequity, program failure, or negative condition for which action is needed. The major influence on the priorities of corporate objectives is that of determining the number and characteristics of the clientele to be served. Other prime considerations are the magnitude of the need/problem, what position must be defended, probable consequences if nothing is done, and the basis for all these judgements.

2. Objectives

Objectives are precisely defined statements of intended accomplishments. They relate directly to the program goals and specify the "what" and "when". Objectives should be realistic and attainable, focus on a single key result, and specify a target date for completion. They objectives should be prioritized and developed in conjunction with line department heads and program/project team managers, as well as assigned for individual responsibility and accountability, even in joint efforts. Furthermore, the objectives need to be easily understood, and consistent with operating policies and the present or future resources available. Often, they are the criteria by which research performance is judged. Establishing the necessary program objectives is a critical part of the planning effort, because they are the building blocks for program work and the source of identification of program projects. The objectives, along with strategies, determine the solution(s) to a problem.

3. Strategies

Strategies are statements which combine the "how", "where", "who", "how much", and "how many" resources necessary to accomplish a program objective. They specify the means for achieving single results. A program strategy is made up of various tasks, the completion of which will result in the attainment of stated program objectives. For example, in R & D the considered tasks within a strategy may include (1) the compilation of standards and regulations, (2) the implementation of technological advances, (3) the distribution of information, (4) the development of a specified dosage form, and (5) the training of certain personnel in specialized skills. The development of strategies requires that department heads and project managers work with the administrative and technical personnel under their direction to accurately define the resource needs. Only the person actually doing the work can precisely define the supplies and equipment and give the time requirements for a specific task. Further, it is very important to have staff input in a "team" effort to gain the commitment needed to meet schedules and overcome difficult problems. Identifying the various tasks to be accomplished is critical to establishing an activity/task sequence for implementation of a program project.

4. Resource Summary

While discussing strategies it is important to mention the resource summary. As the objectives and strategies (including all tasks required) are set in priority, a complete assessment of current and anticipated facilities, personnel, equipment, supplies, and so forth must be documented along with cost estimates by project. Through the assessment of resources and time estimates for each task, two essential elements are developed in order to attain program implementation which would include the formation of a schedule[3,4] and a program project budget.[7]

5. Evaluation

A program evaluation should be set up in the planning stage to monitor and control implementation activities and the program performance assessment when a project is completed or an objective is reached. Various measures exist which are helpful in providing a quantitative summary of a program. The success an entity achieves in reaching state objectives is measured by determining the *actual* vs. the *planned* results. Program managers should use various types of program measures to determine how closely an operational unit comes to meeting stated program objectives.

The following measures are often used:

Input measure — A statistic which indicated the resource employed to operate a program. Resource utilization directly reflects those costs in which management has a high degree of interest at all times.

Work-load measure — A statistic which indicates the volume of work to be done or the magnitude of program coverage or effort.

Output measure — A statistic which indicates the volume of goods and services produced by a program.

Benefit measure — A measure of the value to society of attaining an objective.

One should be careful not to request excessive data and quantitative analysis from the scientific and technical staff. Only data of obvious value should be requested; otherwise time will be wasted, negative attitudes will develop, and overall morale will be depressed. The work load and output measure allow one to monitor the task completion against the project schedule and estimate future project results. Management is highly interested in output measures, along with cost monitoring data; it makes up the guts of project status reports and is usually rendered on a monthly or quarterly basis.

6. Performance Audit

Accompanying the adoption of program management has been the development of performance audit techniques which allow top management to have quantitative, objective evaluations rather than subjective impressions about the success of a program.[6] Such information is very helpful in identifying which managers or key personnel should be rewarded and to what degree. It also tells how well a program was administered or managed and whether or not it should be continued. The performance audit usually consists of a management audit and a program audit.[6] The management audit evaluates the efficiency and economy of a given operation. It frequently involves the evaluation of operations in accounting, purchasing, producing, personnel, and research, but it may also include other activities carried on by an organization. The program audit is an audit of effectiveness by a higher level of authority. Its objective is to determine whether or not the management or employees of an entity have effectively received, accepted, and applies appropriate actions for achieving the desired results.

This type of review is usually undertaken with help from outside consultants. In general, consultants are frequently not welcomed by line managers and scientists, especially if the latter are insecure. One often hears the complaint that a consultant "used my idea" in convincing top management of a particular approach. Actually the consultant's objective is to identify good ideas in order to resolve problems; anyone could be proud if a consultant was used as a vehicle to get their idea approved by management. Planning should be an organizational process rather than an intellectual exercise. Integration of the professional staff and its specialty knowledge and advice with outside specialists is most important. Scientific questions frequently have diverse answers. Advisers can recommend strategies, give technical information, stimulate and encourage in-house staff, identify new projects worthy of consideration, and lend prestige and expertise to confirm and legitimize a program. Consultants realize they are not in the line of authority and they enjoy communicating with the in-house staff. Management must use balance in advisers, achieve the right sequence and mix, and be careful to select consultants who are practical about implementation. Used correctly, consultants can enhance a plan or help shore up the project implementation activities and schedule.

Based on the above elements, a functional, reliable scheme can be made which elaborates a plan for carrying out the R & D corporate objectives more realistically. If this plan is well conceived, it can act as a dynamic, flexible vehicle, with contingency plans if needed, which meet new technical challenges and budget objectives. Above all, a plan is a solid source of information which can act as a vehicle in communication of directions and expectations to personnel at every level of R & D.

B. PROJECT PROBLEMS TO AVOID

The program management approach is not universally accepted as the best management approach to pharmaceutical R & D. Scientists see program management as an attempt to make research a traditional production operation. Many research managers feel that the research contribution cannot be evaluated quantitatively because of: (1) a long-term commitment required of investigators, (2) the possibility of an unanticipated breakthrough in the search for new knowledge, (3) the high dropout rate for research projects for sound scientific reasons, and (4) the general lack of understanding for the complex nature of research operations by nontechnical business managers. Because of the unpredictable nature of drug research, the research manager must balance flexibility of a project plan with the control and quantitative aspects of project management. To gain the proper participation of scientists, and environment must be provided that motivates individual and encourages their creative and innovative talents. Development is associated with creating something new. It is a future-oriented, dynamic process requiring resourceful, innate abilities to resolve unusual, one-time problems intermingled with expected operational difficulties.

Perhaps the best way to support the program management approach to R & D is to discuss the major management reasons for program project failure. Keider[8] has identified a host of management faults that cause project failures. In the *orientation* phase, little or no time is spent in planning, the project is not adequately defined, and short lead times are allowed for estimates. If estimates are made by the wrong people, no standards exist for project duration and no consensus is obtained from the staff concerning critical issues affecting the project. Upon *initiation* of the project, the project leader's responsibility may be undefined, little documentation may exist to identify a work base form, paper flow may be handled poorly, knowledge of "tools" to perform the project more efficiently may be lacking, problem avoidance may not be understood or considered, resource requirements may not be scheduled for the project, and/or the project team's activities may not be clearly presented. Project *implementation* may uncover a lack of project leadership; unanticipated resource requirements; trivial, informal, or insufficient reporting of project information; ill-considered changes of personnel; and failure to inventory available skills. Also, often staff members are considered "universally expert". Their adherence to standards and specifications is frequently either not defined or, if defined, not followed. Thus sometimes there is a lack of project logs, audit trails, check points (thus no monitoring or control) and project estimates, and requirements are not updated. At project *termination* there may be no overall project evaluation, history/statistics may not be determined nor brought together, quality control may not be reviewed, and personnel may not be evaluated. Further, there is little formal turnover, knowledge gained is not usually transferred, and the recommendations for enhancement of future projects are not often documented.

It can be seen by quick review, however, that nearly all of the above-stated management faults may be corrected or greatly improved by utilizing the concept of program planning and the requirement of system management. This probably explains the trend toward program management in pharmaceutical R & D during the 1970s.

C. PROJECT SCHEDULING

Of the many problems associated with program planning, setting the project schedule may be the most difficult. The project manager assembles the activities/task identified in the strategy section of the program/project plan into a logical sequence of events. The sequencing allows as many activities as possible to go forward simultaneously, and ensures that activities required prior to other critical activities have precedent in the sequence. In addressing the logic of project activity, one relies on the objective priorities, strategies and resource summary for technical constraints, availability and application of various resources, and time constraints to optimize a critical task pathway. The planning logic flow chart that result provides a visible display of all project tasks and the interdependencies required to implement the project objectives. Such a precedent network is commonly called Program Evaluation and Review Technique (PERT) or Critical Path Method network.[3,4,9]

Once the optimum activity sequence has been determined, the final planning step of placing time estimates on various activities is needed to develop a project schedule along the network. Governmental regulations requiring specific information on a Notice of Claimed Investigational Exemption for a New Drug (IND) and on New Drug Applications assist in making the basic planning for these types of developmental projects rather straightforward, since the strategy can be defined at the preclinical and clinical level. However, activity time spans are clearly the most difficult variables to estimate and control because of unanticipated technical/scientific problems. Typical unexpected problems include chemical purification method development, raw material manufacture difficulty, metabolite identification, toxicology-teratology problem, and bioavailability or clinical side effect. Experienced pharmaceutical managers recognize that such delays occur, even though one cannot predict exactly where or when. An acceptable amount of slack time is built into critical target dates such as IND submission to account for these delaying events. Some project managers utilize optimistic and pessimistic schedules of dates. The final schedule must be developed collectively between the R & D director, middle management, line managers, and project managers. All these managers and their personnel will have to interact to meet the project schedule. Also, wide discussion of the schedule of project activities will aid in making top management aware of the project complexity, the support services, the technical services, the operational activity required, and the risks involved. Finally, there is a tendency to believe that a plan cannot be changed. It must be recognized that both planning and development are dynamic processes due to technology, new discoveries, problems, or a host of other reasons. Changing a plan for the right reason is a part of the management responsibility and demonstrates the risk of an earlier decision. At this point the plan is defined, scheduled, and ready for implementation.

III. IMPLEMENTATION OF THE PROGRAM PLAN

A. ORGANIZATIONAL APPROACHES

The director is confronted with several difficult problems when undertaking a R & D program. His ability to solve them smoothly and without causing a major loss of morale in the research group is a measure of his skill as a research administrator. Most R & D divisions possess a relatively large number of research skills. These skills are very specifically defined in the pharmaceutical industry. A research director has be devise the best program possible, utilizing the skills available. First, he must be effective in selling his ideas about research programs and the progress of the program to top management. He must also communicate his project needs and plans to company management in order to be able to meet the objectives of the company. Finally, he must present clear directions to his personnel in the R & D division.

There are several key committees that can advise the research director to ensure input for all scientific areas and to utilize specific skills to the best advantage. The research executive committee is composed of top-level research managers who develop policies, recommend therapeutic areas for research, review proposals for exploratory research groups or outside offers of projects, and review summaries of ongoing research projects. The research committee is usually composed of R & D department heads, senior research personnel, and representatives from administration, marketing, and operations. It monitors the progress of research projects and helps decide their fate. A preclinical development committee, composed of specialists in chemistry, pharmacology, biopharmaceutics, pharmacokinetics, toxicology, regulatory affairs, and project management, offers technical advise on preclinical development problems. A clinical planning committee or drug development committee, with clinical specialists in Phase I, II, and III studies, biopharmaceutics, pharmocokinetics, toxicology, regulatory affairs, and project management, technically advises on clinical development projects. There are often other special committees having specific assignments to carry out a given task. These committees coordinate with management in the R & D division, keep management informed, and furnish direction to the program/projects. The organizational structure of the R & D division itself may be in the form of traditional line reporting departments whose functions are based on scientific discipline and are task oriented. In order to carry out the program management approach in this type of organization, project groups or teams must be assembled consisting of scientists and technicians from various departments and a project manager. They take the specific and interdisciplinary actions required to carry out a given task or project. Faust and Ackerman[10] described this type of management approach at Hoffman-La Roche. On the other hand, some pharmaceutical R & D divisions are organized as goal-oriented project units.[11] Each unit has personnel representing disciplines of all areas of development and is charged with the entire responsibility for developing compounds in a designated therapeutic area. This type of organization is ideal for program/project management. Either organizational type requires joint use of the basic support service departments of administration, computing, and biostatistics; library and technical information; regulatory affairs; and patent law and research services. These departments, which include animal care, word processing, purchasing, stockroom, etc., are managed by the research director using both traditional line management and matrix management techniques.

B. COMMUNICATIONS AND TEAMWORK

Employees need regularity and continuity. Management should strive to stabilize the working environment through consistent, clear directives, open communication, and teamwork. Documented, easy to understand and follow operational procedures, and outstanding project managers or product research managers are needed to achieve this result. First, let us consider the operation procedures. These can be prepared at each R & D management level, department, or unit as an operations manual consisting of administrative and technical sections. The administrative section has a brief statement of the essential functions of the unit and outline of the basic area of services to be rendered. It contains a table of organization, indicates reporting lines and areas of authority, and identifies personnel by position with job descriptions for all personnel. Finally, there is a section showing how the unit interacts and communicates with other units within and without the division. Block diagrams or flowcharts are used to show how a request for service is received, what major actions, in sequence, are taken to render the service, and where the output/product goes. This section also contains examples of forms, report formats and informational memos, and the distribution schedule for each communication. The technical section contains standard operating procedures (SOP) for carrying out all operational tasks. The SOP should explain the step-by-step actions necessary to initiate and complete the task required in each job description. SOPs are very important in assuring consistency in an operation, shortening training periods, assuring that correct training is given, and in assuring that all steps — and that the correct steps — are being taken in carrying out a job. SOPs are a key element in quality assurance programs such as good laboratory practices, good clinical practices, or good manufacturing practices.

The project manager handles internal interfaces between the R & D departments to ensure good communication, cooperation, and teamwork, whereas the research director handles interfaces between entities external to a project such as the regulatory affairs office, the marketing division, and top management committees.

As a project progresses through the exploratory to the preclinical to the clinical stages, the mix of managerial, professional, technical, and service personnel changes. Interrelationships between components are usually more complicated than expected. Techniques must be found to provide employees with a sense of contribution and accomplishment. The project manager is the key to success in this area. Project managers are also needed because the project objectives, operational plans, and marketing plans must be reconsidered continuously. Drug development can be filled with unanticipated impediments such as technical problems and changes in regulations, manufacturing, or marketing plans. Management must understand the implications of change in any aspect of the plan in order to select a course of action that will set the balance of power in the system and regulate the flow of resources. The project manager keeps his fingers on the pulse of the project and furnishes the research director with information and advice. Sayles and Chandler[5] describe the project manager using the analogy of a metronome. The project manager deals with time and the organizational process rather than technical judgement. He must see that technical contributions are made on time by: (1) making line and staff aware of priorities, (2) resolving problems in the right sequence, and (3) establishing and updating decision criteria. The correlation of multiple consideration that goes into a decision requires him to have the unusual ability to seek and take advice from line managers and fit them properly into program events and goals. There are always obvious "go" and "no go" decision points along a "critical path" schedule of activities. Great project managers coordinate and correlate the many parallel activities to make certain that the critical activity occurs on time.

The various departments have to evolve reasonably predictable, routine ways of dealing with each other to answer the thousands of questions that are sure to come up. Time can be saved by the project manger finding answers to many of the more routine, procedural questions. It is essential for a good project manager to know what people to contact, the best approach to use, and where to contact them.

A project manager is not a traditional supervisor. Emphasis is on monitoring and influencing decisions — not ordering or making decisions. The project manager's role is heavy in responsibility and light on authority. He must manage a matrix which may mean setting up artificial reporting lines for brief periods of time to accomplish particular technical function. Sayles and Chandler[5] also discuss the major managerial behavior categories for a project manager. These include bargaining, coaching or cajoling, confrontation, intervention, and order giving. Ideally, the project manager is an unbiased observer, but still an accepted member of the project team. He can gain leverage by:

1. Protecting the line managers from outside interference
2. Acting as a mediator among conflicting groups
3. Providing priority access to scarce resources
4. Providing advance warning or coming events or problems
5. Helping justify cost overruns or otherwise securing adequate financial support

To be successful, emphasis must be placed on communications between technical and operational personnel, administration and line staff, and between various levels of management. The project manager constantly uses two essential tools to meet the communications requirement: meetings and reports. The project manager must be expert at: (1) holding productive meetings and (2) preparing lucid, informative reports. Jay[12] has discussed the functions of a meeting, the distinctions in size and type of ways to conduct a meeting to achieve its objectives. He also considers meeting frequency, composition, motivation, agenda preparation, and troubleshooting. All these aspects are important and management needs to consider them and practice good meeting techniques.

Meetings often produce reports, but they also convey plans and project status. During program implementation the project status report becomes an important management tool. Faust and Ackerman[10] outline the contents of a new drug status report which included

1. Project/product identification
2. Research stage (this may also include an updated PERT chart for the project)
3. Therapeutic utility
4. Marketing considerations
5. Patent or licensing status
6. Regulatory (FDA, EPA, etc.) status
7. Bulk raw material status
8. Pharmaceutical development
9. Biological activities of pharmacology, toxicology, biopharmaceutics/ pharmacokinetics, etc.
10. Clinical investigations and comments of special interest on unusual events and critical concerns such as project cost, schedule, significant problems, or breakthroughs

These reports are usually issued quarterly. They give the project team and management an opportunity to reexamine the operational plan and approach and to establish new or additional activities.

IV. CONCLUSION

Project management must stress detail, that priorities are set, that schedules are rigidly adhered to, that specifications are clear, and that activities are carefully monitored. This is not a popular approach with many old-line managers and, unfortunately, some of the more enlightened top managers as well. Line managers tend to be conservative and may be disturbed by the tight schedules that depend on others not under their control or a plan that identifies them as responsible for a critical activity in the corporate mission. To manage in the 1990s with high development costs and severe competition from other companies and other countries such as Japan and the European Economic Community, all aspects of corporate activities will have to be evaluated and newer, more promising management techniques attempted. Corporations should strive to give their scientists opportunities to gain knowledge of new management techniques on operation, planning, system analysis, organization, personnel, and budgeting. This will be imperative if R & D is to give a reasonable return on investment in the 1990s and beyond.

REFERENCES

1. **Faust, R. E.,** Assessing research output and momentum, *Res. Policy,* 3, 156, 1974.
2. **Helms, R. B., Ed.,** *Drug Development and Marketing,* The American Enterprise Institute for Public Policy Research, Washington, D.C., 1975, 3.
3. **Beer, S.,** *Management Science — The Business Use of Operations Research,* Doubleday, New York, 1967.
4. **Hansen, B. J.,** *Practical Pert Including Critical Path Method,* America House, Washington, D.C., 1964.
5. **Sayles, L. R. and Chandler, M. K.,** *Managing Large Systems Organizations for the Future,* Harper & Row, New York, 1971.
6. **Herbert, L.,** *Auditing the Performance of Management,* Liftime Learning Publications, Belmont, CA, 1979.
7. **Pyhrr, P. A.,** *Zero-Base Budgeting — A Practical Management Tool for Evaluating Expenses,* John Wiley & Sons, New York, 1973.
8. **Keider, S. P.,** Why projects fail, *Datamation,* 20(12), 53, 1974.
9. **Rogers, L. A.,** Guidelines for project management teams, *Ind. Eng.,* 6(12), 12, 1974.
10. **Faust, R. E. and Ackerman, G. L.,** Organizing and planning for effective research: program/project management at Hoffman-La Roche, *Res. Manage.,* 17(1), 38, 1974.
11. **Weisblat, D. I. and Stucki, J. C.,** Organizing and planning for effective research: goal-oriented organization at Upjohn, *Res. Manage.,* 17(1), 34, 1974.
12. **Jay, A.,** How to run a meeting, *Harv. Bus. Rev.,* 54(2), 43, 1976.

Chapter 3

PROJECT COST MONITORING

David E. Jones

TABLE OF CONTENTS

I. INTRODUCTION

Project costs are the costs incurred to carry an identified project from one level of development to a more advanced level of development or to completion. The need to identify individual project costs within total research organization expenditures has given rise to the use of project cost-monitoring systems, particularly when many projects are worked on concurrently by numerous departments or groups within such research organizations.

The approach to project cost monitoring described in this chapter provides a systematic method for assigning the total research and/or development costs to those projects on which manpower or money was expended. Thoughtful planning and flexible program design will make possible the generation of project cost data in numerous formats and by various criteria. The manager who initiates and supports the installation of a project cost monitoring system will be rewarded with a powerful information resource which provides a multipurpose management tool.

II. USES OF PROJECT COST INFORMATION

Project cost information can be used for many purposes:

1. Data derived from a project cost monitoring system can provide a ready source of background data on which the cost of a new project can be estimated.
2. Cost estimates can be grouped by time intervals and, thus, become an integral component of the research budgeting process.
3. Actual expenditures on projects can be compared to budget as a basis for a project cost control function.
4. Knowledge of the cost to do specific development work on a project within one's research group is one key element in determining the desirability of contracting for such work rather than employing in-house resources; this is analogous to a "make or buy" decision in production management.
5. Project cost monitoring can also provide an excellent tool for research management. The amount of expenditures, coupled with their timing, reflects the activity on projects and, when compared to the project plan, facilitates comparison of intended and actual results.

III. PLANNING A COST MONITORING SYSTEM

A. IDENTIFY INFORMATION NEEDS

The generation of project cost data should be a response to a need for such information. Therefore, the ideal system for capturing and reporting cost information is the one that will provide the required information on a timely basis for the lowest cost and the least disruption of research personnel. The information to be collected and reported will depend, in part, on the level of detail that research management or corporate management needs to direct research activities.

Project cost reports can be generated weekly, monthly, quarterly, semiannually, or yearly depending on needs. Experience shows that monthly or quarterly reports represent a good compromise between the cost of producing reports and the value of the information provided. Project costs can be tabulated by project totals or by project totals by organizational units, i.e., by division, department, section, group, etc., depending on the need for information. A properly designed cost-monitoring system can serve the organization at many levels and in several ways depending on the flexibility of the program and the detail entered into it.

By using predetermined identification codes, project costs can be subgrouped by type of project, that is, the reason the project was initiated. Such codes allow one to distinguish between the cost of technical service on an existing product from the cost of efforts to develop a new product. This approach can be taken at least one step further by identifying product improvements undertaken for the commercial benefit of the product vs. those imposed by regulatory demands. Likewise, basic research can be distinguished from applied research, applied research from development, etc. Possible codes might be 01 = basic research, 02 = applied research, 03 = new-product development, 04 = product defense in response to regulatory demand, 05 = product improvements, and 06 = services rendered to other divisions, to name a few.

Project costs can be identified by therapeutic category so the efforts directed at specified areas of inquiry can be determined. This code can be broad or narrow as use dictates, i.e., as broad as "anti-infectives" or as narrow as "amoxicillin", "tetracycline", or "erythromycin", etc. Simple codes can be arbitrarily assigned, but if a complex code structure is required, a review of categories used by syndicated market research organizations will prove helpful.

In many companies, marketing units must bear the cost of research done at their request. Originator codes are used to identify project costs by requestor to allow for this tabulation and chargeback.

Determine which research organizational units should be identified in the cost-monitoring report. These are the departments, sections, or groups whose project activity should be included in the report. One approach is to separate organizational components by their roles. Chemistry, pharmacology, toxicology, and clinical research are operating groups; management, administrative services, information services, and data management are, with few exceptions, support groups. Research groups are those that ultimately appear in the computer-generated cost-monitoring reports. Support groups are allocated to the research groups as overhead, prior to entering cost data into the computer (unless a sophisticated computer program accepts overhead costs and allocates them).

Cost-monitoring can be as rudimentary or as sophisticated as needs dictate and costs justify. Careful planning will prevent the omission of desirable report capabilities. It is not uncommon to discover that many unanticipated uses are made of cost-monitoring data. Therefore, identify the cost data at the entry level in every manner that may have useful application; it will be easy to delete unneeded detail, but difficult to add detail latter.

B. STAFF AND SUPPORT REQUIREMENTS

To minimize interruption of the work of research personnel, i.e., those who staff laboratories, it is suggested that administrative personnel perform most of the tasks necessary to capture costs. Unless the research organization is very small, the job of monitoring project costs can periodically require much of the time of an individual or a small team. Because it is necessary to understand the interrelationship of the organizational structure, budgeting units, and the actual work flow within the research organization, it is often beneficial if the same individual or team has responsibility for both research budgeting and cost-monitoring. The logical integration of the two functions provides continuity because they are, ideally, mirror images of one another. Both are closely tied, on a functional basis, to research project managers.

Computer systems support is a necessity to fully exploit the various capabilities of the approach described herein. Early in the planning process, the assistance of computer systems personnel should be enlisted to determine the most cost efficient computer and program support, produce a tentative plan for such support, and, perhaps most important, determine how much storage and retrieval capacity will be needed to provide the desired flexibility. The widespread availability of personal computers, electronic spreadsheet software, and data base management software offer alternatives to program design. Allocations can quickly be made using a spreadsheet, and data can be stored as records in a data base. While the primary purpose of this chapter is to outline an overall approach to cost-monitoring, suggestions will be made on how various pieces of information might be entered into a computer program dedicated for project cost information.

C. PROJECT COSTING APPROACH

This chapter is not intended to argue the merits or disadvantages of direct costing compared to fully absorbed costing as they apply to project cost-monitoring. However, it will be helpful to review the basic differences between the two. Direct costing, simply defined, considers only those costs that are "directly" related to the work on a specific project; direct personnel cost, materials, and outside expenditures, such as consulting service or contract research. This is a widely accepted and widely used approach. However, these costs, when totaled, do not equal the total operating expenses of a research organization or subgroup because many operating expenses, e.g., physical facility costs, support services, and research management, to name a few, are omitted. However, direct costing is accurate, assuming that direct personnel costs are correctly determined, because all such costs are "directly" related to specific projects.

Fully absorbed costing starts with the readily identifiable, i.e., "direct" costs, and then, through analysis and appropriate rationale, allocates the balance of total organizational costs to individual projects. Therefore, a project cost for any period is comprised of its direct costs, as defined above, plus some portion of the cost of running the research organization, i.e., costs for the physical facilities, fringe benefits, support services, and management. While this system compromises precision to some degree because "overhead" expenses are allocated, some feel it more accurately identifies the total cost of a research project. Thorough analysis will suggest criteria whereby such allocation errors may be minimized.

The approach selected for use by a research organization is the one that best supplies the desired information. Although the approach described herein uses a fully absorbed costing method, the reader can nonetheless use the outlined procedures as a guide to cost-monitoring system using only direct costs.

IV. IMPLEMENTATION

Once the planning process has determined what information will be sought from the project costing system and which research groups will be reported in the data base, several steps are necessary for implementation. The goals of the system should be communicated to research personnel, and responsibilities for cost-monitoring should be assigned.

There are five essential steps in producing a cost-monitoring report:

1. Determination of the expenditures incurred by or applicable to the research organization and its component units (i.e., research groups) during a designated period
2. Adjustment of the basic operating expenses of each research group by the allocation of overhead and staff support
3. Analysis of the effort reports from each research group and assignment of costs to individual projects
4. Coding of cost data to ensure that each record is complete
5. Computer entry and calculation so that totals can be reconciled and reports can be generated

While the following example of fully absorbed research costs is admittedly unrealistically simple, it will serve to illustrate the basics of the system. A hypothetical research group consists of ten chemists who are paid the same salary, receive the same fringe benefits, occupy equally sized and equipped laboratories which require identical energy and utilities, have identical outside service expenditures, and are managed by a single superior who divides his time equally among the chemists. In this example, project cost-monitoring is greatly simplified because the total operating expenses for this entire organization could be divided by ten to arrive at the total cost per chemist for the period selected. If, in this period, each chemist worked a single but different project, the cost for each project would be the cost per chemist derived above; the sum of the costs of the ten projects would equal the total operating expenses of the example research organization.

The same basic approach also applies to more complex organizations in which one seeks to arrive at total research group costs which subsequently must be allocated, by appropriate criteria, to individual projects. It's a complex task and requires a systematic approach to ensure accuracy. Each project within each reported operating unit is the basis for each record that will be entered into the computer system or data base with appropriate characterization codes.

A. DETERMINE BASIC OPERATING EXPENDITURES

The basic operating expenditures of a research organization may be readily available from existing accounting systems if monthly operating statements for each budgeting unit are generated. Overhead and support costs will be determined from a review of total organization costs and will subsequently be allocated to those research groups which will be reported in the cost-monitoring reports. It is necessary to identify all of the direct operating costs of the various units in the research organization. If such costs are not available, the design and use of an accounting system designed to capture and report them should precede other steps in the development of a project cost-monitoring system.

B. ALLOCATION CRITERIA

The addition of overhead costs to the basic operating expenses of organizational units requires analysis and a stepwise approach. Allocation criteria should be reviewed periodically and modified when appropriate.

Because research is characteristically labor intensive, research personnel efforts represent a large portion of most research organization costs. Personnel costs plus various readily identifiable outside expenditures, i.e., clinical study grants, consultants, raw material purchases, and contract analytical services, comprise the majority of research costs. These costs can be assigned to specific projects or, at least, to areas of scientific inquiry. It is the identification of the remaining one quarter to one third of total research organization expenditures, i.e., overhead and support costs, that must be identified and appropriately allocated to the research groups to achieve fully absorbed costs.

1. Management

Research management can be allocated to various component operating units as a part of administrative overhead. This allocation is based on the proportional time that management spends directing each of the operating units, e.g., 50% to the chemistry group, 20% to the information services group, 15% to the biological research group, and 15% to the clinical study group. Management time will likely vary from period to period. Thus the cost of research management per se does not appear in a cost-monitoring report but is reflected as a part of the cost of each project reported in the system.

2. Physical Facilities

Physical facility overhead includes all aspects of operating the laboratories and offices in the research organization and includes, at least, depreciation, real estate taxes, utilities and maintenance, and custodial service. Review each operating unit, both reporting units and support functions, in the research organization to determine if a share of total physical facilities costs would be accurately represented by allocation proportional to (1) square feet occupied by each unit or (2) by the total number of employees in each unit. One of these approaches is usually a good starting point which can be modified by unusual circumstances to arrive at appropriate allocation criteria.

3. Employee Benefits

Employee benefits are often tied to direct compensation, and this relationship is even more pronounced when viewed on an operating unit basis which encompasses numerous employees at various salary/wage levels. Included in this group are life and health insurance, social security contributions by employers, and any other benefit program underwritten by the company. If the total benefit package cannot be rationally allocated in total, then each benefit must be allocated separately.

4. Administrative Support Services

Administrative support (personnel, office services, budgeting, and accounting, etc.), information services (library, literature search group, data analysis, and computer support), and the laboratory stockroom generally require more sophisticated allocation which necessitate periodic surveys of users. After determining the total costs of operating these various departments, allocations should be made on a usage basis.

a. Office Supplies and Services

Charges for office supplies may be indicative of how administrative support should be allocated, i.e., large departments may use proportionately more supplies and services. A periodic tabulation of the number of photocopies produced for each research group will provide a basis for the allocation of photocopying service. There may be other measurable services which would offer better guides to the allocation of the other supplies and services. Analysis will determine this.

b. Information Services

One of the most challenging support services to allocate is the information services department or group. Whether all information services, as defined earlier, are in a single department or individual reporting units, usage can vary from period to period which necessitates frequent surveys to determine use of services. The number of requests received for literature searches may be a fair basis for allocating this support service if the effort per request is comparable. Library services are particularly difficult to allocate, but document requests (which may be charged to requestors) may offer a clue. (Note: if the research library also provides library services for corporate entities other than the research organization, this proportional cost can be reflected as an extradivisional service and should not be allocated to research projects.) Statistical analysis is usually related to a project that is being tracked by the cost-monitoring system; these costs should be assigned directly to the project. Because of these project costs, "statistical analysis" becomes a reporting unit which will appear in the cost-monitoring report. Patience coupled with an analytical approach will reveal much about the use of support services.

Table 1 shows how an information services department might be allocated by section to operating units after it is burdened with management, physical, fringe benefits, and other overhead. Once the total cost for each support unit has been identified, it is allocated by selected criteria to each research group that uses such services. The stepwise allocation of such overhead and support departments will determine how a spreadsheet should be designed.

5. Laboratory Stockroom

The costs of operating a laboratory stockroom, which are not reflected in the costs of materials charged to appropriate operating units, can be allocated to users on a proportional basis. The flow of materials, documented by charges to operating units, is one indicator of how these costs should be allocated, or it may be more equitable to allocate shares of this cost proportional to the number of people served in each operating unit. The approach that best represents operating reality should be used to allocate these costs.

TABLE 1
Examples of Allocation of Information
Service to Research Groups

	Computer services	Statistical services	Library	Literature analysis	Totals
Chemistry	804	0	856	980	2640
Microbiology	0	0	240	626	866
Pharmacology	1035	0	985	2173	4193
Toxicology	821	0	730	321	1872
Drug metabolism	0	0	845	185	1030
Clinical investigation	1247	0	847	738	2832
Formulatiton research	657	0	547	0	1204
Analytical research	0	0	685	110	795
Direct code to project	0	8879	0	0	8879
Extradivisional research	0	0	1457	0	1457
Totals	4564	8879	7192	5133	25,768

6. Example of Allocating Support/Overhead Costs

When approached manually, the use of a worksheet like the one shown in Table 2 will facilitate both the allocation of support costs as well as reconciling the "basic unit expenses" with the "adjusted unit totals". Although just an example, it does demonstrate the flow of costs that would be applicable to an even more complex organization.

Support services and overhead costs are allocated to the management/general administrative group. This adjusted total of $15,875 for the period is, in turn, allocated to operating units by appropriate criteria. Because management/general administrative costs are allocated, information services costs are not allocated to management/general administrative, but instead only to other users in the hypothetical organization. Support services and overhead costs become fully absorbed into operating units. On this worksheet, totals are accumulated by row and allocated by column.

C. ANALYSIS OF ADJUSTED UNIT TOTALS

Overhead and support service costs are assigned to those operating units which will be identified in project cost reports. This procedure yields adjusted unit totals that represent the full cost of performing all the work done on identified projects in each reporting units. Restated in simpler terms, the cost of operating a selected organizational unit for a given period is identified. Now to answer even more important questions: On which projects were these operating costs spent and how much was spent on each?

1. Direct vs. Allocated Costs

Identify direct costs in each reporting unit, i.e., expenses which were related to specific projects, and subtract all such direct costs from the adjusted unit total; allocate the balance to specific projects based on the manpower expended on the project. To facilitate the processing of project cost-monitoring and to standardize nomenclature, the use of numeric and alphanumeric project designations is recommended. Whether combined manually or by computer, direct and allocated expenditures for each project are added to yield the total cost of each project within a research group for a reporting period. The cost of a project for the entire research organization is the total of the project costs within each research group for the identified project. Direct costs and indirect costs should be entered as separate records within each research group for each project. Consider the example: the clinical research unit in the example in the Appendix

TABLE 2

Examples of Allocation of Overhead/Support Costs to Research Groups

Unit identification	Basic unit expenses	Management G/A	Physical facilities	Employee benefits	Office supplies/services	Information services	Lab stockroom	Adjusted unit totals
Management + G/A	12,577	-15,875	858	1,470	970	0	0	0
Physical facilities	17,285	0	-17,285	0	0	0	0	0
Employee benefits	14,792	0	0	-14,792	0	0	0	0
Office supplies/services	9,685	0	400	490	-10,575	0	0	0
Information services	18,629	1,590	1,887	1,487	2,175	-25,768	0	0
Lab stockroom	8,785	830	859	400	307	0	-11,181	0
Chemistry	24,895	1,580	1,730	1,621	681	2,640	3,485	36,632
Microbiology	9,187	2,025	1,580	575	219	866	985	15,437
Pharmacology	20,178	1,590	2,085	1,550	503	4,193	1,759	31,858
Toxicology	11,895	1,980	1,590	1,285	329	1,872	457	19,408
Drug metabolism	14,924	1,890	2,079	1,523	401	1,030	2,121	23,968
Clinical investigation	29,879	2,580	2,075	2,103	3,785	2,832	0	43,254
Formulation research	9,974	905	1,071	1,055	602	1,204	879	15,690
Analytical services	7,878	905	1,071	1,233	603	795	1,495	13,980
Direct code to project	0	0	0	0	0	8,879	0	8,879
Extradivisional services	0	0	0	0	0	1,457	0	1,457
Totals	210,563	0	0	0	0	0	0	210,563

incurred basic expenses of $29,879 plus overhead and support services of $13,375 for an adjusted unit expense total of $43,254. According to outside service invoices, travel reports, receipts, etc., $22,703 of the total can be directly charged to individual projects; the balance of the adjusted unit total is allocated by manpower to the effort projects. Manpower effort is determined, and costs are allocated accordingly; records are then entered into the research data base for each project. The process is repeated for each group. Once such a data base is in computer storage, individual project costs can be tabulated by reporting unit, by direct or indirect costs, by period, or by the total of all reporting units for one or more periods as desired.

The reports that can be generated are limited only by the number of ways each project cost data entry is characterized, the flexibility of the program, and the capacity of the computer.

2. Allocation by Manpower Effort

Matching manpower efforts to projects requires a procedure to capture this information. A variety of methods, each with advantages and disadvantages, are in use. The most accurate and the most expensive method requires frequent reports by individuals on their project activities measured in hours or fractions of days. Daily or weekly reports are proportionately less expensive, but also somewhat less accurate. The accuracy of project cost data is dependent on accurate manpower reporting. If time data are collected individually and pooled on a research group basis, consideration of differences in individual salary/wage levels may not be required, as mixtures of various salary/wage levels form a composite for the research group. However, if salaries/wages vary significantly within a research group and project work is not distributed homogeneously throughout such a group, adjustments must be made to compensate for the value of one man day for a highly paid employee vs. that for a less-highly paid employee.

D. CODING DATA FOR COMPUTER PROCESSING

The coding of the cost data for entry into a computer data base depends largely on the information desired and how a particular program is designed. A record will likely contain at least the following fields or categories:

1. Period date
2. Research group code (and subcodes for components within the reporting unit)
3. Project identification
4. Expenditures on the project (in total or by both direct and allocated expense components)
5. A "type of project code" to distinguish between new projects, maintenance projects, or other designation
6. A therapeutic category code
7. A source or requesting group code (to identify who requested the work)
8. A record number which identifies this entry as a unique one (optional, depending on the program)

The use of numeric or alphanumeric codes will condense the number of characters required for data entry, but the use of a dictionary file, also in the computer, allows reports to show both project name and project number. Once the dictionary file is built, it will require periodic maintenance to keep it current as new projects are added. Hard copies of the dictionary files provide the codes necessary to identify each project appropriately when records are prepared. Prior knowledge of the projects is required to correctly assign certain codes, namely "type of project" and "therapeutic category" codes.

If the area of research to be reported involves numerous candidate compounds and the objectives of the research are not yet relegated to a particular therapeutic approach, a series of "basic research" codes will be useful. Their use will circumvent the entry of numerous candidate compounds, most of which will be soon dropped and all of which take up computer storage space. A series of project numbers that are different from those used for discrete projects can identify basic research into various broad areas. This approach is both effective and efficient. Candidate compounds which survive early scrutiny may eventually become specific projects and will be identified by a project or a compound code number.

The use of various "type of project" codes allows the system to more fully reflect the dynamics of drug development. Work on a formulation or a series of candidate compounds which shows promise and will require additional development are now coded "new product development". Once marketed, support for the product can be reflected as "product enhancement" or "product defense" depending on why the work was initiated. However, the use of a consistent project number will allow the cost history of a project to be traced easily.

V. REPORTING CAPABILITIES

The suggested approach to project cost-monitoring is flexible in the reports it can generate. Here are some examples of the types of reports that may be helpful:

1. A standard organizational total report shows only projects (no component units) by various periods such as total spent this period, total spent to date this year, and the total spent to date since the project started (this may be 5 to 7 years for new drugs).
2. An annual total of all expenditures by therapeutic category will allow management to determine if it is spending its resources in the areas and in the amounts that are consistent with long range objectives.
3. Reports for each research group can assist the group management in identifying existing or potential scheduling problems or alert them to budgetary problems.

The project cost reports also provide a complete list of all projects being worked on in the research organization — a compilation that project managers and senior research managers find helpful.

APPENDIX: 1
CLINICAL INVESTIGATION REPORTING UNIT PROJECT COST REPORT

Operating expenditures + overhead & support services = adjusted operating expense total

$29,879   + $13,375   = $43,254

Adjusted operating expense total	-	Direct project costs	=	Balance to be allocated by effort
$43,254	-	$22,703	=	$20,551

Project	Direct costs	+	Allocated costs (share of effort x balance to be allocated)		=	Total project cost
A-1	2,050	+	(15%	x $20,551 = $3,083)	=	$5,133
B-2	5,227	+	(7%	x 20,551 = 1,439)	=	6,666
C-3	8,000	+	(25%	x 20,551 = 5,137)	=	13,137
D-4	1,145	+	(30%	x 20,551 = 6,165)	=	7,310
E-5	0	+	(20%	x 20,551 = 4,110)	=	4,110
F-6	6,281	+	(3%	x 20,551 = 617)	=	6,898
				Total		$43,254

Chapter 4

INFORMATION MANAGEMENT

Richard L. Chamberlain

TABLE OF CONTENTS

I. INTRODUCTION

The "product" of drug development is the summarized and analyzed output in written or graphic form of all of the projects undertaken in the development of a new chemical entity. Pharmaceutical companies expend a great deal of effort organizing and managing this information.

This information must be clean, accurate, and accessible. There are basically two types of information that are involved:

1. The scientific information being gathered in support of claims to be made to the FDA
2. The project control information being generated to assure that the research is conducted in an organized and accurate way

Both types of information are critical to the success of drug development. The first because that is the real objective of pharmaceutical R & D, and the second because it is what controls the processes.

There are two requirements for the management of scientific information:

1. Document new properties of compounds and mechanisms of action that are relevant to the discovery programs under development.
2. Organize and assimilate the various results of the research.

As both types of information are being generated there is also a requirement to be able to share this information. The production of the "final product" requires a great deal of team work. No single department can stand on its own and produce an investigational new drug (IND) or new drug application (NDA). Therefore the outcome of documenting properties and assimilating results must be sharable with nearly all other areas of R & D. This information is a corporate asset just as much as a production plant or other facility.

The central tool used in the management of this information is the computer. It is critical to the scientific and the administrative management of any R & D organization. In many ways the development and use of computer systems is different for the development of new drugs than it is for other areas of pharmaceutical companies. That is, the requirements for dealing with change introduce a new set of requirements that are either nonexistent or of much less importance, for example, to the production or manufacturing areas of these same companies.

We will look at the processes and requirements in each of the following areas:

- Drug discovery
- Drug safety
- Clinical
- Records management
- Administrative management
- MIS organizations
- Information integration

II. DRUG DISCOVERY

Looking at this area in perhaps an oversimplified way, the goal of the chemist is to synthesize compounds with specific properties. These properties could involve interactions with other compounds or with certain cells in the body. They work with the medicinal chemist or microbiologist to somehow optimize or tailor compounds with certain predictable behavior. In reality this process leads to a series of related compounds, all with certain good and bad properties. These synthesized compounds are then subjected to screening experiments in animals or tissue samples to verify the desired properties. This process cycles, learning more about the compounds and synthesizing more.

This iterative process is very long and generates a great deal of information. Historically this information has come from instruments in the lab, research of the literature (both internal and external), and various analyses and summaries of this data. In recent years, however, the volume of data has increased significantly because of the ready availability of computers for storing and retrieving some of these data as well as for emulating some of the processes that had gone on in the lab. There are several ways computers are used to generate this additional information.

A. COMPUTATIONAL CHEMISTRY

The properties of individual compounds can be derived mathematically on the computer. For large proteins and other complicated molecules this can save a great deal of time. To determine many of these properties in the lab or library could take months if it is possible at all. Perhaps more importantly, the computer can determine these properties as the molecule is subjected to other forces or chemical reactions. Although a specific chemical reaction may occur faster in the lab than on a computer, the computer can be stopped and then restarted so that the reaction can be monitored. It is also possible to have the computer calculate some of the myriad properties of molecules, parts of molecules, bonding energies, and other necessary aspects of the reaction as it is being emulated.

The computational programs required to accomplish this tend to be very large and require a great deal of computer resources. Many of these programs will run for days, it could take years to reproduce this in the lab.

B. GRAPHICAL PRESENTATION

Another useful contribution of computers is in the graphical representation of these large molecules. A visual representation of the properties of a compound can be very helpful to the trained eye in determining and understanding how the compounds we deal with really work. In the area of mapping receptor sites, for example, being able to see a representation of the surface energies of a molecule can be very helpful and would be nearly impossible to construct on any kind of dynamic basis in the lab.

C. ORGANIZING RESULTS

The results of the work in the discovery area are basically a set of properties of the various compounds that are studied. Over time a company will look at thousands of compounds. Some will be well known, others will be entirely new. The collection of all of this information is a resource to that company. It costs money to generate this information in the first place and would cost more to regenerate. Therefore it is important that it be assembled in a place and form that is accessible by the right persons and also useful to them.

Even compounds that were studied years ago and rejected for some reason could be worth looking at with new techniques. If this information is lost (or stolen) it can be very expensive in terms of money and time to replace.

Most pharmaceutical companies use data base management systems to store and retrieve this information as it is generated. In many cases the information can be fed directly form the lab instrument to the computer. These systems must be made to interface to other areas so that other scientists can have access to it.

III. DRUG SAFETY

The need in drug safety is for the management and retrieval of the data collected during the animal studies. This data is collected during the "in-life" portions of these studies through to the pathology findings.

A. "IN-LIFE"

Typically, the data collected here is body weight, food consumption (generally the source of the drug), and clinical signs. Most pharmaceutical companies and contract labs have extensive computer systems for collecting this information on-line in the animal rooms. Balances for weighing the animals are interfaced directly to computers so that the technician does not type any information, thereby eliminating a major source of error. Even clinical signs are generally selected from a menu of possible signs.

B. NECROPSY

During necropsy the information regarding organ weights and gross findings is also collected in the necropsy rooms. Weights are collected automatically from balances that are interfaced to computers, and gross signs are selected from menus.

C. HISTOPATHOLOGY

More and more companies are implementing systems that allow the pathologist to record microscopic findings as they are observed in the microscope. In this case the interface is somewhat more difficult. Most systems use menus of tissues and abnormalities where the pathologist can select the desired finding by means of a terminal keyboard, a light pen, a bar code reader, a mouse, or in some cases by voice recognition. The size and complexity of the vocabularies can cause problems for some computer systems.

In all cases the goal is to minimize the time between when the observation is made and when it is entered in the computer, and to minimize the amount of actual typing that an operator has to do. The requirement is that the data be as accurate and complete as possible.

It is also vital that this information be available to all of the scientists involved. The pathologist, for example, must have access to the toxicology data when he is reading slides. Delays in providing these data adds to the already long time required to complete animal studies.

D. STUDY MANAGEMENT

Perhaps the biggest impact of information management systems in drug safety is in the area of study management. That is, with most of these systems it is the computer that is controlling the flow of the study and is monitoring the operators to assure that the proper animals are being weighed in the proper order, that the data are complete and "reasonable", and that in general the study is progressing according to some protocol.

The impetus for the development of many of the information management systems in this area was the "Good Laboratory Practices" regulations (GLPs). These have been implemented over the last 10 years in an effort to correct certain reporting problems found in the collection and recording of this information. The response of most companies to these regulations was to replace many manual recording practices with automated procedures.

These automated procedures can be applied to virtually any lab in drug safety. Regardless of where this information comes from, almost all of it should be accessible by the scientists involved in these studies.

E. CLINICAL CHEMISTRY LAB

In many organizations, the drug safety area is responsible for the clinical chemistry lab. This lab generally has 15 to 20 instruments that are used to analyze blood, urine, and other samples from both animal and human studies. It must be prepared to handle a high volume of samples quickly and reliably. It is in many ways an ideal application for a lab information management system. The data not only need to be collected and fed directly to other systems for reporting and analysis, but there are many quality control checks that need to be performed, and usually the same system is used to schedule and track samples through the tests.

This lab is covered by the GLP and is subject to FDA inspection. In many cases the same lab could be used to analyze samples from the manufacturing area. If this is the case then the lab is also subject to the good manufacturing practices (GMP) regulations. This is not generally an overwhelming problem, but the lab management has to be aware of the overlap in regulations.

F. STATISTICS

The final source of information in drug safety is biostatistics. The demands for ad hoc statistical analysis in drug safety is far less than it is in other areas such as clinical. Many of the statistical analyses can be automated or standardized. Typically, the analyses are made part of a toxicology or pathology report and only need to be reviewed by the statistician. In cases where an analysis is needed, the software generally used is Statistical Analysis System (SAS), BMDP, or in some cases Statistical Package for the Social Sciences (SPSS). In all cases the results of analyses need to be included in reports that become part of the collection of information about a project. This means that these processes need to be interfaced to the other sources of information in R & D.

IV. CLINICAL

Perhaps the least automated area of drug development is clinical research. This is not because people are not trying. It is simply because it is a difficult area to automate. Patients in a clinical trial cannot be locked in cages with bar codes on them for 2 years while they are observed. They move away, go on vacations, and drop out of studies. Humans are in many ways more difficult to study.

In spite of that there is a recognized need for better information management in the clinical area. Many companies that developed their own systems several years ago are trying to update them. They recognize the inefficiencies in the manual handling of paper case report forms. Although we will probably never see the end of paper forms, there are many ways to deal with the paper more efficiently than we do.

A. CASE REPORT FORMS

After the preparation of a protocol, the first step in the execution of a clinical trail is the development of case report forms (CRF). Virtually all companies use some type of word processor or typesetter to prepare the camera-ready copy for a printer.

B. CLINICAL SUPPLIES

Generally, a computerized system is used to help prepare and distribute clinical supplies. These supplies require special labels that may contain a blinding pouch for blinded studies. There is very specific information that needs to be printed on each label. There are computer systems and services that provide for blister packaging that is computer controlled with bar codes preprinted on each package so that all drugs can be tracked and accounted for. Because of the sensitive nature of the contents of these packages, the process of packaging, labeling, and distributing the experimental drug is covered by the GMP regulations.

Both of these applications require and generate information that needs to be interfaced to other parts of the clinical area.

C. CLINICAL DATA PROCESSING

Perhaps the oldest area to use information management in a clinical trial is the data processing area. This group has the responsibility of taking CRFs that have been filled out by an investigator or study director, reviewed by a monitor or clinical research associate, and building a computerized data base of the information. Generally, each study generates a data base. When the study is complete these data are summarized and reported. The largest problem facing the staff in clinical research is making sure that the data entered into the system are an accurate representation of what the investigator observed in his office. This is a difficult and time-consuming problem for everyone in clinical research.

The data are accumulated across the life of the compound and then summarized for the NDA. Generally the data base management system (DBMS) will have either a report writer or programming language for preparing these reports.

D. STATISTICS

In addition to the DBMS, most pharmaceutical companies use SAS for much of their reporting and nearly all of their statistical analyses. The combination of SAS and BMDP constitute far and away the majority of systems in use in this area.

E. REMOTE DATA ENTRY

More and more companies are either adopting or experimenting with "Remote Data Entry". Using this notion, a PC is configured to collect and transmit the data for a study. The PC is placed in the investigator's office and the study nurse or other such person is trained to enter the data shortly after they are observed. Then on a periodic basis the data are transmitted over telephone lines to the sponsor where they are merged into a study data base and reported on.

This provides several opportunities to improve the overall process. It collapses the time from when data are observed to when they are entered into the computer. This should produce cleaner data faster. It means that it is accessible to medical and biostatistics sooner — as the study is progressing. Done properly, it should also help the investigator to comply with the protocol.

The experience with this technique seems to be mixed. It appears that for some study/ investigator combinations it works well and for others it does not. In virtually all cases the company is having to implement two systems — one for their remote data entry and one for their normal data entry — and then go through the steps involved to interface the two systems. This can produce a large manpower load on an already overloaded area that will probably negate any savings that might have been realized. This will probably not move forward in a general way within the industry until a system is available that helps the investigator with the conduct of the study and is *one* system for the sponsor to learn and operate.

V. RECORDS MANAGEMENT

Most pharmaceutical R & D divisions will have a Records Management or Central Records Group. This department will have the responsibility of managing the actual copies of all records of research in the division. Typically, there is some conflict between this staff, whose job it is to be thorough in collecting all records, and the other scientist who naturally feel an attachment to the information they are developing.

Regardless of these issues, all scientific reports that are generated within the company must be cataloged and stored for easy reference and retrieval. A new drug application requires extensive references to outside literature that applies to the compound being submitted for approval. Therefore, the company also must maintain bibliographies of outside literature or have access to such bibliographies.

References to internally generated documents are kept in computerized catalogues. In most cases all documents relating to a particular drug are microfilmed and in some cases stored in computer-retrievable racks. This process is, however, being replaced with more efficient optical disk technology. This newer technology also makes it easier to interface the records area to other areas of R & D.

In most cases *all* information relating to a compound must be gathered and tracked. This includes protocols, correspondence, CRFs, reports, drug shipment records, interim reports, and any other documents that might be relevant. Most pharmaceutical companies also have access to several outside services that provide references to the drug in the published literature. In many cases copies of the articles in the published literature are collected and will be submitted with the application to the FDA.

In addition to managing the information during the research, all of the appropriate information must be assembled and prepared for submission to the FDA. This can be a monumentous task. There are very specific guidelines for the assembling and packaging of a submission. In addition to a specific form, any copies must be legible and page numbered properly. The trend is to install computer systems to take all of the original information and print originals on some high-quality output device, such as a laser printer, so that it is page numbered and ordered — ready to be bound to go to the agency as soon as the last piece of information is finalized.

VI. ADMINISTRATIVE MANAGEMENT

All of the areas mentioned above have certain common needs that are met with information management systems.

A. WORD PROCESSING
Most companies have implemented word processing systems that are used throughout R & D. These systems are not only used for the normal correspondence requirements, but are also used for preparing protocols and study reports. In the drug development environment it is important that everyone be using the same (or highly compatible) systems. In most cases the magnetic versions of these reports are kept and assimilated into a submission to the FDA.

Computer generated reports, tables, and graphs can be fed directly to the word processing system and included in scientific reports. The goal should be to reduce the paper flow and automate the preparation of a submission.

B. BUDGETING
In addition to word processing, there is a need to computerize the budgeting process. More and more the R & D divisions are being asked to manage their resources, both people and finances. This can only be done by budgeting along with the rest of the corporation. In most cases, the budget is prepared and tracked on computers. In some places, this is done with internally developed programs, in other cases spreadsheet programs are used. This will vary depending on the format and procedures used in the budgeting process.

C. PROJECT SCHEDULING
Perhaps the most active area recently has been in the area of project management and scheduling. Although it is at best difficult to schedule "Research", it is quite possible to schedule "Development". The development part of Research and Development includes drug safety, clinical research, and IND/NDA preparation.

In these areas specific projects can be identified and schedules using PERT or CPM methods. A drug project can be divided into subprojects that can consist of specific studies that have start dates and finish dates. Resources can be assigned and tracked. The secret to successful implementation of such a project scheduling system is to choose the right level at which to do the scheduling. In other words, if the schedule is too detailed, then managers and supervisors lose their flexibility to manage and supervise and will spend all of their time updating the schedule. They must be free to change assignments and make adjustments to keep on schedule. None of these systems are perfect for scheduling. They are simply aids to management. If the scheduling is not detailed enough, then it is not helpful in identifying trouble spots and the exercise becomes useless.

Scheduling to the department (or one level lower) is about as detailed as one can get. For example, in clinical data processing, schedule to the data coordinator and data entry level. Only schedule on job classification, not by person's name. For a typical clinical trial divide the trial into about ten different tasks (any more than ten becomes too burdensome). These should be tasks such as:

1. Protocol preparation
2. CRF production
3. Clinical supplies preparation
4. IRB approval
5. Study execution (dosing)
6. Data processing
7. Data base completion
8. Statistical summary preparation
9. Medical summary preparation

For each of these tasks only assign broad job classifications, not individuals' names.

When these tasks are defined make sure that there are clear definitions of what constitutes a start date and finish date. These definitions must be agreed to by everyone.

For each task identify the required resources and the projected duration of the task. Let the system assign the actual start and finish dates if possible. This will make it much easier to update in the future. After the tasks have been input, it is possible to get the computer to summarize resource requirements across time — both money and people. It is also possible to have the system look at the number of available people and reschedule some tasks based on priorities. Although it is often not practical or possible to delay some tasks, this technique can be useful for indicating where additional resources are needed or where work can be "farmed out" to an outside service organization.

Figure 1 is a sample Gantt chart showing several studies that have been input as described above. There are several systems available for PCs and mainframes that do this type of analysis. (The examples here are from TIME-LINE™.)

Figure 2 is a sample report showing the resource requirements by month for the various tasks.

Just as the information collected during the conduct of a clinical trial can be used to better manage the trial, this information can be used to better manage the departments involved.

VII. MANAGEMENT INFORMATION SYSTEMS (MIS) ORGANIZATIONS

All R & D organizations either have their own group that supports computer applications, or they rely on a corporate group.

A. STRUCTURE

The computer support areas of R & D tend to report to one of two places. Either to the management of R & D, or into the corporate MIS organization. Of course given the right priorities either of these will work successfully. There are pros and cons to both relationships. The biggest complaint of having the support for R & D reporting to the corporate MIS group is that it is sometimes difficult to get high enough priority on R & D projects to even get them done. The difficulty of having the systems support group report to the management of R & D is that it will usually be a smaller group and therefore has fewer resources to bring to bear on large projects.

Another organizational trend in some companies is to divide up the systems support group and have each area of R & D with its own programmers and developers. This makes them directly answerable to their users, but also leaves them with no career path and can mean they are stuck working on the same system for the rest of their natural life.

Given the right environment any of these organizations can be made to work. The most common structure is to have the systems support group — with their own hardware — reporting to the management of R & D.

35

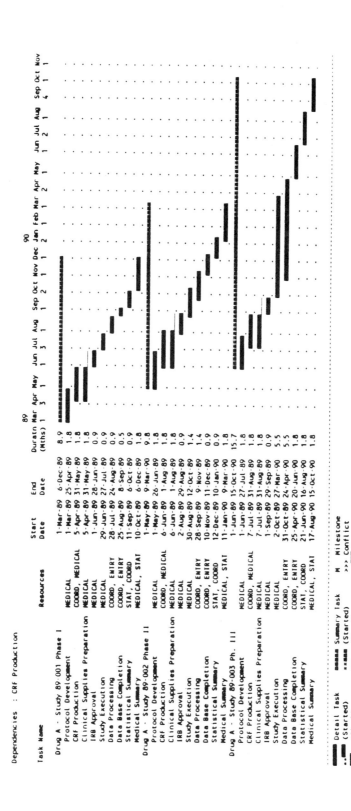

FIGURE 1. Gantt chart.

```
Schedule Name : Typical Drug Project
Responsible   : Project Manager
As-of Date    : 11-Jan-89  9:00am    Schedule File : A:\DRUGA
```

	Mar-89	Apr-89	May-89	Jun-89	Jul-89	Aug-89	Sep-89	Oct-89	Nov-89	Dec-89	Total
Drug A - Study 89-001 Phase I	2.3	5.3	4.4	1.5	6.5	25.5	22.5	21	20	4	113 *
Protocol Development	2.3	1.7									4
CRF Production			2.7	3.3							6
Clinical Supplies Preparatio			0.9	1.1							2
IRB Approval				1							1
Study Execution				0.5	4.5						5
Data Processing					2	18					20
Data Base Completion						7.5	7.5				15
Statistical Summary							15	5			20
Medical Summary								16	20	4	40
Drug A - Study 89-002 Phase II			2.2	5.6	4	1.7	7	23	26.5	23.5	93.5 *
Protocol Development			2.2	1.8							4
CRF Production				2.9	3	0.2					6
Clinical Supplies Preparatio				1	1	0					2
IRB Approval						1					1
Study Execution						0.5	5	2			7.5
Data Processing							2	21	7		30
Data Base Completion									19.5	10.5	30
Statistical Summary										13	13
Medical Summary											0
Drug A - Study 89-003 Ph. III				2.2	5.2	4.6	1	6.2	25	25	69.2 *
Protocol Development				2.2	1.8						4
CRF Production					2.5	3.4					6
Clinical Supplies Preparatio					0.9	1.1					2
IRB Approval							1				1
Study Execution								5.2	5	5	15.3
Data Processing								1	20	20	41
Data Base Completion											0
Statistical Summary											0
Medical Summary											0
Total	2.3	5.3	6.6	9.3	15.7	31.8	30.5	50.2	71.5	52.5	275.8 *

TIME LINE Task vs Time Report showing Total ManDays

FIGURE 2.   Table of required resources.

B. HARDWARE

The most prevalent hardware in pharmaceutical R & D is the DEC VAX line of computers. They are good for doing interactive work and offer a great deal of flexibility when it comes to expanding the configuration or installing departmental computers that can be integrated to other computers so that information can be shared. Since the common sharing of information is very important to the overall goals of R & D, this is a very strong attribute. In addition to VAXs, there are, of course, IBM mainframes, and more and more PCs in use today. It is common to see IBM-compatable PCs and Apple Macintosh PCs in the same organization. The trend is definitely toward networks of different size computers interconnected, sharing the information being managed.

This direction requires that the various groups within R & D cooperate in the selection of hardware and software or the resulting conglomeration of information systems will turn to quicksand and in the end hurt efforts to improve the drug development process.

C. SOFTWARE

We have already mentioned much of the software that exists in pharmaceutical R & D. The MIS organization usually is responsible for the purchase and maintenance of the larger software packages in use.

Most organizations will try to standardize on one or two DBMS. This makes support of these packages much more manageable.

D. VALIDATION

Another relatively recent trend in the information management area has been toward validation of computer systems. As companies have replaced manual procedures with automated systems, the FDA has begun to question the accuracy and maintainability of such systems. This has led to a considerable effort on the part of the industry to develop validation procedures for its computer systems.

Currently, manufacturing and drug safety are the two major areas where this effort has been concentrated. It will undoubtedly spread to other areas as well.

These validation procedures are designed to assure that the documentation exists to demonstrate that these systems in fact do what they purport to do and that they will continue to do so in the future.

An extensive report on computer system validation has been published by a group made up of professionals from the industry and the FDA. This report is available from the Drug Information Association.

VIII. OTHERS

There are other groups that have need to interface with the information generated in R & D.

A. REGULATORY AFFAIRS

Most pharmaceutical companies have a group that has the responsibility of interfacing with the FDA. It is generally better for all concerned if the agency deals with the same people each time some issue surfaces. It is unreasonable to expect that most of the scientists have the know-how and experience to deal effectively with the agency.

These people have to have a detailed knowledge of any new products, their status, and their attributes.

B. QUALITY ASSURANCE

Most research organizations will also have a QA group whose responsibility it is to audit and otherwise oversee the accuracy of information and adherence to procedures. These people also have to have access to certain types of information within the R & D organization.

IX. INFORMATION INTEGRATION

Effective integration of the information generated during the drug development process should be the goal of every company involved in this work. There are tremendous pressures on R & D organizations to be more efficient and productive. Gone are the days of viewing R & D as a black hole that continues to suck up money with little or no justification for its existence. This is forcing management of these divisions to be smarter in the way they manage their tasks, people, and money. It is virtually impossible to make improvements without better information systems. Management cannot function without information. The more successful companies will make their information management systems work for them in an integrated way (Figure 3).

The information must flow into systems that are integrated so that the appropriate scientists or manager can access and interrogate it. As the project progresses the information management systems must be designed so that a minimum amount of work must be done to put a final FDA package together. The time after the research is complete and before the package is submitted is very expensive time. It is time that is square on the critical path. Any of this time or delays to completion go directly on the time to market the drug. For most drugs this will be millions of dollars per month.

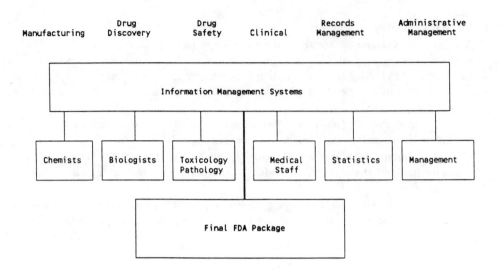

FIGURE 3.   Overall goal of information management systems.

The final step in the integration of this information is to integrate the information system of the company with that of the FDA reviewer. Many of the requirements of the scientists in the pharmaceutical company are also requirements of a reviewer of such a package.

There is currently a great deal of activity in this area. Companies are working with the agency to integrate their information systems to improve the kind of review that can be done and hopefully to shorten the time required for approval.

X. SUMMARY

Information management plays a major role in the drug development process. It must be implemented and maintained in such a way as to optimize the preparation and production of any submissions to the FDA. It must provide information to *any* scientist or manager who needs the information to contribute to the development of the base knowledge of the drug.

If implemented properly these systems can make our jobs easier and not be an added burden.

REFERENCE

1. **FDA Working Group,** *Computerized Data Systems for Non-Clinical Safety Assessments — Current Concepts and Quality Assurance,* Drug Information Association, Philadelphia, 1988.

Chapter 5

DRUG DESIGN

Alfred Burger

TABLE OF CONTENTS

I. INTRODUCTION

A drug or medicinal agent is a chemical that exerts a biological action in animals or people. Usually one will look for curative, prophylactic, or therapeutic properties in such an agent. Some people think of drugs as dangerous, toxic, or potentially harmful substances. The wide proliferation of drug abuse during the last 25 years, from alcoholism and marijuana smoking to amphetamine and narcotic abuse, has associated psychotropic drugs and even drugs in general with destructive and criminal activities in a segment of the population.

As in so many definitions, the truth lies somewhere between these extremes. All known drugs used in the cure, prevention, or treatment of diseases also have toxic properties. Indeed, toxicity toward some cells or body chemicals underlies the medicinal action of all drugs. Since useful drugs are much less toxic — but never completely nontoxic — toward normal cells or tissues, a drug may be called a selectively toxic chemical with hopefully a wide enough margin of safety. The ratio of toxic vs. effective doses is the therapeutic index of a drug. The greater this index, the safer the medicinal agent. Drug design is an attempt to devise substances effective in a given pathological condition and with as favorable a therapeutic index as possible.

II. THE PATH OF DRUG DISCOVERY

The first step in drug discovery is to ask what a drug may be expected to accomplish in a given disease. The pharmaceutical industry from which the great majority of useful drugs emanates poses the following questions. First, does medical expectation justify the search for such a drug, and what improvement in the health, humane, and economic advantages of the patients may be anticipated from the use of the drug? Second, is the state of the art and of biomedical science adequate to risk funding of the research? In other words, will the planned concerted effort have a chance to solve the problem within a specified limited time? Third, are there enough patients afflicted with the disease to justify the scientific and economic effort? It is a tragedy that some severe but rare disorders or diseases occurring in developing countries are not attackable because of the low or even nonexistent economic return on the immense research expenditures. Lately, such "orphan drugs" have received much attention, and in a few cases the manufacturers of such agents have made them available provided that some other medicinal or veterinary activity of the drug balances out the orphan drug properties.

When these questions have been sorted out, a team of experimental biologists and medicinal chemists will look for some "lead" compound that may set the stage for the development of a suitable drug.

III. THE DISCOVERY OF "LEAD" COMPOUNDS

The discovery of a new "lead" drug is still the most frustrating step in drug development. Until the late 1960s the discovery of totally new drugs depended largely on accidental observations, fortuitous findings, hearsay, and the screening of large numbers of candidate materials. A conservative estimate of the success rate of such screening procedures is that one compound out of 5000 advances to clinical trial, with the vicissitudes of subsequent clinical failure due to lack of specificity and mutagenic potential still unresolved.

This random trial of this or that chemical for the treatment of a given disorder has deep roots in the history and aspirations of human society. Since its existence, tribal "doctors" have searched for materials which might lessen pain and alleviate the symptoms and the fatal or crippling course of diseases in people and domesticated animals. They also searched for poisons with which to coat the heads of their hunting arrows, and for stupefying or stimulatory products that would make tribal people forget the burdens and sorrows of their primitive existence, the pain of labor, and premature death. The random discovery of such materials led to a therapeutic folklore of plants and other natural products in many parts of the world, and this still surfaces in the discovery and rediscovery of natural medicinal products.[1] Of course, man is no longer the first test animal for unknown biological actions, but model systems for many preliminary tests have been worked out using laboratory animals. Neither is therapeutic folklore reliable; ignorance of adequate medical diagnosis has often assigned a new natural medicine to a wrong use.

With the advent of synthetic organic chemistry 160 years ago, the number and availability of synthetic compounds soon overtook that of natural products. Both types continue to be screened against various model conditions in cell cultures *(in vitro)* and in laboratory animals *(in vivo)*. The most active and least toxic agents are advanced to controlled clinical trials. The revolutionary development of organic chemical methodology and especially of the use of spectroscopic instrumentation has led to rapid recognition of the molecular architecture of organic compounds. In medicinal chemistry it has reduced the randomness of substances to be chosen for screening tests. If a new chemical bears a relationship in its molecular shape, distribution of positive and negative electrical charges, and overall structure to a known compound, it will be selected more readily for "targeted" screening in the general area in which the earlier prototype had been of biological interest.

Such reasoning relies in some measure on chemical or physical analogy. This theme of comparing chemicals on purely theoretical grounds and drawing conclusions from such comparisons about their potential biological utility is the basis of medicinal chemistry, especially of planned molecular modification. The term "drug design" implies more than comparisons; it indicates some plan which starts with an idea and may furnish a selectively toxic agent for a given condition. Barely ever will the first compound thus designed satisfy the requirements for a clinically useful medication. The first few analogs of a "lead" compound usually support the premises on which their conceptual design was based and at best point the way to further improvements by systematic molecular modification.

In practice, drug design resembles design as it is performed in art. It involves a preliminary sketch and an outline or pattern of the main features to be executed. The final form of a planned drug molecule or preparation has to be filled in later. The detailed course of research will be governed by the individual experience of the medicinal chemist and by rules and preferences similar to those of an artist's vision at a given period of time, style, and innovative experimentation.[2]

In art one can anticipate the size and setting of the proposed painting or sculpture and adapt one's conceptions to these parameters. In music one can choose between a sonata or a symphony and draw on the style appropriate for the composition. In sports, one tries to adjust one's speed and thrust to the visible size and height of the target. In medicinal chemistry one is up against a poorly understood dimension. Most drug molecules are relatively small, with molecular weights between a few hundred and a few thousand daltons, seldom more. All such molecules can do is to react chemically with other chemicals by forming some bonds with them. This is done by sharing or transferring valence electrons between the reacting molecular species. If the target molecule is also reasonably small, the reaction product can usually be purified, isolated, and identified rigorously.

Alas, the target molecules of medicinal compounds are not small; they are cell constituents and biochemicals such as proteins, enzymes, nucleic acids, and lipids usually of macromolecular size. Their molecular weights may range from 10,000 D up, with sizes in the hundreds of thousands and even millions of daltons not at all uncommon. Biochemists are just barely beginning to understand these enormous and convoluted structures which may be folded in such a way that the interior of their molecules is exceedingly difficult to observe. Only in very few cases have the details of the reaction between drug and biochemical target molecule revealed themselves, and the meaning of the chemical chains surrounding the reactive area (the "active sites") is still relatively obscure. Active sites reacting with drugs are called receptors.[3-8] No doubt

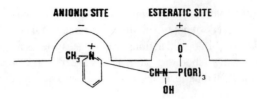

FIGURE 1.   Schematic reactivation of organophosphate-poisoned cholinesterase by 2-PAM. The pyridinium group is anchored at the negative anionic site of the enzyme and enables the aldoxime function to attack the blocking phosphate and thereby to dislodge it from the (positive) esteratic site.

they exist because one can replace a few of the atoms of a drug by radioactive atoms of the same kind and let such labeled drugs react with cells or animal tissues. The binding sites of the labeled drugs can be spotted by radioautography, by exposure of an X-ray film. The location of drug accumulation will be visible on the X-ray photograph, but nothing is revealed about the chemistry of the receptors. Thus drug design resembles shadow boxing; the target is there, but can barely be discerned.

The biochemical mechanism of action of only a few drugs has become known — how these drugs react with enzymes. In a few cases, the reactions are governed so completely by the chemical properties of the drug that one can predict whether or not the drug will have biological activity without too much biological experimentation. However, biological testing remains the final proof of activity and specificity.

Proposals to replace testing in laboratory animals by computer programs have not led to acceptable conclusions. Even the most advanced computers do not simulate the complex and interconnected reactions of the animal body to a foreign drug. For the foreseeable future, animal testing of drugs will remain the precondition to clinical trials in humans.

An example of such *de novo* drug design is the reactivation of organophosphate-blocked acetylcholinesterase (AChE) by 2-pyridinealdoxime methiodide (2-PAM). AChE is a widely distributed enzyme which catalyzes the hydrolysis of its substrate, acetylcholine (ACh) to hormonally inactive choline and acetate. ACh is an important neurohormone which transmits the message to muscles and vessels to contract, among them the bronchies. Persons or animals (including insects) which cannot destroy unwanted ACh almost immediately, through the action of AChE, may die of suffocation. Any inactivation of the enzyme AChE produces this result. Organophosphorus compounds are widely used for pest control on crops and in gardens; they kill insects by blocking their AChE, thereby increasing their ACh content and thus paralyzing their respiration. The same paralysis occurs, unfortunately, if the operator of the pesticide sprayer inhales some of the organophosphate. Quick action to revive such an individual is of the essence. This problem assumes even more ominous dimensions if organophosphates are used as nerve gases in military operations.

It had been known that organophosphates can be displaced from ester derivatives by nitrogenous compounds called hydroxylamines and oximes. The phosphate-blocked enzyme AChE was shown to be such an ester derivative, and application *in vitro* quickly reactivated the enzyme to its original catalytic form. However, this action was too fleeting to be of therapeutic use. Therefore an oxime was chosen which could fasten itself to the surface of the enzyme molecule by a quaternary ammonium group as it also occurs in the natural substrate, ACh. Now the liberating action of the oxime portion became prolonged, the enzyme was reactivated, excess ACh was destroyed, and respiration was restored to normal (see Figure 1). The lesson of this example is the need to understand ever more biochemical mechanisms of diseases. Only few cases of such specific inhibitions have become known and *de novo* drug design is therefore still in its infancy.

Another way of discovering a new therapeutic "lead" is to observe carefully any side effects of an existing drug that have no relation to the originally planned or accepted medicinal action of the agent. If these side effects have a bearing on some unrelated medical condition, they may be exploited by molecular modification.

The best-known examples for this experience are side effects of some of the sulfonamide ("sulfa") drugs. These drugs were the earliest clinically effective bacteriostatic agents and are still employed for antibacterial chemotherapy. In the course of their use, it was observed that some of them also lowered blood sugar and caused diuresis, properties not related to their bacteriostatic activity. Patient molecular modification and synthesis of thousands of analogs removed from their molecules the aromatic amino groups needed for bacteriostasis, altered or enclosed other groups, and created totally new structures which now emphasize antihyperglycemic properties in the oral antidiabetics, or diuretic activities in the well-known thiazide drugs. As a bonus, the thiazides were found not only to be diuretics, but to lower the blood pressure as well in certain types of hypertension.

IV. "LEADS" FROM DRUG METABOLISM

Like the constituents of our food, drugs are also metabolized in the animal body. Drug metabolism takes place primarily in the liver, but other body organs, the kidney, brain, etc., are also able to metabolize some drugs.[10,11]

The most important metabolic reactions are oxidation, reduction, and conjugation. Conjugation involves the conversion of a drug to more soluble, polar, more easily excretable derivatives, in other words, detoxication of the original selectively toxic agent. Oxidation, reduction, and several additional reactions usually also convert drugs to less toxic materials which can then be flushed out of the body. Occasionally, however, the products resulting from these biochemical reactions may be more toxic than the parent drug, or even have new and unexpected biological properties. In this case, the new compounds may become "leads" for activities unanticipated for the original drug. An example for this is the antimalarial drug, chlorguanide. The structure of this agent is changed radically by a chemical ring closure in the course of its metabolism, and the metabolite is the actual cause of the antimalarial activity of chlorguanide; the parent drug is inactive unless it is altered metabolically. The metabolite of chlorguanide was not ideal as an oral antimalarial, but served well as a "lead" for molecular modification which in a roundabout way led to the useful drug, amodiaquine.

Many drugs with unsaturated or aromatic double bonds are epoxidized enzymatically. The resulting epoxides are highly reactive compounds which "alkylate" nucleic acids, prevent separation of their double helix, and induce mutations which can lead to malignant cell growth.

V. PHARMACEUTICAL MODIFICATION

The discovery of a chemical compound with a biological action in a pharmacological test does not often mean this compound will be clinically useful. In rare cases the new compound will have an acceptable therapeutic index and thus be eligible for clinical trial. However, in the vast majority of cases the new compound will need further modification and development. If the properties of the compound are almost acceptable, although not quite so, and if the drug is unique enough, it may be possible to make it more suitable by pharmaceutical manipulation.[12] One of the many ways of doing that is by coating the drug with a plastic capsule which dissolves in some body liquids and not in others. In this way, a drug that is destroyed by stomach acid may be encapsuled in an acidic plastic and slip into the alkaline duodenum where the plastic can dissolve and release the drug for absorption by the intestinal wall. If it is desirable to release hormonal medications in small doses without repeated injections (as with insulin, anabolic steroids, etc.) some sparingly soluble hormone derivatives can be injected intramuscularly as a depot from which the active ingredient is liberated and released over a period of days or weeks by slow diffusion into the circulation. Such timed-released applications require careful pharmaceutical art, but have been standardized and can be accomplished readily.

VI. MOLECULAR MODIFICATION[13,14]

Much more research is involved if the "lead" compound has to be modified by synthetic alterations leading to derivatives and analogs whose exact biological properties are largely unpredictable. The most common scientific motivation for such molecular modification is to enhance potency and specificity, and to lower untoward side effects and toxicity. In the case of insoluble substances, chemical modification may be necessary to make them more soluble without impairing their inherent biological properties.[15-17]

In the pharmaceutical industry, the motive for molecular modification is often one of economics and commercial competition. If the sales of a given drug are substantial and if that drug is monopolized by a company under existing patent and trademark laws, other companies may wish to produce similar drugs, perhaps even with some medical advantages. They will therefore start with the marketed agent as a "lead" compound and search for ways to alter its structure and some of its chemical and physical properties, at the same time retaining the medicinal properties of the "lead" compound or hopefully improving them. Simultaneously the company owning the patented drug usually continues to synthesize analogs in order to protect its patent position and to stay ahead of the field of expected competitors. Thus, molecular modification has become the most widely practiced occupation in the initial phase of drug development. It is now possible to foresee the overall effects of molecular modification on biological activity, although toxicity, mutagenicity, and teratogenicity still defy reliable prediction. In some cases it can be used deliberately to minimize drug toxicity. For example, hydrazines containing the NH–NH structure, and azo compounds having unsaturated N=N groups are so often hepatotoxic that they should be avoided. One can say that molecular modification has become the core of legitimate drug design.

If the "lead" compound contains well-defined functions such as acidic or basic groups, ester, amide, keto groups, etc., it is possible to trim away extraneous portions of the molecule and leave behind skeletal structures with the same functional groups at comparable intramolecular distances. This is the classical route by which synthetic local anesthetics have been conceived based on the structure of cocaine, the benzomorphan analgesics based on morphine, etc. In pinpointing a useful drug, one no longer randomly synthesizes one homolog of an ester, ether, alkylamine, etc., after another, or substitutes one halogen after another in nuclear positions to go from a "lead" to its analogs. Since the early 1930s an expanding set of rules and chemical and physical guidelines has been developed to take at least some of the guesswork out of drug design. These rules are not laws of nature and like other rules are beset with unexpected exceptions. To avoid these exceptions requires all the skill of the medicinal chemist. This also implies that one synthesizes those compounds which offer the optimal prospects of suitable activity and not those that are synthesized most readily. The medicinal chemist must be well grounded in all modern techniques of organic chemistry for this purpose.

Molecular modification relies on structure-activity relationships (SAR). Compounds exhibit similar biological activities if their molecular shapes (stereochemistry) and valence electron distribution and other electrical charges of their molecules are similar. Such compounds are called bioisosteres.[13,18] The greatest confidence can be placed on SAR in structurally closely related series of compounds, but this is no longer a *conditio sine qua non*. As an example, the carboxyl group can dissociate into a negatively charged carboxylate anion and a proton. Similar schemes can be written for sulfonamide groups. Since both produce protons, they react as

$$- C - O - H \;\leftrightarrow\; - C - O^- + H^+$$
$$\quad\;\; \| \qquad\qquad\qquad \|$$
$$\quad\;\; O \qquad\qquad\qquad O$$

acids, and to some degree (depending on the rate of proton release, that is, their acidity) can replace each other in isosteric molecules. Such a replacement will almost certainly furnish a pair of compounds, one with COOH, the other with SO_2NH_2, which exhibit biochemical activity in the same test system. Indeed, p-aminobenzoic acid (PAB) and sulfanilamide (SA) both act on an enzyme needed in

$$H_2NC_6H_4COOH \qquad\qquad H_2NC_6H_4SO_2NH_2$$
$$PAB \qquad\qquad\qquad SA$$

the biosynthesis of tetrahydrofolic acid, an important vitamin as well as bacterial growth factor. PAB is a substrate of this enzyme, while SA is an antagonist blocking the biosynthesis. In other cases, carboxylic acids and structurally similar sulfonamides act in a similar rather than antagonistic manner. The predictable result of an exchange of the two groups in a molecule is therefore some action in the same biological test, either pro or con; at least complete indifference in such a test can be ruled out. This is a simple example of the application of bioisosteric guidelines in drug design.

In 1899 the observation was made that the activity of many hydrocarbons, alcohols, halogenated hydrocarbons, and other rather unspecific cell-life depressants is proportional to their partition coefficient between blood and lipids.[19] These test materials have since then been replaced by more standardizable model systems such as water and the water-insoluble 1-octanol.[20] From thousands of experiments in these solvents it can now be concluded that the activity of many unspecific cell-life inhibitors depends on the ratio of their distribution between water (i.e., hydrophilicity and polarity) and water-immiscible media, i.e., lipophilicity. Since cell membranes consist of layers of lipids and (hydrophilic) proteins, a compound must have a high degree of lipophilicity in order to penetrate cellular and subcellular membranes. Many drugs exist as ionized salts and must therefore be buffered in the biological environment to the respective undissociated acids or bases if they are to traverse membranes readily. Laboratory technicians can determine partition coefficients and ionization constants of several compounds per day and thereby improve the predictability of biological activity. In this manner, measurements of these and other physical properties of drugs contribute to drug design.

By pooling the interpretations of biochemical SAR and of the effects of physical properties on biological activities and subjecting them to statistical analysis, the new science of quantitative structure-activity relationships (QSAR) was born.[20] Most major pharmaceutical firms and academic faculties have added physical biochemists and biostatisticians to their staffs to explore the scope and methodology of QSAR. This has made drug design and development much more complex and expensive than it had been 30 to 40 years ago, but has raised the hope that disease problems which could not even be discussed intelligently then can now be researched in a systematic way.

VII. BIOCHEMISTRY OF DISEASE AND DRUG DESIGN

Diseases arise ultimately from biochemical disorders. These can be brought about by deterioration of the internal environment of the body as in the failure to synthesize essential substrates and biocatalysts for their normal reactions. Aging, nutritional deficiencies of essential amino acids, vitamins, starting materials for essential substrates, inorganic ions, etc., genetic failures, environmental toxicity, and infections are among the causes of those deteriorations.

The biochemistry of diseases has not been studied until recent decades, because analytical methods for the recognition of small though important deficiencies had not been known. Now incredibly sensitive spectroscopic methods have become generally available, and have enabled biochemists to capture previously unattainable minute quantities of aberrant chemicals. The most important instrumentations to make this possible have been the mass spectrometer, nuclear magnetic resonance spectrometers, electron spin resonance, X-ray spectroscopy, column chromatography, and gas and thin layer chromatography. Some of the instruments for such work are still expensive and require mechanics and electricians for continuous trouble-free operation. Nevertheless, most major research laboratories are now fully equipped with these instruments as well as the older and cheaper ultraviolet and infrared spectrometers, fluorospectrophotometers, and other analytical aids. Many of them are computerized to average out individual readings.

Armed with this instrumentation, dozens of endocrine and neurohormones, peptides of every length and complexity, kidney factors, brain and hypothalamic chemicals with startling functions, and hundreds of tissue constituents and normal and abnormal metabolites have been isolated, and their structures have been elucidated in record time. Many of them have been synthesized so that one is no longer dependent on the minute amounts that can be extracted from animal tissues. Some of these metabolites, vitamins, and hormonal factors are useful in medicine for replacement therapy where natural sources in the body are inadequate. Most recently, genes of bacterial and mouse cells have replaced genes from animal organs that induce the production of complex peptide hormones such as human pancreatic insulin and growth hormone. Several pharmaceutical industries have translated these early genetic successes into marketable products. That means that genetic engineering and fermentation methods will take the place of some extraction and synthetic procedures. Genes are regions in the polynucleotide chains of nucleic acids and determine the assembly of amino acids into specific proteins. Thus, molecular biologists and geneticists begin to make their appearance on research staffs concerned with drug development.

VIII. METABOLISM ANALOGY IN DRUG DESIGN[21]

Hundreds of natural metabolites of normal and pathological cells are known, and they pose the intriguing question of whether or not synthetic structural analogs of these metabolites could not take their place or antagonize them in biosynthetic reactions. The number of such analogs a chemist can dream up is very large, but an intelligent selection of priorities can be made based on the guidelines of molecular modification described earlier. A few of the analogs synthesized have shown agonist activities, i.e., they act like biologically useful metabolites although usually less potently. The greatest benefits have been reaped from analogs of those metabolites which participate in biochemical aberrations that lead to diseases. Some of these analogs have become prominent chemotherapeutic agents and represent the intellectual apex of drug design. A few examples shall illustrate these findings.

Hypoxanthine (6-hydroxpurine) is a metabolite which is oxidized in the body to xanthine and hence to uric acid (4,6,8-trihydroxypurine), a chemical sparingly soluble in water. Its salts are also quite insoluble, and deposition of uric acid or urate salts causes pathological damage since these compounds are not easily excreted. If they are deposited in the kidney they may crystallize as kidney stones. Concentration of uric acid in joints leads to a painful condition called gout.

Hypoxanthine is oxidized to uric acid by serving as the biochemical substrate of an enzyme, xanthine oxidase. An analog of hypoxanthine called allopurinol contains one carbon and one nitrogen atom interchanged. It is oxidized much more slowly than hypoxanthine, that is, it is a poorer substrate of xanthine oxidase, but allopurinol interferes effectively with the enzymatic oxidation of hypoxanthine by attaching itself to the active site of the enzyme and denying the normal substrate access to the catalytic site. The result is that formation of uric acid is brought to a standstill, and the amounts already deposited can be washed out by slow dissolution in blood serum. The sequence has made allopurinol valuable in the treatment of gout.

The 6-hydroxy (OH) group of hypoxanthine as well as the amino (NH_2) group of the even more important metabolite, 6-aminopurine (adenine), can be replaced synthetically by isosteric groups, among them thiol (SH). The compound containing the SH group is 6-mercaptopurine (6-MP). Like adenine, 6-MP can be incorporated into polynucleotides, but, unlike adenine nucleotides, the unnatural polynucleotides containing 6-MP cannot function in nucleic acids. Since nucleic acid molecules contain the gene regions which regulate the biosynthesis of many cell chemicals, 6-MP will interrupt cell multiplication ("cell growth"), and the first cells to suffer are those that proliferate in an uncontrolled fashion, that is, cancer cells. Thus, 6-MP can be used in cancer chemotherapy. Unfortunately, normally but rapidly multiplying cells such as bone marrow cells are also depressed by 6-MP and this limits the administration of larger, more effective doses in the treatment of malignancies.

A second example of drug development based on metabolite antagonism is the design of the antiulcer drug, cimetidine. It had been known that among the causes of excessive formation of gastric hydrochloric acid and the concomitant ulceration of the gastrointestinal wall was a hypersecretion of histamine. Classical antihistaminics counteract other damaging manifestations of histamine such as allergies and hay fever, but not hyperchlorhydria in the stomach. Therefore, it had to be assumed that histamine acts on two different types of receptors. Those receptors blockable by antiallergenic drugs were called H_1 receptors, the others H_2 receptors. The H_1 receptor antagonists — the antiallergenic antihistaminics — do not, on the whole, resemble histamine, but contain bulky molecular blocking groups which deny histamine access to the H_1 receptor area. In planning the design of H_2 receptor antagonists, the principal structural features of histamine were chosen as a starting point, namely an imidazole ring carrying a basic side chain. Adoption of the imidazole system as a basic unit was followed by patient modification of the side chain, lengthening it, making it more basic or less basic, studying the effect of bulkier basic groups, replacing carbon by other atoms, etc. A total of 700 compounds was synthesized by 50 chemists over the period of a decade. Two compounds were chosen for extensive clinical trial, and both had to be abandoned because of detrimental side actions. Finally, a third backup drug, cimetidine, was tested. It incorporated an ingenious avoidance of the side effects of the earlier (thiourea) analogs, planned on the chemical drawing board. Later, the role of imidazole as an essential unit in such drugs was questioned, and the imidazole section was replaced by furan and basically substituted groups. Several agents containing these alterations, such as rinitidine, have been introduced into ulcer therapy.

The moral of these examples is that an ever increasing amount of defendable rationale can be brought to bear on drug design by molecular modification, but that much empirical work with its inherent inevitable errors still has to fill in the final details. Application of metabolite analogy, bioisosterism, and some aspects of QSAR have already shortened the initial phases of drug design, but have not had much impact on the cost of this work. An estimated $6 million for chemical and preliminary biological work in the design of a new drug is probably on the conservative side. Imitative drugs patterned on closely similar and therapeutically successful agents will require somewhat less effort and expense. On the other hand, the intellectual challenge of independent and novel drug design rewards the participating investigators, and the joy of being a creative medicinal scientist contributes more to this effort than any other consideration.

IX. CURRENT TRENDS IN DRUG DESIGN

Trends in drug design and development vary with the demands or suggestions of the medical profession, and with the discovery of new biochemical and biological observations that open up paths of investigation of diseases hitherto unapproachable by more traditional methods. Two such examples are the attacks on retroviral infections, especially herpes and acquired immunodeficiency syndrome (AIDS).

Feverish efforts to find chemotherapeutic agents for herpes simplex and HIV infections have been based on the realization that some enzymes essential for the proliferation of malignant cells (cancers) are similar to those that are needed for the multiplication of viruses, e.g., RNA polymerase. The drugs developed at this writing, acyclovir for herpes simplex, and azidode-oxythymidine for AIDS, were designed as antimetabolites in cancer chemotherapy. Although not curative, they have pointed the way future drug design should pursue or, perhaps in some aspects, should avoid.[22]

The aim of drug design to align potential therapeutic agents to the active sites of enzymes and receptors is advancing slowly toward realization of this long-held dream. Receptors for hormones, antibodies, and drugs are beginning to be recognized as proteins and often as glycoproteins, consisting of subunits of molecular ranges of 100,000 to 300,000. Many receptors need a lipid environment. They appear to span cell membranes, with a hydrophobic end on the inside and a hydrophilic terminus on the serum-based outside. Receptors have been isolated, sequenced, cloned, and reconstituted from many relevant organ tissues in quantities of 1 to 100 pmol/g tissue, for example, from brain.[23] Their chemical structure can be studied by the general precepts of protein structure, such as X-ray diffraction spectrometry. Until more is learned about molecular details of their active sites, their folded structures and their functions are being correlated to their biological response and the rate of their response, their stereospecificity, and the relationship of substrates and antagonists. This field of research, together with recombinant nucleic acid and protein work, is generally regarded as the most innovative and promising in drug design. These topics and many more traditional ones are being publicized in a new journal, *Drug Design and Delivery* (Harwood Academic Publishers), which made its appearance in 1986.

REFERENCES

1. **Balandrin, M. F., Klocke, J. A., Wurtele, E. S., and Bollinger, W. H.** *Science*, 228, 1154 (1985).
2. **Burger, A.,** *A Guide to the Chemical Basis of Drug Design,* John Wiley & Sons, New York, 1983.
3. **O'Malley, B. W. and Schrader, W. T.,** The receptors of steroid hormones, *Sci. Am.*, 32, 1976.
4. **Gund, P.,** Pharmacophoric pattern searching and receptor mapping, *Annu. Rep. Med. Chem.*, 14, 299, 1979.
5. **Bindra, J. S.,** Drug receptors, *Annu. Rep. Med. Chem.*, 8, 262, 1973.
6. **Mautner, H. G.,** Receptor theories and dose response relationships, in *Burger's Medicinal Chemistry, I*, 4th ed., Wolff, M. E., Ed., John Wiley & Sons, New York, 1980, 271.
7. **Kuntz, I. D., Jr.,** Drug receptor geometry, in *Burger's Medicinal Chemistry, I*, 4th ed., Wolff, M. E., Ed., John Wiley & Sons, New York, 1980, 285.
8. **Kollman, P. A.,** The nature of the drug-receptor bond, in *Burger's Medicinal Chemistry, I*, 4th ed., Wolff, M. E., Ed., John Wiley & Sons, New York, 1980, 313.
9. **Richards, L. E., and Burger, A.,** Mechanism-based inhibitors of monoamine oxidase, *Prog. Drug Res.*, 30, 205, 1986.
10. **Low, L. K. and Castagnoli, N., Jr.,** Drug biotransformations, in *Burger's Medicinal Chemistry, I*, 4th ed., Wolff, M. E., Ed., John Wiley & Sons, New York, 1980, 107.
11. **Nelson, S. D.,** Chemical and biological factors influencing drug biotransformation, in *Burger's Medicinal Chemistry, I*, 4th ed., Wolff, M. E., Ed., John Wiley & Sons, New York, 1980, 227.
12. **Sinkula, A. A.,** Prodrug approach in drug design, *Annu. Rep. Med. Chem.*, 10, 306, 1975.
13. **Burger, A.,** Relation of chemical structure and biological activity, in *Medicinal Chemistry*, 3rd ed., Burger, A., Ed., Wiley-Interscience, New York, 1970, 64.
14. **Schueler, F. W.,** Ed., *Molecular Modification in Drug Design*, Advances in Chemistry Series, 45, American Chemical Society, Washington, D.C., 1964.
15. **Higuchi, T., Finger, K. F., and Higuchi, W. I.,** Pharmaceutics and biopharmaceutics, *Annu. Rep. Med. Chem.*, 1, 331, 1965; 2, 340, 1966.
16. **Guillory, J. K.,** Pharmaceutics and biopharmaceutics, *Annu. Rep. Med. Chem.*, 6, 254, 1970.
17. **Fung, H. L.,** Pharmaceutics and biopharmaceutics, *Annu. Rep. Med. Chem.*, 8, 332, 1973.
18. **Friedman, H. L.,** Influence of Isosteric Replacement upon Biological Activity, National Academy of Sciences — National Research Council Publ. No. 206, Washington, D.C., 1951, 295.

19. **Cohen, P. J.,** History and theories of general anesthesia, in *The Pharmacological Basis of Therapeutics,* 5th ed., Goodman, L. S. and Gilman, A., Eds., Macmillan, New York, 1975, 57.
20. **Hansch, C.,** Quantitative structure-activity relationships in drug design, in *Drug Design,* Vol. 1, Ariens, E. J., Ed., Academic Press, New York, 1971, 271.
21. **Rogers, E. F.,** The antimetabolite concept in drug design, *Annu. Rep. Med. Chem.,* 11, 233, 1976.
22. **Robins, R. K.,** Synthetic antiviral agents, *Chem. & Eng. News,* 64 (4), 28, 1986.
23. **Snyder, S. H.,** Brain receptors — the emergence of a new pharmacology, *Trends Neurosci.,* 9(10), 455, 1986.

Chapter 6

APPROACHES TO SCREENING COMPOUNDS FOR PHARMACOLOGICAL ACTIVITY

Alfred Burger

TABLE OF CONTENTS

I. INTRODUCTION

The epitome of the U.S. Food and Drug Act and similar laws in other countries is that a drug must be safe and effective for use in medicine. The purpose of pharmacological testing is to measure effectiveness, safety, and relative freedom from unwanted side effects including carcinogenicity and teratogenicity. Every drug is studied first in animals and only after it has been found safe and effective in these tests, is it tried in humans. This chapter will deal with an outline of the testing of experimental drugs *in vitro* and *in vivo* under laboratory conditions and will exclude clinical pharmacology which is essentially a branch of experimental internal medicine.

II. DRUG REGULATIONS

Throughout the second half of the 19th century the U.S. Congress became concerned with the evils of useless and even harmful patent medicines and with food adulterations that were foisted by unscrupulous operators upon a confused and often ignorant public. More than a hundred bills to curb adulteration of food and the sale of patent medicines were considered from 1879 on, but were not enacted because of a reluctance to impose federal controls on states' rights and police powers, and because of effective lobbying by powerful manufacturers and distributors of such chemical products against what they saw as unwarranted extensions of government authority over private business.[1] In 1927, a Food, Drug and Insecticide Administration was split off this Bureau and became the direct predecessor of the present Food and Drug Administration (FDA) of the Department of Health and Human Resources. The Sherley Amendment of 1912 banned false or fraudulent statements about the effects of proprietary drugs.

The next legal updating occurred in 1938 as a consequence of a therapeutic catastrophe. A pharmaceutical company in Tennessee marketed an "elixir of sulfanilamide" with diethyleneglycol as a solvent without testing this liquid clinically. Some 80 patients treated with this mixture died, and the resulting public outcry forced Congress to amend the law, requiring safety as a prerequisite for marketing. In 1960 several European firms brought out a hypnotic drug, thalidomide, which was soon reported to have pronounced teratogenic effects when taken during the first trimester of pregnancy. American women were saved from the dangers of this drug by an alert FDA pharmacologist upon whose recommendations the drug was shelved. Congress again sharpened up the Food, Drug and Cosmetics Act by passing the Kefauver-Harris Amendments of 1962. Requirements for efficacy were added to safety regulations, and the preclinical and clinical trials of each drug were tightened by the FDA.[3,4] Additional amendments include the Comprehensive Drug Abuse Prevention and Control Act (1 May 1971), the Durham-Humphrey Amendment (Section 503 B, 1952), which defines drugs which may not be sold over the counter, but only with a prescription, and the Delaney clause (1958), which bans the use in food of any chemical that has been found to act as a carcinogen in man or animals when ingested in any amount.[5]

The FDA has issued directives which guide all phases of drug development, from the identification of a chemical as being of potential interest in therapy, through all animal tests and clinical phases.[6] Additional information on the nomenclature of drugs, their literature, and general attitudes of physicians towards drugs may be gathered from the treatise by Fingl and Woodbury.[5]

III. SCREENING PROCEDURES

The purpose of screening is the discovery of new drugs which might be of use later in clinical medicine. Screening has the advantage over other more efficient procedures of uncovering unexpected chemical structural types as agents active under the test conditions. Such unanticipated compounds can then serve as starting points for further elaboration of suitable drugs.

All pharmacological screening depends for its justification and eventual success on the use of test methods which have a significant bearing on the disease they are to emulate in the laboratory. Without such significance screening is, and has been quite often in the past, a waste of time. It is not easy to develop screening methods that must be interpreted for disease conditions in other species, especially in humans. The greatest difficulties are encountered in devising behavioral psychopharmacological animal tests which are to simulate human mental disorders. Here the border line between physiological aberration and deviations from learned behavior is not yet clear enough to base test methods on one or the other of these two components.

Screening of random compounds (blind screening) is always a wasteful operation, but remains a necessity if no "lead" is at hand for a given disease syndrome. As mentioned in Chapter 5, most plans for drug research are centered around physiological defects for which some biochemical abnormalities are known. This makes it possible to select candidate compounds that bear a functional or structural resemblance to the abnormal metabolite(s). Such a selection reduces the number of compounds to be screened and injects a note of rationality into an otherwise repetitive operation (see Chapter 5).

If the number of compounds in a screen is still very large, a test must be chosen which can be performed routinely by skilled technicians under the supervision of an experienced pharmacologist who will be alerted by any unusual observation of activities in the test system. *In vitro* testing lends itself best to this type of biological reconnaissance.

For greater in-depth information, a drug will always need to be tested *in vivo*. This takes more skill, effort, time, and expense, and exposes the animal to a risk. Some emotionally overly sensitive individuals oppose *in vivo* experiments in laboratory animals, even in mice and rats, and have been known to aggravate experimental biologists by their efforts to obtain legal injunctions against *in vivo* experimentation. Fortunately, their threats have remained unsuccessful so far. The latest and most serious organized opposition to animal testing is based on the assumption that computerized information should yield *in vitro* answers comparable to actual animal data. There is no evidence that biostatistics has reached the stage where this needs to be discussed further.

IV. *IN VITRO* SCREENING

In vitro means "in the glass"; experiments are carried out in laboratory ware in the absence of a living animal.

If a drug is supposed to inhibit some enzyme which is associated with a disease, the drug is added to a buffered aqueous solution of the enzyme in predetermined concentrations. It is incubated with the enzyme and the substrate is added. After another period of incubation the remaining substrate or the resulting reaction product is titrated or determined spectroscopically. The inhibitor will decrease the amount of reaction product as compared with a control run without the inhibitor.[7]

Purified enzymes are obtained for such experiments by extracting cell cultures or tissues and concentrating the catalytically active protein by chromatography. The cell culture itself in suspension can also be used as a source of the enzyme; however, most investigators prefer some stage of enzyme purification.

It is only a step from a cell culture to the use of surviving isolated animal organs. Isolated hearts, intestinal strips, and other organs can be immersed in a bath containing nutrients and the test drug, and the effect of the drug on their rate of contraction, relaxation, paralysis, etc., can be measured readily and recorded by amplifying devices. Such screening is called *"in vitro-in vivo"* testing. It represents a transition to tests in whole animals and furnishes results more meaningful than cell culture and enzyme preparations.

V. SCREENING FOR ANTIBIOTICS

The screening for antibiotics from microorganisms follows essentially the processing of natural products for evaluation of biological properties. However, the raw materials are not botanical as a rule, nor even cell cultures of the microbes, but soil samples that contain the microorganisms. Literally millions of soil samples from all over the world, starting in one's backyard, have been screened for antibiotic activity. The soil is leached out and the extract dripped into the center of a petri dish charged with several bacterial or neoplastic cultures or other pathogens in culture media radiating from the center of the dish. Inhibition of the growth of the microbial or neoplastic cell colonies can be spotted after an elapse of diffusion time. The microbes or cell strains responding to the inhibition are then isolated by culturing and can be "grown" in suitable nutrients for further study.[8,9]

This simple screening method can be carried out expeditiously by technicians. However, it must be interpreted with caution. The same microbes, especially some widely found Streptomyces species, have been "discovered" time and again in different soil samples and have thus given rise to "false positives".

When the structure of an antibiotically active drug — whether from cell cultures or synthetic — has become known, molecular modification may become indicated. The best-known case is that of the penicillins and cephalosporins, both beta-lactam antibiotics. Fermentation of natural benzylpenicillin under controlled conditions leads to 6-aminopenicillanic acid, the parent amino acid of all the penicillins. Acylation of the 6-amino group with thousands of acid chlorides or acids under the influence of a dehydrating agent has yielded over 10,000 semisynthetic penicillins which have been screened against dozens of pathogens *in vitro* as described above. Similarly, over 2000 acyl derivatives of 9-aminocephalosporanic acid have been screened. Some of these semisynthetic antibiotics have oral activity while the first-generation penicillins and cephalosporins had to be injected into the bloodstream. In addition, screening against antibiotic-resistant strains of pathogens has sorted out those molecular variants which, as least for some time, can overcome this resistance.

It goes without saying that antibiotics selected for *in vitro* activity must be tested for effectiveness and toxicity in laboratory animals infected with the drug-sensitive pathogen. This holds also for chemotherapeutic agents to be used in viral infections and in cancer.

VI. *IN VIVO* SCREENING

The animals used most widely are rodents (mice, rats, rabbits, hamsters), most of which are raised commercially to offer the pharmacologist uniformity of genetic, nutritional, sex, and health standards. One can also purchase animals after they have undergone and recovered from surgery such as hypophysectomy, thyroidectomy, castration, kidney artery ligation, etc., again under controlled and standardized conditions. The proverbial guinea pig is also used widely.

Larger mammalian species include cats, dogs, rhesus monkeys, and minipigs, as well as entirely different animals for special purposes such as amphibians (frogs, toads), fish, sheep, cattle, armadillo (for leprosy), and others. For uniformity, purebred strains are generally demanded; purebred beagle hounds have superseded randomly selected dogs from municipal pounds. Standardization of amphibians, fish, etc., is much less expensive.

The health, handling, and care of all laboratory animals is protected by law.[10] All surgery is performed under anesthesia, and so is all experimentation that causes pain except when pain thresholds are to be measured directly, As a rule, animals are not reused in subsequent tests because that might prejudice the reactions to the new test even after a lapse of adequate time. Animals no longer needed in the laboratory are usually killed by gentle injections of narcotics, and their carcasses are incinerated. Dogs and other large animals that have not been impaired by a pharmacological experiment may be returned to domestic life.

VII. *IN VIVO* TESTING

Tests in intact animals *(in vivo)* are the ultimate criterion of potency, selectivity, oral activity, and toxicity of a drug under laboratory conditions. They must precede similar procedures in humans during clinical pharmacological experiments.

Most test compounds are available only in very small quantities, either from the extraction of natural sources or as end products of often complicated, multistep chemical syntheses. Since the effect of a compound is proportional to the weight of the test animal, the smallest laboratory animals, i.e., mice, are used in the first tests. If there is a cogent reason to suspect that the drug might be metabolized in the mouse in a manner that would preclude use of this species even for preliminary experiments, other species will of course be used, but this is barely ever necessary.

The first test is usually a tentative trial of effective and toxic dose ranges. About five mice matched for weight, sex, and genetic homogeneity are injected with the drug in increasing amounts until an effect is noted. That may include excitement, restlessness, stupor, catatonia, exophthalmia, piloerection, rigidity, and other symptoms which can be interpreted as definite areas of pharmacological activity. Toxicity symptoms such as nausea, vomiting, vertigo, convulsions, etc., can also be observed. Administration of the drug can be altered, from the i.p. to i.v. or oral route, the latter by stomach tube if the drug has to be conserved, or by incorporating the drug in the animals' food or water supply.

For particular tests, specially prepared animals may have to be used. If, for example, hormonal effects are to be studied, rats and mice surgically pretreated to remove various endocrine glands can be purchased. Animals made diabetic or hypertensive are also available. Some species are, of course, more suitable than others to give a good picture of a given condition. Thus, dependence liability resembling human addiction is demonstrated impressively in primates.

VIII. EXTRAPOLATION OF ANIMAL TEST DATA TO HUMANS

The activity and potency of a drug depend on a number of factors. These include intrinsic activity of the drug at its receptors, and this is believed to be more or less identical in different mammalian species. In other words, a cholinergic drug applied directly to strips of isolated gut of different animal species is expected to produce the same force of contraction; an inotropic agent applied to a surviving isolated heart should cause the heart to beat similarly in various species.

Differences in activity arise from the transport of the drug in the animal body. This includes absorption, distribution, blood levels, metabolism, and excretion. The sum of these properties is called pharmacokinetics. Tests for qualitative and quantitative data on the pharmacokinetics of a new agent always follow the primary establishment of activity and toxicity.

For some drugs, the pharmacokinetics in the rat resemble that in humans, for other drugs the dog is a better model. Of all animal species studied, the pig is perhaps most comparable metabolically to humans. Since pigs are large and would consume too much of an experimental drug (activity is proportional to kilogram body weight), a species of minipigs has been bred that has analogous metabolic requirements.

IX. ABSORPTION AND DISTRIBUTION[11]

Absorption is fastest and most complete if the drug is placed directly in the organ to be treated; this is usually not practical and therefore i.p. or i.v. injection is commonly preferred. The drug is carried by the blood, hopefully to its destination, but membranes of vessels along the way permit some of the drug to cross over into other organs. Some portions of the drug may also be absorbed on the surface of serum protein molecules ("sites of loss"). Only a fraction of even the best-absorbed drug reaches the receptors.

For most medicinal purposes, oral administration of drugs is mandatory, especially if medication at repeated intervals and over prolonged periods of time is required. The drug is thereby exposed to salivary, gastric, and intestinal digestive enzymes as well as to gastric acid before it is absorbed across the stomach or intestinal wall, usually into the portal circulation. It is then transported to the liver, the body's principal metabolic organ. Only a small percentage of an orally administered drug will remain available for action at its receptors.

Analysis of various tissues will determine the degree of absorption. In many cases, radioactively labeled drugs are used for this purpose, the radioactivity of tissues being monitored at set time intervals. Spectroscopic tests will confirm whether the drug or its metabolites display the radioactivity in the tissues. These tests also measure the total time needed to clear the organism of the drug. Further discussion of these parameters is found in Chapter 13 on biopharmaceutic and pharmacokinetic studies.

X. BIOTRANSFORMATION

Most drugs are metabolized, mainly in the liver and kidney, but also in other organs; few are excreted unchanged. Biotransformation is studied in conjunction with screening and drug development.

The primary metabolic pathways of foreign compounds are oxidation, reduction, methylation, dealkylation, and some minor other reactions.[11,12] Secondary biometabolism is called conjugation; it serves to solubilize and detoxify compounds as a prerequisite to excretion. Hydroxylated compounds are conjugated as esters of sulfuric acid, amines, or acids as amides of metabolic amino acids, as glucuronides, etc.

A minority of drugs are bioactivated, the metabolites being more active or more toxic than the parent drug. The occurrence of such activated metabolites is suggested by delayed pharmacological activity. Thus, the antidepressant, imipramine, is *N*-demethylated to its more active desmethyl derivative, desipramine. In a similar way, the local anesthetic, lidocaine, is *N*-deethylated to a more potent secondary amine. Activation by ring closure and other major structural changes have also been observed.

Some unsaturated and aromatic compounds are epoxidized, and the epoxides can react with nucleic acids, starting a chain of events that can lead to mutations.

XI. EXCRETION[12]

The major routes or excretion of drugs and drug metabolites are the kidney, the bile, feces, the lung, and the skin. Urinary excretion is the most important route of ridding the body of metabolites as well as foreign materials. Drugs are excreted by the various filtration mechanisms in the kidney. Excretion from the liver by means of the bile leads foreign substances into the intestinal tract. The lungs excrete CO_2 and other gases as well as volatile metabolites (acetone in diabetic coma, mercaptans, etc.). The skin accumulates and excretes various drugs; this can be observed macroscopically in the case of dyestuffs which color the skin as an undesirable side effect of their action.

XII. MUTAGENICITY TESTS

It has become axiomatic to test all drugs for mutagenicity before clinical trial. Existing law requires such tests for food additives only, but in the course of the protracted study of a New Drug Application by the FDA questions concerning mutagenic properties are always raised, and the industry performs the tests in anticipation of such inquiries.

A positive test for mutagenic potential does not necessarily imply that the compound is carcinogenic. However, a positive test is a warning that carcinogenicity — which follows alteration in cellular metabolism, i.e., mutation — may be a danger and it is generally regarded as a suggestion that the compound should be abandoned. The most widely approved mutagenicity test is an *in vitro* procedure by Ames et al.[13] A positive Ames test also warns of teratogenic potential, but this must be confirmed by studying the effects of the drug on rat or murine fetuses. Even if abnormal fetuses result from such experiments, a definite prediction of analogous activity in human pregnancy cannot be made. Nevertheless, apprehension of teratogenic carry-over into humans precludes further use in clinical medicine.

XIII. EVALUATION OF TEST DATA

The therapeutic index of a drug is the relationship of toxic to effective dosages. Most commonly, the LD_{50} is defined as the dose lethal to 50% of the animals used. The ED_{50} is the dose effective for a given test in 50% of the animals. One can also calculate LD_{90}, LD_{100}, ED_{80}, and scores of other values, but biostatistically the 50% data are the most commonly used ones. The fractions, LD_{50}/ED_{50} or TD_{50}/ED_{50}, where TD is the toxic dose, are variants of the therapeutic index. There used to be a tendency toward overspecialization among all branches of medicinal scientists. Those interested in antihypertensive, hormonal, and other pharmacodynamic agents could see little connection with the study of chemotherapy, classically defined as the cure or treatment of infectious diseases. When it became apparent that all drugs affect fundamental biochemical processes, be they bacterial, glandular, invasive, hormonal, etc., these artificial barriers broke down. This led to the routine screening of drugs designed as chemotherapeutic agents in pharmacological conditions, and more than once was activity revealed in apparently unrelated areas. One of the best-known cases, diethylcarbamazine, which was designed as an analgetic, fulfilled this prediction, but on further broad screening was found to have potent antifilarial activity in roundworm infestations.

Observations of side effects unrelated to the original test activity are required under FDA regulations as a contribution to the activity spectrum of a drug. From the standpoint of the medicinal chemist such observations serve as take-off positions in developing new agents for other maladies (see Chapter 5 and the discussion in Chapter 7 on biologics as therapeutic agents).

REFERENCES

1. **Skolnik, H. and Reese, K. M.,** Eds., *A Century of Chemistry,* American Chemical Society, Washington, D.C., 1976, 153.
2. **Young, J. H.,** Drugs and the 1906 law, in *Safeguarding the Public-Historical Aspects of Medicinal Drug Control,* Blake, J. B., Ed., The Johns Hopkins Press, Baltimore, MD, 1970, 147.
3. U.S. Department of Health, Education and Welfare, Food and Drug Administration "New Drug" Regulations, Washington, D.C., 1962.
4. Food and Drug Administration, Use of drugs for unapproved indications; your legal responsibility, *FDA Drug Bull.,* 1972.
5. **Fingl, E. and Woodbury, D. M.,** General principles, in *The Pharmacological Basis of Therapeutics,* 5th ed., Goodman, L. S., and Gilman, A., Eds., Macmillan, New York, 1975, 42.
6. **Gordon, A. J. and Gilgore, S. G.,** The art and science of contemporary drug development, *Prog. Drug Res.,* 16, 194, 1972.
7. **Lowe, C. R. and Dean, P. D. G.,** *Affinity Chromatography, Enzyme Analysis,* John Wiley & Sons, New York, 1974.
8. **Hollstein, U.,** Nonlactam antibiotics, in *Burger's Medicinal Chemistry, II,* 4th ed., Wolff, M. E., Ed., John Wiley & Sons, New York, 1979, 173.
9. **Gottlieb, D. and Shaw, P. D.,** Eds., *Antibiotics,* Vol. 2, Springer-Verlag, New York, 1967.
10. Committee on Care and Use of Laboratory Animals, ILAR, NRC, Guide for the Care and Use of Laboratory Animals, DHEW Publ. No. (NIH) 78-23, U.S. Government Printing Office, Washington, D.C., 1978.

11. **Gillette, J. R. and Pang, K. S.,** Drug absorption, distribution, and elimination, in *Burger's Medicinal Chemistry,* Part I, 4th ed., Wolff, M. E., Ed., John Wiley & Sons, New York, 1980, 55.

12. **Low, L. K. and Castagnoli, N., Jr.,** Drug biotransformations, in *Burger's Medicinal Chemistry,* Part I, 4th ed., Wolff, M. E., Ed., John Wiley & Sons, New York, 1980, 107.

13. **McCann, J. E., Choi, E., Yamasaki, E., and Ames, B. N.,** Detection of carcinogens as mutagens in the *Salmonella*/microsome test: assay of 300 chemicals, *Proc. Natl. Acad. Sci. U.S.A.,* 72, 5135, 1975.

Chapter 7

BIOLOGICS AS THERAPEUTIC AGENTS: PITFALLS AND PROMISES

Michael Williams

TABLE OF CONTENTS

I. INTRODUCTION

Biotechnology, the driving force in the biological sciences in the latter part of the 20th century, is destined to be an important factor in efforts devoted to new drug discovery well into the 21st century. Yet, the potential contribution of this new branch of science, a mixture of biochemistry and cell biology, is controversial.

Keen interest from the financial community in funding biotechnology companies suggests that products derived from recombinant DNA (rDNA)-based technologies offer the opportunity for a wealth of potential new therapeutic entities. In addition, the basic techniques of molecular biology per se provide a powerful tool to better understand the function of biological systems and the factors related to disease etiology. There is some concern, however, from more experienced traditional drug discoverers, who, while recognizing the potential contributions of the technology, question how the new types of "high-tech" drugs, generically termed biologics, will circumvent the problems of bioavailability, efficacy, and unmet medical need that all new therapeutic entities need to address to be approved by the FDA. These factors are of especial concern, considering that most biologics are peptidic in nature. More optimistically, molecular biologists see their technology as *the* "new pharmacology" and the dawning of a new era in therapeutics where diseases previously untargeted or unresponsive to the "magic bullets" of conventional drug therapy will become amenable to treatment.

The logical and synergistic integration of biotechnology into the drug discovery process is a major challenge for drug discovery. Yet it is only very recently, in the commercial sector, that science, rather than finance, has been the driving force in the use of molecular biology. Access to venture capital funding has enabled many molecular biologists to start their own companies to the extent that it is an exception that a department head from a major university does not have his or her own company. And, based on the phenomenal success of computer entrepreneurs, many such individuals hope to amass vast personal fortunes while discovering drugs. These hopes are fueled by the challenges facing established pharmaceutical companies due to changes in the business environment: increased global competition,[1] compound lines facing patent expiration and generic competition; increased costs of bringing a drug to market and increased financial expectations.[2,3] Drug houses have therefore turned to biotechnology in the hope of finding new ways to remain competitive while maintaining a favorable return on investment.

These conflicting attitudes and the resultant confusion have, however, raised expectations beyond what might be considered reasonable and have delayed the integration of molecular biology, as a research tool, into the multidisciplinary arena that is drug discovery. In addition, many pharmaceutical companies have succeeded in alienating both their pharmacologists and molecular biologists by hiring the latter, with unlimited funding (usually at the expense of existing programs), to do the "real" drug discovery in a total vacuum, not realizing, despite an extensive history to the contrary, that drug discovery is not a simple product of an equation where scientific idea plus money equals drug. This fact has been realized recently by the financial community which has rather hypocritically judged Genentech as being overoptimistic in its financial projections for the antithrombotic biologic, tissue-plasminogen activator (t-PA)[4] when the former itself insisted on ignoring the realities of the marketplace in terms of product acceptance and reimbursement, as well as pricing. Thus, an unfortunate backlash now exists where the inherent promise of the biotechnology has been compromised by overzealousness.

II. OF BIOTECHNOLOGY, MOLECULAR BIOLOGY, AND GENETIC ENGINEERING

The science of biotechnology, defined as "the process of *in vitro* alteration of genetic material for the process of creating new gene combinations or modifications",[5] relies on living systems, prokaryotic and eukaryotic, to produce biological materials. While recent advances in molecular biology, specifically rDNA and hybridoma-based monoclonal antibody production, have provided the basis for the present biotechnological explosion, the underlying concepts can be traced back to the genetic experiments of Mendel in the last century and have been extensively used in the present century in the selective breeding of both plants and animals.

The discovery of the genetic code in the 1950s, followed in the next decade by information related to the cellular factors involved in the control of gene expression and the ability, via the use of restriction endonucleases and various "blotting" hybridization techniques, to derive restriction maps for DNA from various sources has allowed its subsequent sequencing by a variety of biochemical techniques. The discovery that a DNA molecule could be generated with cohesive ends by using the *Eco*R1 restriction enzyme and could then be rejoined by the enzyme DNA ligase provided a means for site-specific genetic recombination. The mixing of *Eco*R1-derived DNA fragments from mammalian DNA with bacteria plasmid DNA that had been similarly treated, followed by DNA ligase treatment, enabled the insertion of foreign DNA into bacterial plasmids, which then acted as vectors for the rDNA thus formed. This technology, developed by Boyer and Cohen in 1973, provided the basis for the founding of Genentech.

The total DNA content of a mammalian cell can be fragmented via the use of appropriate restriction enzymes chosen from the over 400 identified to date and inserted into plasmid vectors to form a heterogenous population of bacteria termed a "DNA library". Using radiolabeled mRNA corresponding to the gene being sought or an mRNA derived from knowledge of the partial sequence of the protein product of interest, oligonucleotide-specific cDNA clones can be identified, isolated, and amplified by growth of the resultant bacteria. Pure mRNA probes are, however, relatively rare. Using reverse transcriptase, however, mRNA can be used to synthesize a complementary or cDNA fragment that can then be used to construct a bacterial cDNA gene library from which single cDNA recombinant molecules can be isolated or cloned by appropriate screening methodologies.[6] The resultant cDNA probes can then be used as a tool to study intact cellular DNA to search for copies in cell genomes or mRNA using radiolabeled cDNA. The potential for altered DNA patterns in individual genomic DNA fragments produced by restriction endonuclease activity can similarly be probed. DNA markers, restriction fragment length polymorphisms (RFLPs) and various oligonucleotide probes can be used to identify the genes responsible for genetically based diseases. Such predictive diagnosis allows the identification of individuals who are likely to develop diseases such as cystic fibrosis and muscular dystrophy. "DNA-fingerprinting" has also proved to be a powerful tool in the forensic sciences, and while equally important in determining the consequences of reproductive activity in genetically disease-prone individuals, it has disturbing and unresolved social implications, not the least of which relates to the ability of the insurance industry to remove a large element of chance from its actuarial tables. RFLPs have allowed the determination of over 50 genes involved in genetic disease states as well as permitting the detection of transforming *ras* genes in various human cancers.[7] In concert with oligonucleotide hybridization techniques that permit detection of oncogene translocations, RFLPs may prove to be important in cancer prognosis and diagnosis.

Recombinant DNA plasmid expression vectors in prokaryotic or eukaryotic cells can be used to mass produce gene products, providing a relatively inexpensive source of proteins that have biological or therapeutic importance. The cells are allowed to divide and grow in fermenters, resulting in peptides and proteins that are theoretically purer than those obtained by fractionation of human or animal tissue sources.[8] In addition, since the expression vectors are usually derived from human cells, the protein products are usually nonimmunogenic and thus do not give rise to antibody production.

rDNA expression systems are not without their problems, however. In bacteria, the gene product is often unstable and is rapidly degraded. In addition, incorrect folding, leading to biologically inactive molecules, can occur in peptides dependent on disulfide bridge formation, the intracellular environment of most bacteria resulting in the reduction of the critical S-S bond formation. This problem has been overcome by either engineering *Lac-Z* inclusion bodies that stabilize the protein or by genetically attaching secretion/affinity "handles" to the rDNA gene product, which permits secretion of the peptide/protein from the bacterium. The use of an immunoglobin G (IgG) handle forms the basis of KabiGen's EcoSec system for the production of insulin-like growth factor-1 (IGF-1), secretin, and various recombinant vaccines.[8] Altered posttranslational modification and anchoring of the gene product in unicellular systems may also result in protein that lack the biological activity of interest.

Another facet of biotechnology is the fusion of antibody-producing lymphocytes with immortalized myeloma cells resulting in the production of hybridoma cells. Such immortal clones permit an unlimited supply of monoclonal antibodies, which have revolutionized conventional disease diagnosis techniques, in terms of specificity, rapidity, reproducibility, and speed. Monoclonal antibodies may also be useful in the site-specific delivery of bioactive materials.[9]

DNA constructs may also be made where alterations in the cDNA are made *in vitro* via the use of genetic engineering. These are then transfected into mammalian cells or embryos and their effects on differentiation and function are studied. Similar alterations in the DNA may be used to engineer improved versions of the protein expressed by a given gene.[10]

Joining the promoter sequence of a highly active mammalian gene with that of the coding sequence for a protein of interest results in a transgene that when transfected into an embryo can be used to produce large amounts of that protein — in essence a protein factory. Transgenic mice capable of producing milk containing t-PA are one result of this approach,[11] and it is anticipated that transgenic dairy animals may be used to provide a variety of therapeutically useful milk products. Transgenic mice with the activated *ras* oncogene (OncoMouse/DuPont) are available as carcinogenic models for cancer research.[12]

III. BIOLOGICS AS DRUG ENTITIES

A biologic is a therapeutic entity, usually an endogenous hormone, autacoid, or homeostatic mediator, that has the potential to produce a beneficial effect on mammalian tissue function when the status quo is compromised such as usually occurs following trauma or disease. While such entities are often viewed as replacement therapy, vaccines are also representative of this class of therapeutic agent. Recombinant hepatitis B vaccine and recombinant insulin represent two of the first biotechnological drugs, while vaccines against another 15 or so infective organisms are undergoing clinical trials.[8]

In addition to hormones such as insulin, glucagon, thyrotropin, and oxytocin, which are amenable to extraction from animal or human tissues, or calcitonin, adrenocorticotropic hormone (ACTH) 1-24, and secretin, which may be synthesized, biologics encompass other naturally occurring peptides and proteins that can only be obtained by rDNA methodologies. These include t-PA, blood Factor VIII, interferons, interleukins, erythropoietin, human growth hormone, granulocyte macrophage colony-stimulating factor (GM-CSF), adhesion factors, hirudin, and various growth factors. Biotechnology has thus provided the means to produce biologics that were previously prohibitively expensive or unobtainable by extraction of synthesis.

Such rDNA products represent the first generation of peptide products and have provided a means to treat disease conditions that lacked effective therapies. Limited successes with biologics in the area of immunology, oncology, and inflammation have led to major conceptual changes in therapeutic targeting for such disease states with conventional treatments such as nonsteroidal anti-inflammatory agents and chemotherapy being viewed as transition treatment measures subject to replacement by biological response modifiers that are selectively active at disease-related targets. This view may be considered naive based on the limited successes to date, unacceptable side-effect profiles, and limited therapeutic applicability having been observed for the various cytokines that have been clinically tested. It is, however, an important new perspective for the pharmaceutical industry inasmuch as drug discovery efforts are being redirected from finding "improved" analogs of indomethacin and cisplatin to discovering agents that may have direct effects on the disease process with a marked increase in specificity and reduction in side-effect profile.

The second generation of rDNA products offers considerably more promise as therapeutic entities in that these peptides are being genetically engineered to have an improved pharmacological profile. The elimination of amino acid sequences susceptible to proteolytic attack or alterations in receptor/enzyme binding domains may improve oral activity, bioavailability, and target-site specificity as well as reducing the side-effect profile and duration of action. t-PA and single-chain urokinase-like plasminogen activator represent second-generation rDNA products[10] that, while more selective than urokinase or streptokinase as antithrombotics, appear to offer little in the way of clinical advantage.

The third generation of rDNA products is that of chimeric molecules where a transgene utilizing discrete sequences from the coding domains of two or more genes results in the production of what are known as "designer peptides". These entities may combine the catalytic domain of an enzyme with the recognition sequence of a cell-specific receptor that allows the vectored delivery of the enzyme. A t-PA hybrid consisting of a disulfide link between the A chain of plasminogen and the B chain of urokinase is twice as active as urokinase.[13] Bispecific antibody conjugates recognizing fibrin and t-PA epitopes increase the potency of t-PA fivefold, presumably due to an increase in the effective concentration of t-PA in the proximity of the fibrin deposit. Hybrid-hybridoma bispecific antibodies to fibrin and t-PA are 11 times more active than t-PA *in vitro*, and, in contrast to the chemically linked conjugates, are most homogenous and stable as well as easier to produce.[10]

IV. THERAPEUTIC INNOVATIONS IN THE AREA OF BIOLOGICS

A. IMMUNOMODULATORY AGENTS

Many of the biologics currently targeted as drugs are immunomodulators involved in inflammatory responses. The lymphokines and monokines affect cell growth and differentiation, and, while effective in preserving host function in response to tissue injury or infection, are major contributing factors to autoimmune diseases such as rheumatoid arthritis.

The seven interleukins, the α and β forms of tumor necrosis factor (TNF), and γ-interferon (INF-γ) have a complex and synergistic relationship modulating both B and T cell differentiation, growth, and function. Interleukin-1 (IL-1) and TNFα stimulate production of INF-γ and enhance IL-2 and IL-6 release, while IL-5 can induce IL-2 receptor expression in activated B cells. In light of the involvement of these agents in a variety of autoimmune disease states, considerable effort is being expended in finding ways to reduce their activities.[14] Strategies include receptor antagonism, transcriptional and posttranscriptional control, and inhibition of protein processing. The use of the factors themselves, INF-γ, TNFα, and IL-2, as biologics has focused on tumor therapy with mixed results in the clinic that may be obviated by combination therapies.

B. BLOOD FACTORS AND HORMONE REPLACEMENT THERAPY

The use of rDNA technology to produce blood factors such as erythropoietin (EPO), GM-CSF, and Factor VIII has provided new tools to treat patients with anemia and hemophilia. These biologics act as replacement therapies or to enhance the function of endogenous blood elements. Human growth hormone and insulin are other hormones that provide benefit in the treatment of various clinical situations.

C. ACQUIRED IMMUNODEFICIENCY SYNDROME (AIDS)

AIDS is one of the major targets for pharmaceutical intervention in the immediate future and is probably the most amenable to biologic-related drug targeting despite its many drawbacks. The causative agent of AIDS is the HIV-1 retrovirus, which specifically destroys CD4$^+$ T cells. The retrovirus has three enzymic activities pertinent to its infectivity: reverse transcriptase; integrase; and proteinase. Azidodeoxythymidine, AZT, the only effective treatment to date, inhibits the reverse transcriptase. Recently, however, the three-dimensional structure of HIV-1 aspartyl protease has been reported by researchers from Merck.[15] Thus two potential approaches to combating this disease are inhibition of the protease or antibodies that block the CD4 receptor.[16]

D. BONE METABOLISM

Steroid supplementation or the bisphosphonates represent the currently available drug treatments for osteoporosis and bone regenerative therapy. Transforming growth factor β (TGFβ) can augment the activity of matrix-producing cells in bone tissue and this indirectly facilitate bone mass formation. TGFβ is representative of a supergene family that includes three bone morphogenetic proteins (BMPs) that are involved in the initiation of cartilage formation and resultant bone formation.[17] While these factors have been discovered relatively recently, nonrecombinant BMP has been found to have varying degrees of success in the repair of fractures and skull defects in several species.

E. WOUND HEALING

Wound healing is a complex process involving cell-cell interactions in a variety of tissues. A number of biologics can facilitate the process of wound healing including: platelet-derived growth factor, epidermal growth factor (EGF, which is related to TGFβ), IGF-1, TNF and angiogenic factors, and IL-1. These agents appear to synergize with one another to effect an increase in cell density and extracellular connective tissue. In light of the fact that these biologics can be used as topical agents, they should prove therapeutically useful in their first- or second-generation rDNA formats.

F. NEUROLOGICAL DISEASES

Nerve growth factor and EGF, as well as a variety of neuromodulatory peptides, are involved in the differentiation of the mammalian nervous system and nerve regeneration. Because of the latter properties of such agents, there is a considerable interest in the use of such entities as potential therapeutics for a variety of neurodegenerative diseases including Alzheimer's and Huntington's chorea. Research in this area is at an early stage and will be dependent on the availability of such quantities of biological material for clinical evaluation. The presence of binding sites for endothelin and a number of cytokines in the brain and the observed central effects of the latter in clinical trials suggests that these biologics may subserve a modulatory role in brain function. As peptides, such agents may represent biologics for therapeutic targeting in central nervous system diseases. At the same time, the identification of such sites, distinct from peripheral sites targeted for drug therapy, reinforces the probability of side effects.

G. CANCER THERAPY

Chemotherapeutic approaches to the treatment of cancer, while often successful, have "shotgun" side-effect profiles that can only be justified by the seriousness of the disease under treatment. It is only in the past decade that biotechnology has provided the impetus and means to better understand the etiology of cancer and the process involved in the transformation of normal cells into malignant phenotypes.[9] Proto-oncogenes comprise a discrete set of approximately 24 genes with a ubiquitous distribution that can be transformed to oncogenes and are thought to be causative in tumor formation. Proto-oncogenes appear to be essential for normal cell function. For instance, the *ras* gene product p21 has GTPase activity and is involved in cellular transduction mechanisms in concert with a protein, glyceraldehyde phosphate (GAP), that activates GTPase activity and terminates the signaling process. Mutated p21 products have a reduced ability to interact with GAP as well as reduced GTPase activity. Oncogenes are formed from their respective protogenes by various transcriptional mechanisms including chromosome translocation, gene amplification, derepression/transactivation, hypomethylation, and proviral insertion and activation. Posttranscriptional mechanisms may also be involved in the metastatic process. These entities are currently being exploited as therapeutic targets in the cancer area with a variety of potential approaches including activation of oncogene suppressor genes and antisense oligonucleotides. CSF and other immunostimulants may also have potential in the treatment of cancer as may gene therapy.

V. BIOLOGICS AS COMPARED TO CONVENTIONAL THERAPEUTICS

In contrast to the process of drug discovery, the challenge in producing biologics in sufficiently high purity and quantities adequate for use a therapeutics is one comparable to pharmaceutical production rather than the discovery process per se. Thus, the traditional approaches involving screening and optimization of lead compound activity play little part in the development of biologics as therapeutic agents.

After identification of a therapeutic target at which the biologic produces a beneficial effect, the challenge is to engineer a system to produce sufficient material for patient use. However, "high tech" is insufficient to make a biologic a "blockbusting" new chemical entity (NCE). Market forces exert considerable influence on the potential of new biologics and underline the need for caution in treating such entities as distinct from those in conventional use. A case in point is recombinant t-PA, which at $3,000 or so per treatment appears to offer little benefit over the similar use of streptokinase at less than a quarter the cost.[4] Similar comments have been made in regard to the use of peptidic bradykinin analogs as pain killers.[18] Certainly, high tech per se cannot dictate market conditions, especially in an era of continuing emphasis on health cost containment.

These considerations are further impacted by the poor bioavailability of the biologics currently available. Most situations in which biologics are currently used involve systemic delivery and subsequent action in the vascular and reticuloendothelial systems. As with traditional drugs, however, biologics need to be targeted to specific sites to produce their effects. The additional costs in designing drug delivery systems may be anticipated to have a further negative impact on biologics in the marketplace unless such entities offer unique properties to meet unmet medical need.

The development of biologics as pharmaceutical agents may be considered in terms of four distinct phases. The first is the use of first- and second-generation rDNA products. The second, comparable to the third phase of rDNA technology, will involve the use of chimeric molecules, bifunctional antibody systems, and vectored, protected drug delivery systems. These phases, taken within the context of feasibility, represent a new wave of therapeutic agents that, irrespective of disease focus, may be generically termed biological response modifiers and which, given freedom from immune reactivity and unknown side effects, represent a totally new approach to human disease therapy.

The third phase of biologics will, however, be the most critical to the drug discovery process. This will entail the melding of basic research findings on the structure of the molecular targets at which the various biologics produce their effects with clinical data on the effects of the existing biologics with the tools used for the discovery and development of conventional therapeutic agents. This phase will represent the melding of biotechnology with the traditional approach to result in the fourth phase, that of "organic biologics", traditional pharmaceuticals synthesized by the organic chemist, optimized and directed to defined molecular therapeutic targets.

In order to achieve this situation, the major disadvantages of each of the technologies will need balancing with their inherent strengths. Available evidence suggests that biologics may cost half as much or less to bring to market as compared to conventional pharmaceuticals.[19] In comparing the two processes there are, however, inherent contradictions and assumptions that negate potential synergies between biotechnology and conventional drug discovery processes.

A. STRATEGIES

Much of the effort in conventional drug research is focused on the use of chemicals that antagonize the effects of natural mediators. Indeed, with few exceptions, most of the drugs currently in use are either receptor antagonists or enzyme inhibitors. In the hypertension area, for instance, the β-blockers act by antagonizing the effects of norepinephrine on heart function, while the angiotensin converting enzyme inhibitors act to prevent the formation of the pressor substance, angiotensin II. In contrast, as already discussed, the area of biotechnological drugs relies on the use of bioengineered biologics that duplicate the effects of known effector agents. In the light of the discovery of drug-specific receptors for the opiate analgesics and the anxiolytic, diazepam, it is possible that endogenous agents exist that function in a manner analogous to the biologics. Although antagonist function, based on the blockade of the effect of a given agonist in a defined biological system, may be considered somewhat reductionistic, it is evident based on the clinical efficacy of drugs such as the histamine H_2 receptor blockers and the various neuroleptics that receptor antagonism is a bona fide mechanism for therapeutic intervention.

The mechanistic focus of conventional drug discovery may therefore be distinct from that of the biologics, although, with the reporting of inverse receptor agonists that have negative efficacy,[19] it appears likely that drug therapies relying on receptors as their molecular targets need not necessarily conform to any discrete agonist/antagonist profile. Accordingly, the argument that engineered biologics are cheaper, easier and quicker to produce than conventional drug molecules, and that the approach to the latter, by implication, is less intellectually rigorous fails to take into account both the successes in the conventional drug arena as well as inherent differences in the types of product resulting.

B. SIDE-EFFECT PROFILES

It has also been suggested[19] that biologics, because they are genetically engineered natural products, are more efficacious and freer from side effects than conventional drugs. While this may be the case in situations where biologics are administered at doses thought to be within the "normal" range, when rt-PA is used as an exogenous thrombolytic agent, it is given in doses that far exceed this "safety zone". While this particular biologic is used as an acute therapy, in those cases where biologics are given on a chronic basis, the method of administration can result in pharmacokinetic profiles markedly distinct from the availability of the endogenous factor. Phasic availability of biological material following bolus administration may then affect the target tissue to alter receptor functionality and organ responsiveness.

The proposal that biologics have limited side-effects profiles as compared to conventional drugs appears inconsistent with a further suggestion[19] that biologics have a broader therapeutic advantage because they affect more basic cellular processes. While this may be the cause for biologics such as growth hormone, there is little evidence at the present time to suggest that this will be the case for all biologics unless they are all found to have a tonic, homeostatic influence on cell function. GM-CSF, during clinical trials for use in anemia, was found to be an extremely effective cholesterol-lowering agent.[21] This action, while viewed as beneficial, is a side effect nonetheless.

The whole issue of side-effect profiles in drug therapy, irrespective of compound source, is poorly understood. Organic therapeutics that have a limited side-effect profile due to their inbuilt selectivity may have a limitation in their "breadth of useful indications" when compared to biologics. By definition, however, breadth and selectivity appear incompatible. The CNS-related side effects and hypotension seen during clinical trials with the interleukins and INF-α, respectively,[14] would suggest that there is at best a very fine line between "breadth" and side effects for biologics. Efforts in making third-generation chimeric, bifunctional rDNA products are inherently "polypharmic" with more, rather than less, biological activity being anticipated. This approach is not dissimilar from having different activities in a single chemical molecule that then contribute to its efficacy in a synergistic fashion. The novel antipsychotic risperidone, which has potent activity at three monoaminergic receptor systems, is a case in point.[22]

Based on currently available clinical information, it would appear that few biologics are side-effect free. It seems unwise, therefore, to theoretically ascribe inherent benefits to these agents that have yet to be proven to any great extent in man. As with conventional therapeutics, the mechanistic basis for side-effect profiles is poorly, if at all, understood.

VI. BIOAVAILABILITY ISSUES

A. DRUG DELIVERY

Biologics as DNA products are peptidic in nature and thus subject to proteolysis en route to their site of action. For this reason, such entities have little, if any, oral efficacy and short half-lives. To circumvent these problems, the industry has invested heavily in drug delivery research.[23]

For biologics, as with peptides, these systems comprise three main approaches: noninvasive methods that circumvent degradation in the gut and avoid skin reactions at the injection site; administration via controlled delivery systems or in a "packaged" protected form; and vectored, site-specific delivery.

With the exception of the third approach, which is still the subject of considerable basic research efforts, the delivery of biologics depends on the administration of heroic quantities in the hope that sufficient amounts will reach the site of action in a biologically active form. This approach, especially with chronic administration, increases the potential for initiation of an allergic reaction. Even when administered intravenously, considerable amounts of peptidic molecules undergo degradation, first-pass metabolism, and binding to plasma proteins. Nasal administration, as in the case of ACTH, has similar problems, while controlled-release systems (osmotic minipumps or mechanical pumps) can result in dose dumping as well as pharmacokinetic profiles that are inconsistent with optimal therapeutic activity. Liposomes, red blood cell ghosts, and nylon microcapsules have been used as packaging systems for drug delivery. None has as yet been shown to be practical or consistently useful.

B. STABILITY

In addition to problems with bioavailability, peptides are also inherently more unstable when stored than chemicals. They are sensitive to light and temperature fluctuations as well as moisture and can easily lose their biological activity upon hydration, spontaneous reduction, or oxidation. While these problems may be circumvented by appropriate storage conditions and continued bioassay of activity, neither solution is comparable with the ease of use of the majority of drugs currently in use. Furthermore, in addition to the expense of monitoring the potency of peptidic drugs and controlling their shelf life, drug companies will also have to determine whether or not biologics have the capacity to become immunogenic as they age.

When the therapeutic use of such entities relates to either life-threatening situations or within an adjunct situation to cancer therapy or surgery, the single-dosage forms necessary and their need for ongoing quality control may be acceptable in terms of cost. Should such agents be positioned as more selective nonsteroidals or diuretics, their cost-benefit ratio will be prohibitive. Ideally, the organic molecule that acts at the same target as the novel biologic would be an ideal situation.

VII. MONOCLONAL ANTIBODY STRATEGIES

The use of monoclonal antibodies has principally focused on their potential for disease diagnosis. Over 150 monoclonal antibodies have been approved for use as diagnostic tools to detect a variety of disease indicators. In addition to quantifying the traditional analytes measured by radioimmunoassay, monoclonal antibodies can be used to image the degree of tissue damage resulting from a heart attack as well as in the treatment of septic shock (Centoxin).

Anti-idiotypic antibodies may represent a new class of drugs based on hybridoma technology. Monoclonal antibodies can be made to a drug. These are first-generation antibodies that can then be used to raise second-generation antibodies or "anti-ids", which theoretically should resemble in three-dimensional structure the original drug molecule.

Monoclonal antibodies can also be used to purify proteins, as cofactors in enzymic catalysis,[24] to enhance the production of peptidic drugs as well as to act as targeted drug-delivery systems for conventional drug therapies. This latter approach has been especially useful in the area of cancer therapy where immunotoxins such as abrin and ricin can be targeted to tumor-specific epitopes to spare normal cells from toxin actions. Adriamycin, daunomycin, INF, formyl-methionyleucylphenylalanine (fMLP), chlorambucil, and cobra venom factor, a functional analog of C3/C5 convertase, have also been targeted using monoclonal antibodies.[25]

VIII. MOLECULAR BIOLOGY AS A TOOL IN DRUG RESEARCH

rDNA and cDNA technologies have vastly altered the ability of the research scientist to study the functioning of biological systems. Techniques such as *in situ* hybridization, frog oocyte receptor expression, receptor isolation, cloning and sequencing, and the preparation of monoclonal antibodies have all facilitated research efforts in the areas of peptide effector agents.[26]

rDNA technology, in concert with the availability of cDNA libraries, has resulted in an exponential increase in knowledge related to receptor structure and function. Many receptors have been identified as part of supergene families with common structural elements suggestive of similar functionality. The ability to point mutate receptors and express these provides an additional vantage point for the determination of structure activity relationships for receptor-ligand interactions. Information derived from genetically altered receptors and from chemically or genetically modified receptor ligands can be used to enhance the value of computer-assisted molecular modeling in the drug-discovery process. Recent work using adrenergic receptor chimeras[27] has allowed delineation of the domains involved in ligand binding specificity and G-protein effector coupling.

The ability to express cDNA in frog oocytes has enabled cloned receptors to be identified using electrophysiological techniques. Even a few copies of a receptor that are not amenable to detection by biochemical techniques elicit appropriate electrophysiological responses to selective ligands in the transfected oocyte system.[26] In addition, the ability to select for a single cDNA product provides a unique biological system where individual components of a recognition/transduction/effector system can be studied in a relatively simple and controlled environment. In the area of neurobiology, this represents a major step in being able to understand the complex interactions involved in brain function that have only been amenable to study in the infinitely more complex and consequently more ephemeral whole-animal behavioral models.

In situ hybridization techniques allow the study of gene transcription and, together with monoclonal antibody techniques, facilitate understanding of the role of processing peptidases in the maturation of gene products and protein targeting. Monoclonal antibody technology has also enhanced diagnostic capability. Analytes previously detected by chemical methodologies can now more accurately and reproducibly be identified using antibodies. Thus the effects of new therapeutic entities on cellular metabolites can be more easily studied as can metabolites of the compounds themselves to derive more accurate adsorption, distribution, metabolism, and excretion (ADME) data.

The use of molecular biology in drug research extends well beyond the rDNA "protein factory" concept, providing useful information on drug targets that can be used in concert with traditional computer-assisted and medicinal chemistry approaches to design and test new compounds.

A further benefit of the biotechnology revolution is current focus on ligand-modulated, hormone-responsive elements on DNA as viable drug targets, these being members of the steroid/thyroid hormone supergene family.[28]

IX. GENE THERAPY

The infection of a gene-deficient individual with a functional form of the gene represents the ultimate in biologic therapy.[29] While the ethical issues of this approach have been extensively debated, the possibility of treating cancer, severe combined immunodeficiency syndrome (SCID), AIDS, Down's syndrome, cystic fibrosis, diabetes, epilepsy, and hypercholesterolemia by gene therapy is attractive. Genes can be delivered by liposomes, DNA vectors, and recombinant retroviruses. While the concept of gene therapy is attractive, there are some problems. In addition to the possibility of cellular oncogene activation or viral oncogene infection, another major problem is that the position in which the exogenous gene is inserted cannot be easily controlled. As a result, the exogenous gene can inactivate endogenous functional genes, be itself inactivated by the surrounding DNA, or give rise to new and potentially harmful transgenes. Such problems may explain why introduction of the gene for the enzyme, adenosine deaminase, which is lacking in SCID, using retroviral vector delivery, results in only 10% of the amount of enzyme required for successful therapy.[29]

X. COMMERCIAL AND LEGAL CONSIDERATIONS

Naturally occurring biological materials, by their nature, are difficult to patent. This has led to numerous costly lawsuits and to a growth in the legal profession associated with the biotechnology industry. It is probable that some biotechnology companies spend more on legal fees than on research. From an altruistic drug-discovery viewpoint, this is an unfortunate situation not only because of the complexities of the law that award companies use patents for biologics or for the process technology in some countries but not others, but also because the cost of litigation, however valid, can be more visibly decided on the basis of financial worth than justice. Limitations in current patent law and the financial motivation driving the biotechnology revolution appear to be poor criteria on which to base judgments that have major impact on the future of society as a whole.

Even in those instances where law courts rather than money have prevailed, the decisions have been unusual and often contradictory. For instance, the continuing patent litigation suit between Amgen and Genetics Institute (GI) over EPO initially resulted in Amgen being awarded the patent to produce EPO by rDNA technology in the U.S. with GI being able to market EPO in the U.S. As a result, GI was able to produce EPO abroad and import it for sale. At the time of writing (1989), both companies are making and marketing EPO while readying themselves for further visits to court.

One way to circumvent these problematic and seemingly unresolvable issues (especially when process patents are apparently easy to circumvent) is to produce an unique molecule based on the first-generation rDNA production. In the t-PA area, many companies are using genetic engineering not only to produce improved biologics, but also to produce patentable essentially *synthetic* entities. Such efforts differ little from those in ensuring broad patent coverage for conventional chemicals.

The commercialization of biologics as therapeutic agents has already been discussed in relation to Genentech's experiences with rt-PA and the stability and ease of use of peptidic materials as drugs. In life-threatening situations where no other medications are available; the cost-benefit ratio of biologics will be without parallel, especially when the alternative is surgery. However, in those instances where biologics do not provide discernible advantages over existing (and cheaper) therapies (streptokinase vs. t-PA), it is highly unlikely that they will be acceptable alternatives.

XI. DESIGNER DRUGS

If morphine was unknown and the endogenous opiates, the enkephalins and endorphins, were the only known ligands for the opiate receptors, the situation would be similar in many respects to that for the majority of biologics currently targeted for therapeutic use. Since the discovery of the endogenous opiates in the mid-1970s many millions of dollars have been spent in searching for molecules that mimic the effects of these agents that might also be free of the side effects — respiratory depression, constipation, and addiction — associated with morphine usage. Despite many theories related to receptor subtype selectivity, no such agent, peptide or otherwise, has yet been identified. Morphine, with its known limitations, thus remains the benchmark in pain control and a highly successful therapeutic entity.

From the present discourse, it is self-evident that biologics, while representative of a new and potentially exciting approach to drug therapy, are prototypes that must be replaced by conventional organic molecules that are as selective and potent in their therapeutic actions as the biologics, but have superior bioavailability and stability as well as being nonimmunogenic. In addition, such agents will be cheaper and more convenient to use in practical situations.

The source of such entities will require two separate drug discovery approaches. The first, already described, involves the use of biotechnology approaches in concert with computer-assisted molecular modeling, X-ray crystallography of therapeutic targets using rDNA vectors to obtain sufficient quantities of receptors and enzymes, and traditional medicinal chemistry in concert with conventional pharmacological approaches. The second, akin to the "discovery" of morphine, relies on the screening of natural products from plant, bacterial, and marine sources to find new lead compounds. In the area of immunomodulation there have been some striking successes following this approach. Cyclosporin A and FK 506 are immunosuppressants isolated from natural sources that are used in transplant therapy and act to block transcription of IL-2. Numerous other entities obtained by such "brute force" screening are under evaluation as tumor modulators, anti-inflammatory agents, and immunosuppressants. Inasmuch as these agents are derived from natural sources, they are by definition biologics. In contrast to the agents previously described, such entities appear to be closer to conventional therapeutic agents in that they act to block reactions occurring endogenously. It remains to be seen, however, whether or not "cyclosporin-like" agents may be identified in mammalian tissues.

In incorporating biotechnology into the drug discovery process, it is becoming increasingly apparent that while the technology has revolutionized the conceptual approach to identifying drug targets, the ultimate therapeutics will be patentable, synthetic, organic molecules. These will evolve, as have drugs in the past, by the diligent, methodical identification and development of lead compounds with optimal activity, bioavailability, and cost-benefit ratios.

The clinical evidence accumulated to date on the effects of the biologics currently available indicates that the first-generation products have the potential for all the problems associated with conventional drugs including side effects that limit their usefulness. In addition, their peptidic nature, for reasons discussed above, present additional problems, not the least of which is cost. In this regard, a better strategy than improving delivery methodologies would be to accelerate research efforts in the area of the fourth-generation "organic biologics".

Until clinical data are generated on second- and third-generation biologics, the major benefits of the biotechnology revolution to date are the broadening of research horizons as to viable drug targets and the establishment of a host of research boutiques that are highly motivated and able to evaluate potential new therapeutics free of the conservative approach attributed to the larger pharmaceutical companies. This ability to more rapidly move technology from discovery to therapy phases and the larger skill bases involved in the drug discovery in all quarters has done much to revitalize the industry and provide hope for new therapies that will meet unmet medical needs in an effective manner.

While the legal aspects of this revolution remain problematic, it is at least sobering to acknowledge the fact that while many attorneys are becoming rich in the course of litigation, they at least represent a potential patient population that can help absorb the development costs of second- and third-generation biologics. Assessment of the drug potential of these conceptual entities will be eagerly awaited by all those involved in drug-related research.

REFERENCES

1. **Redwood, H.,** *The Pharmaceutical Industry. Trends, Problems and Achievements,* Oldwicks Press, Felixstowe, U.K., 1987.
2. **Kolata, G.,** Companies searching for next $1 billion drug, *New York Times,* November 28, 1988, D1.
3. **Anon.,** The new world of drugs, *The Economist,* 310, 63, 1988.
4. **Chase, M.,** Genentech, battered by great expectations, is tightening its belt, *Wall Street Journal,* October 11, 1988, A1.
5. Committee on Science and Technology, Issues in the federal regulation of biotechnology: from research to release, House of Representatives, 99th Congress, 14 260 0, U.S. Government Printing Office, Washington, D.C., 1986
6. **Davis, L. G., Dibner, M. D., and Battey, J. F.,** *Basic Methods in Molecular Biology,* Elsevier, New York, 1986.
7. **Watkins, P. C.,** Restriction fragment length polymorphism (RFLP): applications in human chromosome mapping and genetic disease research, *Biotechniques,* 6, 310, 1988.
8. **Josephson, S. and Bishop, R.,** Production and isolation of peptide hormones: a contribution from biotechnology, *Drug News Perspect.,* 1, 271,.1988.
9. **Huber, B. E.,** Therapeutic opportunities involving cellular oncogenes: novel approaches fostered by biotechnology, *FASEB J.,* 3, 5, 1989.
10. **Haber, E., Quertermous, T., Matsueda, G. R., and Runge, M. S.,** Innovative approaches to plasminogen activator therapy, *Science,* 243, 51, 1989.
11. **Westphal, H.,** Transgenic mammals and biotechnology, *FASEB J.,* 3, 117, 1989.
12. **Rosenfeld, M. G., Crenshaw, E. B., Lira, S. A., Swanson, L., Borrelli, E., Heyman, R., and Evans, R. M.,** Transgenic mice: applications to the study of the nervous system, *Annu. Rev. Neurosci.,* 11, 353, 1988.
13. **Robbins, K. C. and Tanaka, Y.,** Covalent molecular weight ~ 92 000 hybrid plasminogen activator derived from human plasmin amino-terminus and urokinase carboxyl-terminus domains, *Biochemistry,* 25, 3603, 1986.
14. **Boger, J. and Schmidt, J. A.,** Immunomodulatory approaches to the treatment of inflammation, *Annu. Rep. Med. Chem.,* 23, 171, 1988.
15. **Navia, M. A., Fitzgerald, P. M. D., McKeever, B. M., Leu, C-T., Heimbach, J. C., Herber, W. K., Sigal, I. S., Darke, P. L., and Springer, J. P.,** Three-dimensional structure of aspartyl protease from human immunodeficiency virus HIV-1, *Nature (London),* 337, 615, 1989.
16. **Capon, D. J., Chamow, S. M., Mordenti, J., Marsters, S. A., Gregory, T., Mitsuya, H., Byrn, R. A., Lucas, C., Wurm, F. M., Gropman, J. E., Broder, S., and Smooth, D. H.,** Designing CD4 immunoadhesins for AIDS therapy, *Nature (London),* 337, 525, 1989.
17. **Wozney, J. M., Rosen, V., Celeste, A. J., Mitsock, L. M., Whitters, M. J., Kriz, R. W., Hewick, R. M., and Wang, E. A.,** Novel regulators of bone formation: molecular clones and activities, *Science,* 242, 1528, 1988.
18. **Williams, M. and Neil, G. L.,** Organizing for drug discovery, *Prog. Drug Res.,* 32, 329, 1988.
19. **Buell, S.,** Designer drugs: biotechnology comes of age, *Pharm. Exec.,* 9, 54, 1989.
20. **Williams, M. and Sills, M. A.,** Quantitative analysis of ligand receptor interactions, *Comp. Med. Chem.,* 3, 45, 1990.

21. **Nimer, S. D., Champlin, R. E., and Golde, D. W.,** Serum cholesterol-lowering activity of granulocyte-macrophage colony-stimulating factor, *JAMA,* 260, 3297, 1988.

22. **Leysen, J. E., Gommeren, W., De Chaffoy De Courcelles, D., Stoof, J. C., and Janssen, P. A. J.,** Biochemical profile of risperidone, a new antipsychotic, *J. Pharmacol. Exp. Ther.,* 247, 61, 1988.

23. **Tomlinson, E.,** (Patho)physiology and the temporal and spatial aspects of drug delivery, in *Site-Specific Drug Delivery,* Tomlinson, E. and Davis, S. S., Eds., Wiley, Chichester, U.K., 1986, 1.

24. **Tramontano, A., Janda, K. D., and Lerner, R. A.,** Catalytic antibodies, *Science,* 234, 1566, 1986.

25. **Upeslacis, J. and Hinman, L.,** Chemical modification of antibodies for cancer chemotherapy, *Annu. Rep. Med. Chem.,* 23, 151, 1988.

26. **Conn, P. M.,** *Neuroendocrine Peptide Methodology,* Academic Press, San Diego, 1989.

27. **Kobilka, B. K., Kobilka, T. S., Daniel, K., Regan, J. W., Caron, M. G., and Lefkowitz, R. J.,** Chimeric α_2, β_2-adrenergic receptors: delineation of domains involved in effector coupling and ligand binding specificity, *Science,* 240, 1310, 1988.

28. **Evans, R. M.,** The steroid and thyroid hormone receptor superfamily, *Science,* 240, 889, 1988.

29. **Marx, J. L.,** Gene therapy — so near and yet so far away, *Science,* 232, 824, 1986.

Chapter 8

PROJECT SELECTION FACTORS IN PHARMACEUTICAL R & D

Richard E. Faust

TABLE OF CONTENTS

I. THE RESEARCH ENVIRONMENT

A. NATIONAL GOALS

Industrial research has contributed greatly to the growth of the American economy over the past 100 years, and the domestic pharmaceutical industry, heavily research oriented, has led the world in the introduction of new drugs. However, technological innovation including new drug development in the U.S. has faltered over the last 10 years. Davis[1] observes that the challenge now is to renew this prime source of industrial strength of the country through a synthesis utilizing the characteristic strengths of industry, academia, and government. To bring this about long-range investments by industry are required, as well as stable, realistic policies by governments to encourage such investments. He notes that industrial research is at the threshold of a new era, but that a new synthesis of national, corporate, and academic resources to sustain innovation is essential. However the broadened and modified interplay between the public and private sectors takes place, it will have a pervasive influence on the nature of pharmaceutical research undertaken by the drug industry and ultimately on the project/program selection process.

People are demanding a greater voice in decision making regarding technology of all types, including how health care dollar resources should be invested for the total good of society; this includes influencing decisions concerning research programs and projects. The Organization for Economic Cooperation and Development reports that in Europe three general positive trends are being recognized:[2]

1. The government should provide fuller information about technological choices or assure that adequate knowledge is available through other institutions.
2. The public must be brought into the process of defining and making choices early enough that those choices are not merely trivial or artificial.
3. Regulation and legislation must be based on social cybernetic principles of foresight, feedback, and flexibility so that timely responses can be generated by an informed public.

B. CORPORATE POSTURE

Project selection within a firm is influenced by the corporate posture toward long-range, exploratory research. Research is by nature a process of risk taking. Many projects offer an unknown and highly variable payoff for an often uncertain expenditure, and this is especially true of those research activities at the exploratory end of the R & D spectrum. As a company grows successful on the foundation of past technology, there is a tendency to close the door on innovation. Yet, in the pharmaceutical business success depends on the replacement of technologies and the kind of corporate planning that encourages an investment in fundamental research supported by a serious commitment from top management to pursue long-term projects.

Dean[3] comments that, "As is well known to every research manager, the time horizon to top management in U.S. industry is one year with occasional exceptions extending out to three, and rarely to five, years" — a fact which has generated a temporal mismatch between the natural pace of innovation and the time horizon of most industrial corporations. According to Dean it has taken an average of 19 years for 10 important innovations to mature from idea to product. Major pharmaceutical innovations now exceed 10 years and some approach the average reported by Dean.

Profits are the only real measure of performance, for they are society's reward to the organization that performs beneficially. However, management must adopt a time horizon for reward sufficiently long to ensure that reward corresponds to long-term profitability. The pharmaceutical industry needs top managers who endorse a long-range corporate strategy and who recognize the real time and money dimensions of innovation.

Project selection and the entire R & D process within a firm are influenced by its long- and short-term business objectives. In some cases top corporate management may decide to have research develop a particular product or line of products, either supporting existing franchises or moving into new marketing areas. When such senior management decisions are made, then project selection criteria become established.

II. THE STRATEGIC RESEARCH PLAN

A. OVERALL PLANNING GOALS

It is axiomatic that no pharmaceutical company can be preeminent in *all* health/medical research fields. Limited resources dictate that each company must expose itself to some risks and pass up opportunities. The research strategy problem is to establish, in light of the best information available, *where* the research operation should (1) concentrate its efforts, (2) remain in close touch with scientific areas, and (3) virtually ignore certain developing technology. To minimize serious technological threats to the existence of the company, research management must recognize positions that will have to be defended at all costs and then saturate these areas with research. Next, the strategic plan should identify areas where optimal new-product opportunities exist and establish programs to move research activities in these directions. Such a plan also must ensure that sudden advances in certain areas of science will not catch the firm unaware and eliminate a major segment of its business. Furthermore, it must minimize the risk of overlooking exceptional exploitation opportunities offered by rapid developments in new scientific areas.

It is important, therefore, that a careful assessment be made of the current technological and scientific strengths of an R & D operation which are then compared to those which are needed to support the present and future business of the company — in other words an evaluation of where the research operation "is" and where it "needs to be". Input form a number of sources is needed to assure that the approach used produces realistic assessments, These sources include scientific management, corporate planning personnel, business/marketing specialists, senior corporate management, and possibly external consultants.

Dohrmann[4] describes a technique for carrying out such an assessment with specific ranking criteria. The 5-year horizon used, however, would need to be expanded to at least 20 for such an analysis within the pharmaceutical field, since discovery and development timetables are so much longer. He emphasizes that ranking the technology needs of the corporation is a difficult task because many of the interacting variables have synergistic effects that must be considered. Some of the variables that need to be considered and that impact on project selection strategies include the importance of the technology (priority), cost of obtaining the technology, expected benefits, magnitude of risk, timing or when required, and importance to business/marketing strategy and goals.

B. A BALANCED PROGRAM/PROJECT APPROACH

Selection of programs and projects must be *balanced* in order to meet research goals and strategies. So many detailed decisions are involved in the planning process that intended program balance may be lost if management does not step back for a careful overview of its research plan. Emphasis must be balanced among the following parameters:

Long- and short-term goals — Balance of fundamental and applied research will result in adequate support for attainment of long- and short-term goals.

Offensive and defensive research — Research must be concerned with giving adequate attention to maintaining the company position in present markets and exploring new areas that may result in new business opportunities.

Operating division supported — Research effort must be allocated to support the various existing and proposed new business operations. Determining the proper balance of effort requires major planning attention.

Scientific areas — Management should ensure, particularly in fundamental areas, the program scope includes key scientific fields presenting major long-range scientific threats or opportunities within the sphere of activity of the company. It is especially important for a firm in such a science-based industry as pharmaceuticals to decide how much to spend on research, how to divide this budget between the different categories, and how much to spend on individual projects. Only in recent years have serious efforts been made to put these decisions on a somewhat more rational basis.

III. BASIC CONSIDERATIONS IN PROJECT SELECTION

A. EXPLORATORY AND DEVELOPMENT PROJECT

Project selection philosophy and methodology differ at various stages in the research process and may be examined at two points, namely at the beginning or exploratory research stage and at the time a compound is selected for development. The exploratory end of the research spectrum includes research activities of a more basic or fundamental nature designed to generate new leads. Some firms use technological forecasting techniques, such as Delphi, to identify areas that afford a promising return on research investment and provide a queue of good projects which can be instituted when personnel and facilities permit. In general, however, the more exploratory or fundamental research within an operation, the more difficult it is to develop a quantitative or highly sophisticated and measured means of selecting projects. Development projects are established when a compound or series of compounds is selected and a decision made to pursue a New Drug Application (NDA).

At this stage the economic characteristics of each project may be evaluated, including technological risk and expected net income, using computerized investing models and related sophisticated quantitative approaches if desired.

One important factor in selecting projects by most methods is the assumption that there is very little chance that a project intended to produce one kind of result will produce a very useful outcome of an entirely different kind. Yet, the history of drug development has numerous examples of drugs that were designed for one use which found utility in entirely different therapeutic applications.

B. CRITICAL PERSONNEL FACTORS

In all R & D operations the role of personnel involved is often a critical parameter in successful conclusions. The so-called "people factor" exerts a vital influence in any project selection system and should be included in the planning process.

1. Available Skills and Talents

Project selection may be influenced by the number and type of scientific personnel that can be assigned to a particular activity. If certain capabilities and skills are lacking, then time will be required to find and hire the specialists needed to institute the project. Thus, in project selection one must be concerned constantly with the capabilities of in-house personnel and the ease with which new personnel with appropriate expertise may be acquired. It is much easier in a rapidly expanding research operation to take on new projects, whereas in a static or shrinking research organization new projects are often added with considerable stress and difficulty.

2. The Project "Champion" Concept

It is wise to involve as many of the scientific staff in the selection of projects as possible, through some sort of participative or peer review process. Some observers go further and feel that major, truly innovative ideas usually do not require rigid, formal evaluation and acceptance by some routine project selection system, but that such ideas emerge logically as most important and begin to gather support by more and more personnel in various areas of research and marketing. Thus, as the number of "champions" increases, the momentum and support propel the idea into active project status and usually one with a high priority.

3. Use of Consultants/Experts

R & D management is often criticized by internal senior management or other corporate functional groups as well as external "experts" (e.g., consumerists, economists, public policy specialists, or politicians) for poor allocation of resources, faulty project selection, and inadequate productivity. To respond to this criticism research managers sometimes seek external expert opinion and advice through one of several approaches. A consulting firm or group may be contracted to perform an audit of R & D operations. A permanent panel of science advisors may be created to assess research programs and projects for relevance and importance to the success of the firm. Another approach involves the research staff itself in the evaluation and selection of research projects.[5] The highly participative technique utilizes an experienced-based resource group of experts in a systematic manner which attempts to minimize impulsiveness, while maximizing careful review and decision making. Through carefully structured brainstorming sessions candidate research projects are generated and then selected based on feasibility determinations and prioritizing. The approach recognizes that selected research projects is ultimately a matter of judgment. Perhaps the greatest weakness in using internal experts in this and other methods is that there is not accounting for the fact that the judgment or experience of some members should be weighted more heavily than that of others.

4. Communications

Because of the increasing tendency toward specialization among scientists, the problem of integrating the communicating research information influencing project selection becomes a very distinct challenge. A free flow of information and open decision-making techniques encourage an integrated organization capable of examining all alternatives and making the best decisions with regard to project activities. The research operation characterized by pockets of isolated units and suboptimization finds it difficult to bring the judgment of its best brains to the challenging problems of selecting the most promising and exciting projects.

5. The "Science-Manager" Concept

As a result of the increasing complexity of research effort and its interdisciplinary and multidisciplinary nature, it is becoming increasingly evident that the management of research, including the vital task of selecting programs and projects, is best handled by individuals who have both a fundamental technical and scientific background as well as knowledge of management principles, including organizational theory, operations research, decision analysis, and personnel development. These "scientist-managers" are especially skilled at maximizing the entrepreneurial spirit of the scientist in a corporate environment that often entails a certain degree of bureaucracy, politicism, and communication difficulties.

6. Management Style

Project selection is influenced by the management style of the top research administrator and his approach to creating a productive research operation. One may feel that the best research result will evolve from hiring the most qualified scientists and giving them maximum freedom to pursue research in their area of expertise consistent with the goals of the group. On the other end of the attitudinal and style spectrum, the director may feel that research is most productive when it has clearly defined objectives which are closely aligned to and influenced by marketing concepts, as well as carefully programmed and controlled by sophisticated decision-making techniques. Although there is a trend toward more quantitative and systematized project selection methods, at present subjective evaluation based on scientific judgment and expertise is still an important factor influencing selection in most large research establishments.

7. Informed Judgment

Because total research resources are limited and obviously will never be able to support all potentially useful investigations, some projects must be denied. No area of pharmaceutical research can be advanced as rapidly as its proponents might desire without affecting other areas. The problem of allocation of resources or of achieving a suitable balance becomes a matter of determining how much one project is worth as opposed to another which might be developed with the same resources. Hence there is need for a good scientific resource allocation methodology. The critical need for such a management decision tool has become more and more pressing as the resources devoted to R & D have soared. However, whatever technique is employed it will not replace informed judgments, nor can it operate in the absence of these judgments. The responsibility for taking decisions always remains with the human decision maker. All of the various techniques and tools for selecting projects are means of providing information needed for the decision maker and not automatic processes.

C. PROJECT INTERDEPENDENCE

The goal of the research manager is to select the portfolio of projects that maximize R & D output in both the short and long term. As long as projects are independent, few problems exist, but when projects are interdependent, which is usually the case in pharmaceutical research, the selection is more complicated. Dependent projects fall into two classifications. If the decision to undertake a second project will increase benefits from the first, then the second project is said to be a complement of the first. If the decision to undertake the second project will decrease the benefits expected from the first, then the second project is said to be a substitute for the first. In the case when the potential benefits derived from the first project will disappear if the second project is accepted, or where it is technically impossible to undertake the first when the second has been accepted, then the two projects are said to be mutually exclusive. Many drug development projects compete for scarce toxicology facilities, limited clinical testing resources, etc., and are therefore of the mutually exclusive type.

D. PROJECT FUNDING
1. Size of the Firm

For smaller firms with more limited research funds, the orientation of research activities is more restricted. Some firms tend to concentrate on certain research areas, a strategy which influences directly project selection philosophy. For example, certain pharmaceutical companies specialize in research associated with drugs for gastrointestinal disorders, ophthalmics, dermatologicals, or products used by patients in hospital settings.

2. The Research Budget

The overall profile of projects and research programs is directly affected by the magnitude of funds provided to the R & D function. Thus, project selection and initiation are often integrated into the annual budget approval process. In order for research operations to maintain sufficient flexibility, however, some method should be in place which allows for the initiation of new projects during the year without formal and difficult approval procedures. Also, research funding should be stable, rather than fluctuating from year to year, for such an unstable and uncertain environment makes project selection and commitments extremely difficult.

E. AUDITING PROJECT SELECTION SUCCESS

In order to assess how well a project selection system is operating within an organization, it is essential to conduct periodic audits of project successes and failures. This can be a difficult task, for it is related to the perplexing management problem of evaluating R & D results. However, some specific data and perspectives can be developed, such as:

1. Were the R & D cost and time projections realistic?
2. Were project timetables maintained?
3. Were sales and marketing predictions substantiated?

In order to gather additional insights on project life cycles, information should be developed on the number of projects initiated, terminated, and underway.

IV. HISTORICAL DRUG DEVELOPMENT PERSPECTIVES

A. TRENDS AND EMERGING PATTERNS

The pharmaceutical R & D process is a dynamic, sensitive, and unique one characterized by increasingly complex inputs, long and costly development cycles, considerable inter- and multidisciplinary teamwork, and a sensitivity to both internal corporate and external environmental forces. To develop a new drug today can take 10 years or more and cost more than $50 million if one includes the cost of research efforts on leads that fail along the way because of toxicity, poor relative efficacy, or related factors, as well as the time value to money.[6]

As a result of costly regulatory requirements and the complexity of modern biomedical research and drug development, some particularly significant changes in recent years reflect alterations in R & D management philosophy which in turn impacts on project selection trends. First, there is more emphasis on "defensive" research projects, those aimed at prolonging the life cycle of currently marketed products through the development of new or improved dosage forms or the generation of new or broadened indications. Even in the large research-oriented firms, as much as 20 to 25% of the R & D budget may be allocated to such defensive research projects.[7]

In many pharmaceutical companies the balance between exploratory long-range research endeavors and short-range development projects has shifted, so that fewer resources proportionally are directed to innovative and more basic research activities. Funds that would normally be invested in exploratory research are now directed to conducting more sophisticated toxicological studies and clinical studies and all the related activities associated with generating the massive documentation needed for the typical NDA.

According to P.M.A. data, R & D expenditures by product class have remained fairly similar over the past decade.[8] The top four categories in 1978 with their percentage share of the R & D dollar were anti-infectives 18.9%; central nervous system and sense organs 16.8%; cardiovasculars 16.6%; and neoplasms, endocrine system, and metabolic diseases 16.4%. Thus, two thirds of the funds went for investigations related to infections, central nervous system, neoplasms, and the heart. These areas, which represent broad market need and opportunity, reflect the result of project selection strategies of the major pharmaceutical companies, However, within this scope many firms have had to reduce the number of areas in which they conduct research and in some cases the number of projects. At the Merck Laboratories, for example, in the 5 years between 1969 and 1974 the number of research projects dropped 10%.[9]

B. RESEARCH RESOURCE ALLOCATIONS

Back in 1966 Mansfield and Brandenburg[10] reported that despite the remarkable increase in the amount of attention directed to the economics of R & D, there were surprisingly few detailed studies of the research and development activities of the firm. They noted that although something about the factors influencing total expenditures of a firm on R & D were known, little information was available about the allocation of funds among projects that were undertaken and the probable outcome of these projects. This was true of pharmaceutical research also at that time, and since then, there has continued to be a paucity of detailed studies focusing on project resource allocation and success in drug development.

In the early 1960s one major pharmaceutical firm evaluated projects using the following 10 points:[11]

1. The nature of the treatment
2. The trend of the disease — is it increasing, decreasing, or static?
3. The diagnosis of the disease — is there a good method of recognizing the disease?
4. Severity of the disease — does it cause a critical illness or only a minor illness?
5. The duration of the disease — years, days, or months?
6. The U.S. incidence of the disease; that is, the actual number of people who have it
7. The export incidence of the disease
8. Competition in the field — are there drugs already available for the treatment?
9. Opportunities — chances for success in the field and magnitude of effort needed to develop a solution
10. Market or sales estimate

V. PROJECT SELECTION METHODOLOGIES

A. OVERVIEW OF FACTORS INFLUENCING SELECTION

Project selection decisions are often influenced by a number of important considerations such as (1) corporate policy, (2) the size of the research budget, (3) the type of research — exploratory, development, or defensive, (4) technical and scientific skills available, and (5) competitive activity.

In a study of the research planning methodologies and approaches of six leading pharmaceutical firms, project selection was found to be influenced by a number of scientific, marketing, and organization factors.[12]

Scientific factors that were found to influence project selection included

1. Interrelationship with other research activities — synergistic advantages or competitiveness with other programs
2. Probability of achieving project objectives
3. Time required to achieve project objectives
4. Impact on balance of short- and long-term programs within research
5. Estimated cost of the project in the coming year and to completion
6. Utilization of existing research talent and resources
7. Value as a means of generating experience and gaining a technical expertise in a field — a foundation for future research activities
8. Need for critical mass of expertise and activity to ensure progress
9. Elasticity of resource input and probable output relationships
10. Patentability or exclusivity of discoveries from project
11. Competitive research effort in the area — in academic and government research centers

Marketing considerations that were found to influence project selection included

1. Projected sales and profits from effort
2. Relationships-to-need as reflected by current state of consumer satisfaction

3. Status and efficacy of current competitive products or means of meeting consumer need
4. Compatibility with current marketing capabilities and strengths
5. Influence of new competitive products under development

Organizational and other elements that were found to influence project selection included

1. Relationship to activities at other research centers of units within the company
2. Timing of project with respect to other activities in marketing, research, etc.
3. Manufacturing capabilities and needs
4. Prestige and image value to the company
5. Effect on organizational esprit de corps and attitudes
6. Impact on governmental, public opinion, and other environmental pressures
7. Alternative uses of scientific personnel and facilities if project is dropped after a few years
8. Moral compulsion to develop drugs meeting medical needs, but having low or no profit potential

All of these various elements are not of concern in every decision influencing project selection and priorities, but the compilation does represent a checklist of items which are often reviewed, sometimes intuitively, before decisions are finalized.

B. QUANTITATIVE APPROACHES

Mathematical programming techniques vary in complexity and have the capacity to consider virtually any variable in the program. These variables include, for example, such factors as the number of possible projects, possible versions of the projects, present value of the expected benefits from projects, number of scientists required, number of technicians required, and capital expenditure required. Such complex linear programs require the use of a computer.

In general, however, precise, quantitative techniques for selecting R & D projects are not widely used in the pharmaceutical industry. As observed by Dean in a study of 40 industrial firms, including pharmaceutical companies, the lack of use of sophisticated methods is based on the shortcomings of the models themselves, many of which ignore factors that are critical in project selection decision making.[13] These factors include the following:

1. Adequate treatment of risk and uncertainty
2. The continuous nature of investments in or expenditures for projects
3. The need for multiple criteria
4. The interrelationships among projects
5. The role of experience and intuition in such decision making

The project selection technique used should not be based on its complexity, but by its value to the research operation and the business enterprise. No matter how quantitative the project selection methodology, there are vital qualitative considerations which must, in the final analysis, be resolved by the experiences and intuitions of the managers making the selection. In fact, the various highly quantitative and sophisticated models which had been popular in recent years seem to have lost their appeal. Decision makers now tend to believe that such mathematical models and formulas tend to mislead by implying that quantifiable information is available that is more reliable and complete than is actually the case.[14] Perhaps the key to the use of any project selection technique is to be flexible and not accept or reject a project based on one particular selection scheme or project ranking approach.

C. FINANCIAL CONSIDERATIONS

There are many criteria and approaches that can be used to rank projects in order of their financial attractiveness or to help decide if a particular project is worth pursuing. Payback or break-even time is a criterion giving the number of years from the beginning of a project before the total expenditure is recovered out of proceeds. Return on investment is the ratio of the net profit in any particular year, or the average profit over a longer period, often the estimated profitable life of the project, to the total investment, expressed as a percentage. The present worth of a project is the sum of the present worths of all net (positive) incomes and (negative) expenditures related to a specific time, usually the date of the evaluation, at a given interest rate. The discounted cash flow yield reflects the interest rate which reduces the present worth of a project to zero, so that the present worths of total expenditure and total income become equal. It also represents the maximum interest rate at which money could be borrowed to finance the project and still break even at the end.

One financial-based project selection system used in a multifaceted research department of a large pharmaceutical company is oriented to those compounds which are approximately midway through clinical testing.[15] The absolute value of the project and the incremental value of bringing each compound to market earlier are determined using a profitability index consisting of the present value of projected income divided by the present value of projected expenses. In order to make these calculations key marketing and research inputs are needed. Research needs to develop a profile for each compound which includes (1) a description of therapeutic effects, (2) possible adverse side effects, (3) the dosage form to be developed, (4) the potential advantages over competitive products, (5) cost of the clinical program, and (6) alternative introduction dates. Marketing research develops a detailed revenue projection for each compound based on (1) the advantages over competition, (2) the market introduction date, (3) the anticipated new product introductions by competitors, (4) the patent expiration date, (5) the market growth rate, (6) the level of promotion required, and (7) the cost of goods.

The technique clearly demonstrates the dramatic income decline over the life of the drug resulting from only a 1-year delay in marketing introduction. Without a system to which everyone is committed, there are often three project completion dates.[15] Marketing usually uses more optimistic dates, whereas research usually tends toward more pessimistic projections. Corporate management uses dates that fall somewhere in between.

The various financially oriented and other quantitative project selection methods employed today are not the ultimate in decision-making procedures. They do, however, offer a way of discounting risk when comparing research alternatives by providing the decision maker with vital perspectives and a statement of attitude toward risk which can be communicated to others.

D. SIMPLE PROJECT RATING SCHEMES

Ranking approaches for evaluating projects are based on the premise that the values of key variables needed for the application of more sophisticated quantitative models cannot be accurately estimated. Several ranking approaches have been designed for pharmaceutical projects. Some of the earlier reports include that of Mottley and Newton,[16] who suggested a scale of "poor", "unforseeable", "fair", and "high" (0, 1, 2, 3, respectively) for rating a project on each of the following five criteria: promise of success, time to completion, project costs, strategic need, and market gain potential. The individual ratings are multiplied together and projects with the highest composite score are chosen until the predetermined budget for the year is exhausted. Obviously, there are difficulties in assigning meaningful numbers to the various criteria for each project and careful attention must be given to who provides the judgment.

Another project selection technique is described as the "innovation potential method."[14] Eight factors are weighted according to their importance based on the experiences of research management, and a total of at least 70 is necessary for a project to be seriously considered. One factor weighted 20 is the quality of communications including technical-marketing, technical-customer, and technical-technical interfaces. The scientific and technological competence of the research organization with regard to the project is weighted 20 also. The presence of a champion, usually someone placed high in the organization and outside the actual working groups who is deeply dedicated to the success of the new project, is given a weighting of 15. Marketing opportunity represented by the project is scored 15. Technical opportunity, which is the measure of the applicability of in-house or newly developed technology to the proposed project, is weighted 10. Top management interest in the project is rated 10, an assessment of the competitive environment affecting the project 5, and the relative importance of 5. The innovation potential model is simplistic, but has been fairly successful in a relatively small, highly selective chemical specialty firm. Variations of the model could easily be adapted to the particular needs of a pharmaceutical R & D operation and provide a valuable approach to the project selection challenge.

One project selection methodology initially developed for use in a major federal research and development laboratory is equally applicable in an industrial setting and could be adapted for use by pharmaceutical firms.[17] The approach does not rely on cost-benefit type calculations, but does require that each level of management examine those parameters important to the conduct and eventual utilization of research results. The primary criteria against which a research program is judged are listed below:

1. The first criteria, impact, is assessed in terms of relevance, authority, and coupling. Relevance reflects the need or utility of the proposed research and is quantifiable in terms of the market affected. Authority related to the momentum and support for the program. The higher up in the organization the project receives support and the more widespread its potential impact, the greater the incentive for its acceptance. Coupling has to do with the interest and relationship of the research to the ultimate user. In the pharmaceutical firm this would be the marketing function which reflects the needs of the physician and patient.

2. Feasibility, which reflects the measurement of risk involved in accomplishing the task, is the second criteria. The feasibility of success depends upon three factors, namely technological risk, technical competence of the research group including the availability of specialized skills and adequate facilities, and management capability necessary to accomplish the task.

3. The third criteria, intrinsic scientific merit, is one which is not usually included in many highly mathematically and computerized evaluation techniques. It is one which any large, long-range research operation in the pharmaceutical field must recognize in the construction of a balanced portfolio of projects. Intrinsic scientific merit involves the ability of the research laboratory to grow and keep pace with and contribute to the advancing front of biomedical science and drug development. It is concerned with the continuing long-term viability of an R & D organization and focuses on developing technological strengths. It fosters opportunities for maintaining intramural expertise capable of assessing and utilizing the broad expanse of scientific knowledge being generated in other research laboratories. Exploratory research is encouraged. Proposed projects are examined not only for intrinsic scientific merit, but also for their synergism with other R & D and how they foster overall research strengths.

The construction of the algorithm involving the three criteria of impact, feasibility, and research merit to evaluate research programs/projects must be tailored to a specific research organization. It is an interactive, iterative experience which must involve all concerned parties. Only after general agreement is obtained as to the more significant parameters and their relative importance can a quantitative scheme be developed. The approach described has potential value in examining and selecting research projects and actively developing a balanced program of research in the pharmaceutical arena.

Mazzoni[18] has developed a simple, yet valuable approach to project evaluation based on a checklist encompassing 32 important variables. These are divided into marketing, R & D, medical, financial, and production elements. In the R & D area, for example, the following variables are assessed; likelihood of technical success, R & D time (end of Phase II), time to document claims (end of Phase III), product stability, R & D cost, and availability of skills.

VI. OTHER KEY FACTORS INFLUENCING PROJECT MANAGEMENT

A. ADVANCES IN THE BIOLOGICAL SCIENCES

The escalating cost and expanding time frame for the development of a drug has made the project selection process even more critical. To assure an adequate return on research investments, drug candidates must have a strong probability of demonstrating clear advantages over existing compounds or of meeting unfulfilled medical needs. Over the past 25 years remarkable advances have taken place in the biological sciences which have not yet resulted in improvements in therapy. The virtual explosion of knowledge in biochemistry, immunology, molecular and cell biology, and neurobiology should result in a new era of drug discovery and development in which agents are designed to interrupt a specific disease process rather than simply treating its signs and symptoms. The traditional approach of screening thousands of compounds for biological activity is gradually changing. Increasingly, the pharmaceutical research scientist is able to design drug molecules to perform specific pharmacological functions with minimum side effects. This has evolved as a result of new knowledge of biochemical processes within the cell, the immune response system of the body, the structure and function of the cell surface and receptor molecules, and a host of related biological mechanisms.

Therefore, one of the clearest trends is that the biological sciences will play a vital role in drug discovery and development which will impact on project selection decisions. Development in biochemistry have encouraged a greater focus on enzymes as specific drug targets. Efforts to identify, characterize, and develop inhibitors or activators for key enzymes involved in metabolic processes are increasing. The use of radioactive ligands has enabled a better biological characterization of various hormone and neurotransmitter receptors. The study of such receptors will permit increased understanding of how hormones and neurotransmitters work and permit the development of specific, potent antagonists (blockers) and agonists (mimics). Conceptual advances are occurring which will lead to novel approaches to inhibit or stimulate immunologic pathways, that is, control individual cellular events in the generation and expression of immune responses. Metabolic pathways will continue to occupy the attention of scientists in the search for new drug leads. As new compounds are isolated which are involved in important physiological processes, the routes of synthesis and degradation and the role of associated enzymes will provide important clues for drug development projects. Neurobiology is another exciting area and the potential therapeutic implications of synthetic peptides will grow substantially as more active peptides are isolated and peptide analogs resistant to proteolysis are synthesized. Molecular biology and gene technology have progressed dramatically, and recombinant DNA technology represents one of the most exciting and potentially productive areas of biomedical research and development.

B. THE RESEARCH-MARKETING INTERFACE

Perhaps one of the most critical interaction and communication links in drug R & D is found at the interface between research and marketing.[19] It is obvious that the impact of marketing in the project selection process varies with the stage of the research process and, indeed, how we define a project. As we move from the exploratory end of the R & D spectrum to the point where leads are identified and a decision is made to pursue a Notice of Claimed Investigational

Exemption for a New Drug (IND) and NDA, projects become better defined and the role of marketing increases. Inadequate or inappropriate marketing inputs or attempts to exert excessive control over the R & D processes at any point can create major problems. However, difficulties also arise when research programs are too unstructured and unattuned to marketing strategies and the near-term concern for increased revenues and profits. When there is a realistic degree of influence over research operations with meaningful common goals established, the interaction between research and marketing is optimized.

A number of valuable marketing inputs to the R & D process and project selection may be identified. First, by examining deficiencies in current therapy, studying competitive developments and marketing strategies, and looking closely at broad medical trends, patterns, and needs, marketing personnel can help mold the direction of exploratory efforts and thus have a positive impact at early stages of the R & D process in the orientation of basic research activities. Marketing should provide an even more direct input into the selection of development projects evolving from these exploratory programs. Once projects are formalized, marketing needs to monitor progress and provide important insights concerning (1) the nature of clinical studies to be undertaken and desired claim structure for the product, (2) dosage forms to be developed and their characteristics, and (3) timing of the NDA submission. Marketing also should exert considerable influence on projects and research activities in support of existing products, including broadened claims, new dosage forms, and overall defensive efforts. The marketing-research interface is one of the most critical elements in the larger corporate technical plan aimed at assuring the technoscientific success of the firm. Highlighting the need for adequate coupling and cooperation at this interface is the necessity for making the whole system work, that is, generating and selecting good research projects and moving them through the challenging developmental stages to successful product introduction.

C. LICENSING AND TECHNOLOGY TRANSFER

Project selection within R & D operations is influenced by the growing interest within the pharmaceutical industry in licensing compounds or products in order to complement internal research leads and ultimately R & D productivity.[20] Because of organizational characteristics and philosophical perspectives, firms approach the licensing task somewhat differently, but in all cases the interrelationships with internal projects and research activities are an important consideration. The licensing effort requires delicate orchestration so that such activities are not viewed as threatening and competitive to internally generated research projects. As one examines internal research commitments and strengths, various areas (e.g., antibiotics, cardiovasculars) may be identified on which the licensing team can concentrate. However, as each therapeutic research area becomes more complex, due in part to increasing regulatory pressures, and as research budgets encounter more stringent assessment, the number of leads that a research group can pursue becomes reduced. Therefore, considerable care must be directed to seeking licensing candidates which are most complementary to internal research projects and which contribute to a balanced output portfolio of products in the near and long term.

D. ADVANCED DECISION ANALYSIS TECHNIQUES

Strategic planning and decision making concerning research programs are often made in the face of considerable uncertainty. The tempo of change and the influence of uncontrollable external factors preclude using the past for firm guidance. However, techniques for decision analysis are emerging and offer promise in enabling decision makers to deal more effectively with uncertainty in planning and allocating their organization's resources.[21] One application of subjective probability involved the R & D portfolio of a leading European pharmaceutical company.[22] Using forecasts made over the previous 7 years, R & D managers were able to study the success of development projects and thus gain insight into project selection.

VIII. SUMMARY

As in many industries, project selection within the pharmaceutical firm is influenced by many diverse factors. However, the scientific orientation of drug research which tends toward the exploratory end of the research spectrum generates project selection approaches which are often less affected by immediate economic and marketing considerations than those followed in many other industries.

Project selection in the pharmaceutical industry is becoming more important due to a myriad of factors and trends, among them:

1. The longer and costlier development cycles
2. The complexity of modern science which requires a large critical mass of experts and skills
3. An emphasis on near-term productivity rather than longer-range exploratory research
4. A multitude of external forces, including mounting regulatory requirements and consumerist pressures
5. The shortening patent life following new product introduction
6. The growing impact of licensing and technology transfer groups
7. The concern for orphan drugs
8. The influence of marketing and financial inputs as R & D "productivity" is scrutinized
9. The shift of certain research overseas and more global approach to project development
10. The R & D management concern for maintaining a motivated and creative staff in an era when research funding is being reexamined and science itself is being questioned for relevancy in today's culture

The pharmaceutical R & D process consists of a number of project management steps encompassing idea generation and processing, project evaluation and selection, project monitoring and control, and project completion or termination. Each of these steps is interrelated, for after ideas are developed and projects initiated, alert managements need to monitor progress to be assured that the company is investing in those projects which will have the most beneficial effect on business success. Whenever a project encounters major technical problems or when it becomes obvious that commercial results will be significantly less than estimates used to justify the program originally, decision makers may elect to drop the project and invest funds in more promising activities.

In the final analysis, the ultimate payoff from good project selection should be to reduce the delay between initial discovery and eventual commercial exploitation of attractive innovations, to improve their chances of success and profitability, and also to minimize the expenditure of money and other resources on potentially unprofitable projects.

REFERENCES

1. **Davis, E. E., Jr.,** Industrial research in America: challenge of a new synthesis, *Science,* 209, 133, 1980.
2. Technology on Trial: Public Participation in Decision-making Related to Science and Technology, Organization for Economic Cooperation & Development, Paris, 1979.
3. **Dean, R. C., Jr.,** The temporal mismatch-innovation's pace vs. management's time horizon, *Res. Manage.,* 17, 12, 1974.
4. **Dohrmann, R. J.,** Matching company R & D expenditures to technology needs, *Res. Manage.,* 21, 17, 1978.
5. **Denny, F. I.,** Management of an R & D planning process. Utilizing an advisory group, *IEEE Trans. Eng. Manage.,* EM-27, 34, 1980.

6. **Hansen, D. W.,** The pharmaceutical development process. Estimates of current regulatory costs and times and the effect of regulatory changes, presented at the Inst. Health Econ. Soc. Stud., University of California Seminars, Los Angeles, September 8 to 10, 1977.

7. **Faust, R. E.,** The 1962 drug amendments: challenge to the research process, *Am. Pharm.,* 19, 11, 1979.

8. Annual Survey Report, Ethical Pharmaceutical Industry Operations, Pharmaceutical Manufacturers Association, Washington, 1978 to 1979.

9. **Sarett, L. H.,** FDA regulations and their influence on future R & D, *Res. Manage.,* 17, 18, 1974.

10. **Mansfield, E. and Bradenburg, R.,** The allocation, characteristics, and outcome of the firm's research and development portfolio: a case study, *J. Bus.,* 39, 447, 1966.

11. **Carney, T. P.,** Problems in research administration, Proc. 16th Natl. Conf. Adm. Res., Denver Research Institute, 1963, 77.

12. **Faust, R. E.,** Project selection in the pharmaceutical industry, *Res. Manage.,* 14, 46, 1971.

13. **Dean, B. V.,** Evaluating, selecting, and controlling R & D projects, *Am. Manage. Assoc. Res. Study No. 89,* 79, 1968.

14. **Paolini, A., Jr. and Glaser, M.,** Project selection methods that pick winners, *Res. Manage.,* 20, 26, 1977.

15. **Clark, P.,** A profitability project selection method, *Res. Manage.,* 20, 29, 1977.

16. **Mottlley, C. and Newton, R.,** The selection of projects for industrial research, *Oper. Res.,* 7, 740, 1959.

17. **Cooper, M. J.,** An evaluation system for project selection, *Res. Manage.,* 21, 29, 1978.

18. **Mazzoni, D. J.,** Rx for the pharmaceutical marketer: preventive marketing, *Med. Mark. Media,* 7, 16, 1972.

19. **Faust, R. E.,** Project selection and research-marketing interactions, *Med. Mark. Media,* 12, 44, 1977.

20. **Faust, R. E.,** Acquisition/licensing strategies for pharmaceutical products, *Drug Cosmet. Ind.,* 112, 48, 1973.

21. **Menke, M. M.,** Strategic planning in an age of uncertainty, *Long Range Plann.,* 12, 27, 1979.

22. **Balthasar, H. V. et al.,** Calling the shots in R & D, *Harv. Bus. Rev.,* 56, 151, 1978.

Chapter 9

THE STATISTICIAN IN PHARMACEUTICAL DEVELOPMENT

Walter B. Cummings and Gerald Hajian

TABLE OF CONTENTS

I. INTRODUCTION

The chemist, the pharmacologist, the toxicologist, and the medical scientist each bear a direct responsibility for a particular phase of pharmaceutical development. The statistician, in contrast, has a supporting role in nearly all of the many phases of this process. This chapter will examine this supporting role of statisticians, and will identify the common element of their contributions in the various phases of pharmaceutical development. It is directed to pharmaceutical development managers in understanding the role of the statistician, thereby enabling a more imaginative and effective use of this valuable resource in R & D.

According to Webster,[1] statistics is "a branch of mathematics dealing with the collection, analysis, interpretation, and presentation of masses of numerical data". Statisticians assist in the collection of data in the various phases of pharmaceutical development through the statistical design of experiments. They perform data analysis through the application of appropriate statistical methods to estimate effects and test for differences while adjusting for other "noise" factors which tend to obscure the effects under study. Statistical interpretation of these experimental results involves the application of probability theory to make inferences to larger populations or settings. And the statistical presentation of data requires the accurate summarization of masses of data while preserving and displaying their salient features.

Because the statistician is concerned with the collection and interpretation of data, he or she necessarily has an interest in data processing and the construction of computer data files. Associated with both the collection and processing of data is the question of data quality, and the practicing statistician soon learns to identify inconsistencies in data. Finally, he or she rapidly becomes quite adept at using the computer as a tool to analyze and summarize experimental results.

The following sections explore how skills of the statistician have application in various phases of pharmaceutical development, including drug synthesis, drug screening, toxicology, and clinical development/evaluation.

II. DRUG SYNTHESIS

The major role of the statistician in the synthesis of new compounds is in the area of structure-activity relationships. Research chemists often know the classes of chemical structures that are effective for the treatment of a particular disease. Compounds in a particular class or type may have a common parent structure, and differ only by several substituent groups at different positions on the parent structure. Some of these compounds may be synthesized and tested in a biological test system. The chemist would like to know in sequence which compound to synthesize from the class of compounds being tested.

If a relationship between biological activity and chemical structure exists among the tested compounds, then the chemist can use numerical techniques to estimate which substituent group and position number will maximize the biological activity. The chemist could then synthesize this new compound for testing in the biological screen. The statistician can assist the chemist by developing appropriate numerical techniques for establishing structure-activity relationships. These numerical and statistical techniques usually involve the use of regression and experimental design theory. An example of this is given by Free and Wilson.[2]

Chemists also use the statistical and numerical techniques of pattern recognition. Pattern recognition data frequently arise from mass spectroscopic examination of a compound. A complex structure-activity relationship is generally needed to estimate biological activity from pattern recognition data. Stuper and Jurs[3] address the problems of using numerical and statistical methods to correctly classify compounds into two classes (active and nonactive) from sets of chemical measurements or pattern recognition data.

Predicting drug toxicity is another example of the use of structure-activity relationships.

Using toxicity structure-activity relationships, chemists may be guided to synthesize drugs that have lower predicted toxicities. Enslein[4] uses chemical structure (fragment keys), partition coefficient, and molecular weight to predict the rat median lethal dose. Again, the statistical techniques of regression and experimental design were used by the same authors to develop the structure-activity relationships.

A chemist is often interested in the number of isomers or analogs of a parent compound that can be synthesized. The number of isomers that can be synthesized from a parent compound is sometimes needed for patent applications. Also, a chemist is likely to develop a class of compounds with a large number of isomers or analogs to increase the chances of finding a biologically active compound. Thus, in addition to structure-activity relationships, statisticians play an important role in isomer enumeration by developing appropriate numerical and probabilistic methods as noted by Rouvray.[5] These methods assist a chemist in determining how many compounds it is possible to synthesize within a class of compounds (parent structure plus substituents).

In the future, the statistician should be increasingly involved in the field of computer graphics as applied to molecular modeling. Interactive computer programs for the three-dimensional visual display and manipulation of chemical structures are used by chemists to find new drugs. An example is the computer program named MACROMODEL by W. C. Still et al.[6]

III. DRUG SCREENING

Following synthesis, new compounds are tested in animal or microbial models to indicate biological activity as measured by some endpoint. For example, a bacteriologist may test new compounds on several bacterial strains for growth inhibition. This is known as drug screening.

Statisticians aid in designing drug screens to ensure that they are accurate and capable of detecting the active compound. Because the outcome of each test varies from animal to animal, the proper number of animals to be tested is important for the accuracy of the test system. If too few animals are used, an active compound may give a negative test result and an inactive compound may give a positive test result. Thus, the statistician is concerned with the misclassification errors of the test system.

The statistician works closely with the pharmacologist/bacteriologist to choose design parameters that minimize misclassification errors and efficiently utilize resources, i.e., number of animals and dosages. If too many animals are used in a screen, then the number of compounds tested is small. Conversely, if too few animals are used in a screen, then the number of compounds tested is large at the expense of a large misclassification error. The statistician can assist the scientist in balancing these criteria and maximizing the utilization of resources, like animal housing. Dunnett[7] has written extensively on this subject.

Biologists also use rate constants from experiments at the molecular level to compare drug activity. Among the molecular experiments are enzyme binding experiments. Again, the statistician works closely with the biologists to choose design parameters that minimize the error in determining the rate constants from experiments conducted at the molecular level. Endrenyi[8] has edited a book on this subject.

In the future, statistical techniques of experimental design and estimation will be applied to the problem of linking DNA and protein sequences with biological activities.

IV. TOXICOLOGY

Toxicologists are involved with the testing of candidate drugs for safety. Animal test systems are used for acute, subchronic, chronic, teratology, reproduction/fertility, and carcinogenicity studies. Also used are mutagenicity test systems, among which are the bacterial Ames test and the mammalian Mouse Lymphoma test.

In the protocol development phase of toxicological testing the statistician assists in planning for studies with respect to experimental design, randomization, and the statistical analysis to be employed. This role has been reinforced with the advent of good laboratory practices.[9]

Each study is initiated by a written protocol. The statistician takes an active part in the development of the protocol by consulting with the study director on the goals, the objectives, and the experimental design. Consulting on experimental design involves a discussion with the study director on:

1. The number of treated groups and their dosages of drug
2. The types of control groups
3. The number of animals per group
4. The observations to be used for statistical comparison between treated and control groups and estimation of parameters (e.g., LD_{50})
5. The time at which observations will be taken during the course of the study
6. The randomization of treatment groups and cage positions
7. The statistical methods to be employed (i.e., tests for differences between the treated and control groups or parameter estimation procedures)

Thus, in the protocol development phase of a toxicological study, the role of the statistician is to assist the toxicologists in (1) stating the goals and objectives of the study and (2) identifying and experimental design (including randomization) to achieve the objectives in an efficient manner.

During the conduct of the study, the statistician assists the study director when modifications to the protocol become necessary. Protocol modifications are reviewed to determine their effect on the experimental design, randomization, or outcome. After a review, the protocol modifications are documented and attached to the original protocol.

At the conclusion of certain studies, the statistician uses the appropriate numerical methods as specified by the protocol to test for differences between the treated and control groups for each predetermined parameter or to estimate parameters (e.g., LD_{50}). Also, numerical methods are used to test for the presence of a dose-response effect due to the drug for each predetermined parameter. These results are incorporated into the final toxicology report.

Because toxicological studies generate large amounts of data, the statistician has an interest in the processing of these data. Typically, a toxicological study contains 20 parameters measured at several time points (5 or more) for about 100 test animals, which could result in 10,000 data items. Usually a laboratory automation system collects and stores the data from instruments. These data are usually stored in an ordered manner according to study, animal number, and date of observation. The laboratory automation system must provide a computer file that is amenable to statistical analysis. At the conclusion of the study, the statistician uses the data stored on computer files to analyze the results of the experiment. Standardized computer programs are available to assist the statistician in the analysis of these data. Thus, the statistician is concerned with (1) the gathering of these data via a laboratory automation system, (2) the storage of these data in an appropriate data base system, and (3) the computer programs or standardized statistical packages needed to analyze these data.

An additional role of statisticians in the toxicology field is in the area of risk estimation. One particular application is the extrapolation of tumor and/or mutagenic risk from high experimental levels of the drug to the low levels of the drug that the patient will experience. Some risk estimation models extrapolate using a linear relationship between risk and dose. Other models use a more complex relationship between risk and dose, and involve complex numerical calculations using computer programs. Statisticians and toxicologists can work closely in trying to improve models for estimating human risk for carcinogenicity and mutagenicity results.

V. CLINICAL DEVELOPMENT/EVALUATION

The clinical development phase is intended to establish drug efficacy and safety including identification of the indication, target population, and optimal dosing regimen. Sponsors need the clinical development program to be sound, rapid, and efficient. Regulators require the program to be scientifically credible and carefully documented. Documentation, validity, efficiency, and speed are all areas where the statistician contributes heavily.

A. PROGRAM RESPONSIBILITIES

The typical clinical development program consists of a carefully planned sequence of studies. Early studies focus on pharmacokinetics and dose tolerance. These are followed by efficacy studies — first exploratory, then confirmatory, and then expanded with additional emphasis on safety. Following marketing, studies are initiated to clarify remaining questions (sometimes a condition of drug approval), to expand indications, to support marketing, and to develop new formulations. Finally, there are postmarketing surveillance studies to monitor drug performance in larger and more loosely defined populations, to detect the rare side effect not easily picked up in earlier clinical development, and to continue to add to the overall drug knowledge base. The statistician is a key member of the clinical development team. He has particular responsibilities in defining, implementing, and adjusting the overall plan of studies, in the design and reporting of the individual study, and in the overall summarization and interpretation of information gathered in the drug development process.

In addition to the development of a plan for a rational sequence of studies, there are other important program-wide planning issues that must be considered. Standardization of case report forms, data bases, analyses, and presentation are factors important to efficient and rapid data processing, analysis, documentation, and interpretation. Within the clinical development team, the responsibility for concerns of this nature rests largely with the statistician.

B. THE INDIVIDUAL STUDY

The successful clinical study requires good planning, careful execution, and clear summary and documentation. The statistician participates at each of these stages. We now examine the statistician's study activities in further detail.

1. Planning

The statistician's role in planning consists of (1) identification of precise study objectives, (2) development of an efficient and robust study design to meet these objectives, and (3) assistance in the development of good case report forms for recording study results.

It is difficult to address an issue so fundamental as the identification of study objectives. Yet often, this is where the statistician makes his greatest contribution. Clear and precise objectives are necessary before study design can be properly addressed. The clinical scientist typically has a lengthy list of questions he would like to answer with a potential study. The interaction between the clinical scientist and the statistician leads to distillation of that list to one or two important objectives and a realistic assessment by both of the roles that the study will play in the overall clinical development process. The adoption of realistic expectations at the initiation of a study is essential.

Objectives vary from study to study in many ways. Early efficacy studies are exploratory in nature. Their purpose may be to obtain estimates of performance or to evaluate methodology and data collection forms. Later confirmatory studies are intended to provide conclusive evidence in support of specific claims. A common mistake in establishing the objectives of a clinical study is to be too aggressive. Enthusiasm for a new drug often leads to a desire to obtain the clinching study to support a favorable regulatory review before the indication or target population is clearly defined, the proper formulation or optimal dosing regimen has been determined, or a suitable measurement instrument or assessment procedure has been developed. Furthermore, the change of several paramenters in successive trials tends to obscure the reasons for differing outcomes. Thus, in developing study objectives it is important to (1) perform adequate exploratory research before attempting confirmatory studies and (2) keep studies as simple as possible.

Just as it is important to recognize the objectives of the clinical study, it is important to clearly state these objectives as part of study plan or protocol. The scientific method consists of (1) exploration or data gathering, (2) hypothesis formulation, (3) independent confirmatory experimentation, and (4) drawing conclusions. A common abuse of this process is to formulate hypotheses and draw conclusions from the same experimental data. In this case the hypothesis test outcomes do not provide the independent confirmation sought. The statement of clear and precise study objectives as part of the study plan, i.e., before the study is initiated, stands later as clear testimony that the conclusions drawn were the independent confirmation sought and were not generated from a post hoc fishing expedition through the study data.

Once the study objectives have been determined, an appropriate experimental design must be developed. This involves the identification of many factors including

1. Response parameters (preferably as objective as possible)
2. Constraints in the clinical setting
3. The treatment structure, i.e., controls (positive or placebo), multiple dose groups, etc.
4. The degree of response regarded as clinically meaningful
5. An assessment of the inter- and intrasubject variability in the chosen response parameters

A broad determination of the general design and required sample size can usually be made from these considerations. However, many statistical issues remain. These include blinding, randomization (including stratification), frequency of assessment, acquisition of covariate data, method of handling study withdrawals, and an analysis strategy to include interim analysis needs, key analysis variables, and general methods.

The statistician also assists in the development of case report forms. Good case report forms allow for the efficient collection of data in the clinic. They guide the investigator through the study of each subject, indicating with clear instructions the data to be recorded and the various decision points in the patient treatment. Case report forms should also be easy to process, i.e., to review, edit, and transfer the data to computer files. Finally, study case report forms should be as consistent with those of other studies for the drug as is reasonable, taking into account differing objectives and data needs. Standardization allows data processing, analysis, and presentation efficiency and facilitates study-to-study comparisons and overall summarization. The clinical scientist, the data processor, and the statistician are all involved in the development of these instruments. The statistician's particular responsibility is to ensure that the data required to achieve the study objectives are obtainable using the data collection instrument.

2. Ongoing Study Support

While an occasional clinical study may be completed in a matter of days, the typical study involves sequential patient enrollment, treatment, and evaluation over a period of weeks or months. During this period the statistician (1) prepares for future analyses, (2) performs interim analyses as appropriate, and (3) reviews and assesses the impact of suggested study modifications.

The clinical scientist has a keen interest in the progress and trends throughout the study. At a minimum he would like a rapid assessment following the study conclusion. To enable the timely reporting of study results, whether intra- or poststudy, the statistician uses the time following the initiation of the study to prepare formats for listings and tables, a more detailed analysis plan, and programs to generate listings, tables, and analyses.

Summarization and interim analysis of an ongoing clinical study is a valuable aid to the clinical scientist in monitoring the study progress, planning new initiatives, and assessing the overall development program progress. Sometimes these activities are included in the study plan and other times they are not. Interim analysis of confirmatory studies in particular has many potential pitfalls. The statistician can evaluate the consequences of such analyses and advise the clinical scientist accordingly. One problem that arises from such analyses is that they potentially provide information to the investigator that affects subsequent patient evaluation and thereby biases the study outcome. Another is that they provide information which could lead the clinical scientist to alter the study design. For example, the study could be prematurely terminated because it was viewed a likely failure or significance had already been obtained. Conversely, the study could be extended beyond the original design because of trends which need additional evidence to reach statistical significance. Such examinations of the data, with a potential for introducing bias or study modification, can raise serious and difficult-to-answer questions regarding the validity of conclusions. Thus, the statistician's interim analysis role is to be prepared and provide them in a timely manner when appropriate, but to assure that the study is not compromised.

In many ongoing clinical studies, adjustments to the design are suggested. For example, patient enrollment may be slow. Inclusion/exclusion criteria could require modification, or a new center might be opened to facilitate study completion. The statistician should be involved in the consideration and development of all design changes and must assess them in terms of (1) the consistency with study objective, (2) the impact on integrity of the study, and (3) the effect on study analyses. For instance, if inclusion/exclusion criteria are altered, can data from patients enrolled prior to the amendment be properly pooled with data from postamendment patients?

3. Poststudy Analysis

If the clinical study has been well planned and carefully executed, the final analysis and documentation is relatively straightforward. The full statistical analysis will cover all areas of data and will explore their interrelationships. It will address study objectives directly, and will simultaneously summarize other features of the study in a descriptive and/or exploratory way. An outline of the full statistical analysis contains detailed patient accountability, compliance, baseline description, dosing summary, efficacy and safety analyses, and listing of data. The statistician works closely with the clinical scientist to produce the planned analyses and subsequent follow-ups that are required. The result of this close collaborative effort between the statistician and the clinical scientist is a joint medical/statistical report which carefully documents and describes the study results.[10]

C. OVERALL SUMMARIZATION

The many studies initiated in the clinical development of a new drug, when considered together, produce a large body of potentially very useful data over and beyond the results of the individual studies. If reasonable standardization is used in the development of individual study data collection forms and data bases, the construction of a drug data base for overall summarization and further analysis will not be overly difficult. Overall summarization of clinical safety and efficacy experience is a "requirement" in the new drug application.[11] Additionally, there are likely to be particular questions that were not or could not be addressed in individual studies. An example might be the response and/or safety of the drug in the elderly. A single study in the elderly might be difficult to set up. However, the overall drug data base is likely to contain information on a significant number of elderly patients and could be used to make the desired evaluation. Thus, the statistician is likely to expend considerable effort in the construction and analysis of the overall drug data base.

D. THE FUTURE

The involvement and influence of statistics and the statistician in the clinical development of drugs has grown at a remarkable pace. This influence has been driven by numerous factors including regulatory demands for stronger levels of evidence and increased documentation, increased sponsor requirements for accurate assessment of the relative benefits and risks as they proceed with development, and sponsor requirements for efficiency and speed in evaluation of increasingly complex and difficult to assess therapies.

Refinements are rapidly occurring in data processing/management systems which make clinical data accessible for summarization much more rapidly than in the past. This generates new demands from statisticians and programmers to provide systems so that clinical scientists can access and assess the available data easily and appropriately without having to rely on support staff. This demand for "hands-on" access to the data is coming from reviewing authorities as well in the form of computer assisted new drug applications.

The association of the statistician with the clinical development team has been made closer by the collaborative joint report-writing process. The interactive nature of the development of study results in the joint reporting process has spawned requirements for additional and deeper levels of analysis and resulted in a greater appreciation for the potential contributions that the statistician can make in increasing the drug knowledge base. These analysis requirements will continue to grow as clinical scientists further realize the possibilities that exist.

The demand for statistical support in the design and support of postmarketing surveillance studies is growing rapidly. The emergence and availability of large data bases constructed by third-party payers and large health care groups will ensure and accelerate interest and growth in this area. Undoubtedly, specialists in linking, analyzing, and interpreting these large data bases will find greatly expanded career opportunities in the pharmaceutical industry.

In summary, the availability of information related to the development of new therapies and their subsequent use after marketing is exploding with respect both to speed and quantity. The statistician is key to the summarization and assessment of this exploding clinical information base, both directly and through the development of systems.

VI. PHARMACEUTICAL DEVELOPMENT

Chemists and engineers must determine the production process from starting materials to finished product before a candidate drug can be manufactured. As with any manufacturing process, quality control methods are employed to ensure uniformity of output from the variabilities of the process. Manufacturing outcomes are frequently probabilistic, such as the amount of the product deposited by a filling machine. Quality control procedures must be applied in determining the "average" amount to be filled, and the "variability" of the filling machine. Besides machine outputs, batches of drug products also have probabilistic outcomes with respect to stability, identity, purity, and strength. Again, statistical and quality control procedures are applied to make statements about the average shelf life, average purity, and their variabilities associated with the production process.

The present role of the statisticians in pharmaceutical development is to (1) assist chemists in planning studies for stability and expiration dating, (2) set up inspection and quality control procedures to assure that batches of drug products meet specification (identity, strength, quality, and purity), (3) aid in validation of processing equipment, and (4) determine validation of analytical methods. Indeed, this role has been reinforced with the advent of good manufacturing practices.[13]

Studies for stability testing and expiration dating require good experimental designs. Before a study can be initiated, the statistician and chemist should agree on a protocol for the conduct of the study. This protocol should give (1) the goals and objectives of the study, (2) the experimental design, (3) the randomization with respect to different sampling times and temperature of storage, and (4) the numerical and statistical methods used to compute the expiration date. In some cases, accelerated stability testing is conducted by the use of higher temperatures. When accelerated testing is used, the Arrhenius equation is used to give the relationship between rates of decomposition and temperature. After the study is completed, the statistician uses the appropriate numerical and statistical methods to compute the strength vs. time curve and the expiration date.

Quality control procedures to assure that batches of drug product meet specificiations (identity, strength, quality, and purity) must be developed prior to production. The statistician works closely with development personnel in determining how many samples will be needed and when they are taken during the manufacturing process. The samples are then analyzed by the appropriate chemical methods for identity, strength, quality, and purity. Using probabilistic methods, the statistician can compute quality control limits for each specification. These quality control limits give the range of specification values expected from an acceptable manufacturing process. Specification values outside these quality control limits indicate that a deviation has occurred in the manufacturing process. Thus, a batch of drug product giving specifications outside the quality control limits indicates that the batch should be rejected for distribution.

Validation of automated equipment requires studies with protocols and good experimental designs. Any machinery will yield a variable output. As an example, the amount of drug placed in a capsule by a filling machine is variable within certain limits. Validation studies are studies conducted to determine the limits of variability of output from a particular machine and the frequency of output that exceeds the specifications.

VII. SUMMARY

We have discussed the role of the statistician in the drug development process from synthesis to product development. This development process is comprised of a lengthy series of scientific investigations. Generally the experimental outcomes are probabilistic rather than deterministic. Because of this, statistical methods must be used in the design and evaluation of experiments to enable unbiased and supportable conclusions with low and known margins of error. At the same time, the application of statistical methods helps to provide the required information in a relatively economical and efficient way.

While the areas for the application of statistics in drug development are diverse, there are strong similarities in the manner in which the statistician supports experimental objectives in these areas. The statistician accomplishes this support through:

1. Aiding in the clear definition and statement of experimental goals and objectives
2. Developing experimental designs consistent with study objectives
3. Assisting in the planning for collection of appropriate data
4. Evaluating the impact of suggested changes to the ongoing study
5. Analyzing the study data
6. Drawing and reporting supportable conclusions from the study

Each of these is important in the successful implementation of the scientific method in new drug development.

REFERENCES

1. Webster's New Collegiate Dictionary, G&C Merriam Company, Springfield, MA, 1976.
2. **Free, S. M. and Wilson, J. W.,** A mathematical contribution to structure activity studies, *J. Med. Chem.,* 7, 395, 1964.
3. **Stuper, A. J. and Jurs, P. C.,** Reliability of nonparametric linear classifiers, *J. Chem. Inf. Comput. Sci.,* 16, 238, 1976.
4. **Enslein, K.,** An overview of structure-activity relationships as an alternative to testing in animals for carcinogenicity, mutagenicity, dermal and eye irritation, and acute oral toxicity, *Toxicol. Ind. Health,* 4, 479, 1988.
5. **Rouvray, D. H.,** Isomer enumeration methods, *Chem. Soc. Rev.,* 3, 4, 1974.
6. **Still, W. C. et al.,** MACROMODEL, Department of Chemistry, Columbia University, New York, 1988.
7. **Dunnett, C. W.,** Drug screening: the never-ending search for new and better drugs, in *Statistics: A Guide to the Unknown,* Tanur, J. M. et al., Eds., Holden-Day, San Francisco, 1972.
8. Endrenyi, L., Ed., *Kinetic Data Analysis,* Plenum Press, New York, 1981.
9. Food and Drug Administration, Nonclinical laboratory studies—good laboratory practices regulations, *Fed. Regist.,* 43, 59986, 1978.
10. Food and Drug Administration, Guidelines for the Format and Content of the Clinical and Statistical Sections of an Application, FDA, Washington, D.C., July 1988.
11. Food and Drug Administration, New drug and antibiotic regulations, *Fed. Regist.,* 50, 7452, 1985.
12. Food and Drug Administration, Submission of new drug applications to the Food and Drug Administration using computer technology, *Fed. Regist.,* 53, 35912, 1988.
13. **Deming, W. E.,** Making things right, in *Statistics: A Guide to the Unknown,* Tanur, J. M. et al., Eds., Holden-Day, San Francisco, 1972.

Chapter 10

TOXICOLOGY

Ralph W. Fogleman

TABLE OF CONTENTS

I. INTRODUCTION

There are many texts on toxicology which describe techniques, give data from literature reviews on specific compounds, or outline protocols suitable to meet the ever changing requirements of federal law and regulations.[1-8] The purpose of this discussion is to examine some basic problems of philosophy and science in understanding toxicology in its broadest sense — examining its purposes, goals, successes, and failures. From this, discussion and controversy may broaden the concepts of toxicology to the benefit of mankind and the environment, and expand our knowledge of how to use the information already available.

In new drug development, the evaluation of safety takes on a different meaning from that implied in the assessment of an environmental contaminant. As Karl Beyer so aptly stated, "To assure safety for all is to deny therapy to any". The key to the safety philosophy is the concept of "conditions of use", taught by Lloyd Hazleton to those of us fortunate enough to work with him over the years. A drug is selected for its ability to alter a physiologic function, and is usually biologically active. Under the conditions of use, limits can be defined, such as dosage level, nutritional requirements, or routes of administration, within which the drug will have a high probability of safety. If those limitations cannot be met within the therapeutic range of the proposed drug, the product is essentially a failure for its intended purpose. Therefore, it is essential to the proper development of a new drug for this important philosophy to be kept in mind, by both the research group charged with developing the drug and by management providing research and development funds for the project. One of the most difficult decisions to be reached by management is the decision to kill a project in the face of adverse data. An understanding of the many factors underlying the development process and the role the toxicologist plays in the decision-making process is essential for sound, efficient, and effective drug development.

II. THE TOXICOLOGIST

Toxicology is a multidisciplinary application of scientific knowledge to the problems of hazard assessment, and therefore is the receiver of the input of knowledge of many scientific disciplines; it applies these facts, phenomena, laws, and proximate causes, gained and verified by exact observation, organized experimentation, and ordered thinking, to define the conditions under which a product may be used safely.[10] The toxicologist thus must be well grounded in many scientific areas including anatomy, physiology, biochemistry, pharmacology, mathematics, genetics, immunology, psychology, and medicine. In addition, the toxicologist must also have some sense of management of people, money, and facilities and be prepared to enter into the management decision-making process.

Toxicologists in most organizations hold responsible positions high in management, serving both line (operational) functions in directing large, well-staffed laboratories, and staff (planning) functions for guidance of management in selecting and developing new products. Both roles are essential, and a lack of expertise in either function is costly, both in terms of dollars and in terms of human health benefits.

Unfortunately, the demand for toxicologists has far exceeded the supply, and one finds many serving as toxicologists who do not have an adequate background of experience and training. This is particularly true in the regulatory agencies, where this lack of experience is the most costly to the consumer. Inexperienced reviewers have rejected data, or requested new studies in situations which should never have been challenged had there been a full understanding of the practical limitations of science. In part, the "working" toxicologist, who is intimately involved in studying the drug, failed to explain to the "reviewing" toxicologist in the agency the significance of the work; there is, however, an antagonistic attitude between regulator and regulated which tends toward an adversary attitude. This attitude alone is costly to consumers, and has delayed the development of new drugs to the detriment of the public health. Management needs to understand this situation and to develop concepts and guidelines to effectively minimize its impact on a research program. This can be done.

III. THE TOXICOLOGY LABORATORY

The toxicology laboratory is a capital-intensive, high-technology operation, which undergoes constant change as new knowledge, new techniques, and new disciplines are integrated into the demands of safety assessment. Staff requirements include pathologists, biochemists, computer scientists, embryologists, geneticists, microbiologists, and other specialists, each with a full complement of technical assistants and special equipment. Few laboratories are completely qualified to conduct all aspects of a complex toxicology study, but there are many specialized laboratories equipped to handle limited portions of a program. Management must utilize contract laboratories and university laboratories to augment the in-house capabilities and staff, if all necessary data are to be applied to safety assessment of a new drug.

IV. PLANNING

From early screening studies, candidate compounds are selected for development. Early screening may provide initial toxicological data such as the LD_{50}, the dose-responses slope, the biologic systems affected, and possibly some indication of duration of action. From these preliminary inputs, protocols may be designed which emphasize the scientific aspects of the problem which are judged important, and delete or deemphasize those aspects which have little or no bearing on safety assessment and are unproductive in terms of time and costs.

Guidelines are available from the regulatory agencies which, when properly used, provide a basis for assurance that all key areas are examined and the study will be adequate for interpretation. Such guidelines are relied upon heavily by the regulatory toxicologists for assurance that data comparisons with similar drugs can be made for regulatory procedures; they have tended to become test requirements, rather than guidelines, in that deviations unapproved in advance result in rejection of the study regardless of the scientific validity of the deviation. On the one hand, the regulated industry can plan for the costs and timing of such studies, but on the other hand, science is stifled, and the consumer is the ultimate loser.

A series of protocols requires an integrated plan for their execution. Use of program evaluation and review technique (PERT) -type planning programs is essential to efficient utilization of money, personnel, and facilities. Case after case can be cited where studies were scheduled only to discover that the chemists were unable to supply sufficient compound, that an analytical procedure was not ready when the tissue samples were available, or that personnel were not available when needed. Several planning programs are needed: (1) an overall integrated plan which includes input from all segments, from inception to final marketing, and is useful to management for financial planning; (2) a segmented plan which details the requirements for each major area of input such as toxicology or chemistry; and (3) a detailed plan for each protocol. The plans must be time-related, financially supported, realistic statements of the goals to be accomplished. Management must follow through to be certain all segments are accurate and, most importantly, are closely adhered to. Any changes must be recognized early and the impact on the overall program assessed. More time and money are wasted by failing to coordinate all aspects of the plan than any other single factor in the development program.

Contacts with the FDA are considerably facilitated through adequate planning. The usual practice is to submit toxicology protocols to the agency for advice and comment prior to initiation. In this step, the role of the toxicologist is very important, and the homework must have been done in advance, not at the conference. The details of the protocol, the justification of the species, the tissues to be examined, and the biochemical parameters to be measured are essential items to be noted. If the protocol differs from the guidelines, the alterations must be justified. Once accepted by the FDA, changes by the sponsor can result in serious delays in the regulatory process. Changes can, of course, be made, but they must be discussed in advance with the FDA and documented in the record, or the study may be rejected by the agency.

V. COSTS

Costs of toxicology studies are difficult to assess, because many studies are interrelated with functional evaluations. However, in general terms, the cost of work done to meet guideline toxicology studies can be estimated at $500,000 to $2 million to $3 million or more, with major commitments of funds coming during the later portion of the development period.

Costs have moderately increased during the period 1980 to 1988, and can be expected to increase at a rate equal to or exceeding the inflation rate, as the demand for laboratory facilities and personnel increases. The requirements for highly trained technologists and specialized equipment necessary to measure and evaluate the various parameters of hematology and biochemistry are only two examples. The use of computers for data collection and assimilation, the requirements for good laboratory practices (GLP) and raw-data archiving have all contributed to the actual costs of toxicology studies. Recent implementation of requirements to update the data base for many pesticides and industrial chemicals, mandated by law, will severely limit the available facilities, and undoubtedly will affect pricing. The contract industry anticipates the situation to continue to be critical for the next 5 to 8 years.

The costs for defining the safety of a drug, while a relatively minor part of the total development costs, should not be taken lightly by management, because well-thought out studies will not only define the risk/benefit limits, but may demonstrate areas of concern in the clinical arena. Conversely, shortcuts usually waste research dollars and hide potential problems.

Management must also recognize that the project can be lost by adverse data only available at completion of the more expensive and time-consuming studies. For example, the carcinogenic potential of a drug may not be detected until completion of the histopathology examination of a 2-year study, or about 3 years from initiation of the study. Effects on the reproductive cycle may not become apparent until the second or third generation, and not known until after a year or more into the study.

Costs of time in the development program are of greater significance to management than dollars. The loss of as little as 2 weeks in the development schedule has created problems which resulted in the ultimate loss of the product for more than one pharmaceutical manufacturer.

VI. LAWS AND REGULATIONS

The Food, Drug and Cosmetics Act, as amended, is the basis for regulating both the safety and efficacy of drugs sold in the U.S. The regulations to carry out the requirements of the law are found at 21 CFR, Subchapters A and C, for general provisions, Subchapter D for human drugs, and Subchapter E for animal drugs. It is essential that management, and the toxicologist playing a management role, be intimately versed in these regulations; otherwise, errors of planning and execution will result. It is beyond the scope of this discussion to detail specifics of the law and regulations, but their impact on planning is considered as an integral part of the philosophy of drug development. Although this may be considered a trite statement, it is always easier to comply with the regulations than it is to fight them.

VII. GOOD LABORATORY PRACTICE

Since 1978, the chemical industry has come to recognize the GLP regulations as a fact of life in the development of safety data. The original final regulations were published December 22,

1978 and became effective June 20, 1979 as 21 CFR Part 58. On September 4, 1987, the regulations were modified, effective October 5, 1987, to "clarify, delete, or amend several provisions of the GLP regulations to reduce the regulatory burden on testing facilities". Significant changes were made in the areas of quality assurance, protocol preparation, test and control article identity and characterization, and in retention of specimens and samples; the change with the greatest impact on the industry deals with test article identity, purity, and stability.

The Environmental Protection Agency has also installed GLP regulations at 40 CFR 160 for pesticide toxicology studies submitted to that agency under Federal Insecticide, Fungicide and Rodenticide Act, and at 40 CFR 792 for data submitted under the Toxic Substances Control Act. There is little difference between the three sets of GLP regulations with the major exception of times for retaining records.

In summary, these regulations define the bases on which the FDA may disqualify a study, a laboratory, a scientist, or a drug, specify the organization and personnel requirements of a toxicology laboratory, identify the facilities and equipment and how they are to be operated, and detail the records to be maintained. Inspections by FDA personnel are authorized, and failure to allow inspection, or failure to provide adequate data, records, and information, can lead to disqualification.

Most laboratories have complied fully with these regulations, and those that were not able to meet the requirements are no longer in business. However, it is prudent to inquire into the results of the last GLP inspection of a laboratory prior to placing a study. Such information is usually readily supplied, or can be requested from the Agency under the Freedom of Information Act. It must be borne in mind that the sponsor of a nonclinical laboratory study retains full responsibility or the integrity and completeness of the study, regardless of where the work was accomplished. To satisfy this responsibility, vigilant monitoring by an outside source is essential to assure management that compliance is maintained. For work conducted within the company-owned facility, the "in-house" quality assurance unit (QAU) is the usual procedure. All commercial laboratories maintain such a unit to assure clients that the GLP regulations are met for each study. Most firms placing work with commercial laboratories also monitor their studies independently, even though this represents duplications of effort and increased costs of technical time and dollars. Monitors may be the sponsor's QAU, or it may be the toxicologist responsible for the study. The purpose is to assure management that the study is in compliance, and may be utilized in the safety evaluation of the drug. Legal responsibility for such monitoring has not been spelled out in the regulations, and while the consensus is that it is the responsibility of the laboratory conducting the study to comply, industry sponsors have taken the informal position that the sponsor also assumes the liability when the data are filed as a part of the official application to the FDA.

The detailed records required to be maintained are probably the greatest source of noncompliance citations issued by FDA inspectors. For example, retention of records for cleaning, maintenance, and inspection of equipment was found to be a major item in early inspections. Protocols, although considered adequate in describing the work to be done, were found to be deficient in that details of the statistical methods to be used were not identified, the study director was not named, the means of animal identification was not specified, and the proposed starting, completion, and reporting dates were not stated. Records obtained during the study were not complete, in that raw-data sheets were not properly signed by the technicians, errors had been incorrectly entered or changed, and no checks were available to ensure that the data had not, or could not, be altered.

Much of the detail for laboratory operations has now been clarified through standard operating procedures and the recordkeeping associated with this phase of the GLP regulations is now generally in compliance. Internal QAUs maintain records and assure that cleaning, maintenance, and inspection meet the regulatory demands.

Protocols have greatly improved with the enforcement of the GLPs. In the past, much of the decision process was the responsibility of the scientist conducting the study, but as toxicology expanded to include the multidisciplinary approach, no one individual was adequately trained to foresee all problems in all areas embraced by a toxicology study. The regulations now require what is basically a sound scientific principle of thinking through the details of the study, identification of those areas which need to be closely supervised, assurance that adequately trained personnel will be available when needed, that equipment and facilities are adequate, and that there is a reasonable expectation that the work will be completed on time and that the data will be suitable for the intended purpose in the development program. Records concerning changes in the protocol are now much better kept than before the advent of GPLs. Most protocols require at least some modifications as the study progresses, and these changes are permitted, of course, when properly documented.

Probably the biggest change that has affected the drug industry, and probably the most significant in terms of drug development philosophy, is the requirement for data on compound stability and bioavailability. Drugs mixed with diet may or may not be stable for the period of time required for mixing, storage, and presentation to the test animal. Unstable drugs may give data totally unrelated to the actual toxicologic effects in man or other animals. By monitoring blood levels, an otherwise stable drug in food may be found not to be absorbed, and the toxicology results are meaningless. Such studies require advance preparation by the analytical laboratory, and must be programmed into the development scheme, but experience has shown that this advance planning and work pays handsome dividends in the final outcome of the project. It has led to more detailed and sophisticated studies of pharmacokinetics early in the development program so that dosages can be selected and scheduled on a rational basis. For example, a 3-month study in dogs, costing $150,000, in which the drug is administered once daily is worthless for its intended purpose if the half-life of the drug is only 3 h. Also, early studies on metabolism coupled with pharmacokinetics may show the test animals can adapt by altering metabolic and excretory pathways which affect the interpretation of drug safety under its proposed conditions of use. Such studies are now implied, if not specifically required, by the GLP regulations.

In practice, data collection and retention are becoming computerized. Data input at the technician level is conducted by portable terminals located in the animal rooms. Programs are available that ensure, through recordkeeping with built-in safeguards, the prevention of alteration. By definition, such electronic data processing (EDP) records are raw data and must be retained by the laboratory. Use of CRTs by the study director allows rapid evaluation of results, timely statistical analysis of data, and current readouts of the status of the project. The key, of course, is adequate planning and programming of the computer. Laboratories without access to computer programs and facilities are operating under a handicap of additional time and costs to maintain, store, and recall the raw data. Many sponsors request monthly reports, and EDP provides an economical means of providing the necessary data, either as tapes or as printouts. The use of EDP in the toxicology laboratory will undoubtedly increase greatly as the GLP regulations are refined and enforced.

The GLPs apply, by definition, only to those studies, both *in vivo* and *in vitro*, designed to determine the safety of the test substance. However, a broad interpretation of the definition has been given in the preamble of the proposed regulations (FR 41; 51210, November 19, 1976) which include those studies which assess functionality and effectiveness. In basic terms, any study which involves laboratory animals or biological systems probably comes under GLP regulations. Only studies conducted on humans, clinical trials in humans, and field trials in animals as well as initial screening studies for potential utility are specifically excluded. Considering that portion of the Food, Drug and Cosmetics Act which requires full disclosure of all data to the FDA, it is difficult to decide which studies are subject to GLP and which are not. In reality, any data which is nonclinical should probably be considered to fall under 21 CFR Part 58, and planning should be accordingly adapted.

VIII. INTERPRETATION OF RESULTS

In developing a new drug, continual evaluation of the data must be done to identify problem areas early. "Safety" is defined as the limits within which a compound is expected to have a beneficial effect with the lowest possible risk. Those limits must be continually probed, and the risks must be evaluated and assigned a degree of hazard. Assessing hazard is difficult because it involves risk/benefit analysis. Factors suitable for assessing hazard for a drug are entirely different from those used to evaluate a pesticide, food additive, or an industrial chemical, for the simple reason that a drug is intentionally taken for a specific purpose, the exposure is strictly defined, and the person is aware of the exposure. Usually, there is competent supervision of the administration of a drug, so that the risks of serious injury are significantly reduced.

Drugs intended for animals, however, offer another kind of benefit/risk evaluation from that required for human drugs. Animal drugs must be safe for use in the animals, which means they are administered under competent supervision for a specific medical purpose. Serious injury has an impact on the benefit/risk evaluation as it relates to growth, food utilization, and general well-being of animals, as much as for human drugs, but with animals, an economic factor enters the calculations. From this point, however, evaluation of benefit/risk of animal drugs enters a totally new phase — that of benefit/risk to humans consuming the edible products of treated food animals which may remain as residues. As with food additives, pesticides, and other components of our food supply, exposure is unknown and unsupervised. It has been aptly observed that the meat from one cow represents about 2400 hamburgers and the unwitting exposure of as many as 2400 people, many of whom are children, to drug residues.

For those risks which are difficult to quantitate, such as for carcinogens, current scientific philosophy and regulatory decision making has altered the rigid interpretation represented by the so-called Delaney Clause. Initially, this clause was interpreted to prohibit the use of a food additive, new animal drug, or color additive which have been shown to cause cancer in man or animals. However, through the "DES Proviso", a legal interpretation was made that a carcinogen could be used in animals, provided "no residue" occurred in the human food from such treated animals. To resolve the "no residue" issue, a process of risk assessment, using statistical methods, has been devised to estimate the level of residue which will result in no more than a 1:1,000,000 increase in cancer in man. The final regulations for implementing this philosophy were published in the Federal Register on December 31, 1987, and became effective on February 29, 1988 as 21 CFR 500, Subpart E. It is also referred to as "Sensitivity of the Method", or "SOM". Its major emphasis is the requirement for early metabolic and pharmacokinetic data to identify metabolites and evaluate the metabolic pathways used by the animal for detoxification and excretion. Those compounds which are suggestive of carcinogenic activity, either from mutagenicity studies and short-term toxicology data, or by structural similarity to known carcinogens, are required to undergo extensive chronic testing in two species. Metabolites may also require chronic testing, if the data suggest they are present as residues in the human food, and were not treated by "autoexposure" in the study with the parent material. Further, a suitable residue method for a "marker" compound may or may not be the parent drug, but might be a more easily detected metabolite. Thus, the development of a drug for use in food animals faces a potentially expensive development cost, if multiple chronic tests, extensive metabolite identification, and residue methodology studies are required under this regulation.

The fate of the biomass from antibiotic fermentation when used as a feed additive form of medication has already led to the development of a Guideline by CVM, which includes, as one possible approach, 180-d feeding study in rats, a 90-d feeding study in dogs, a 2-generation study with a teratology component in rats, and a battery of genetic tests, these latter to be conducted not only on the aqueous and organic solvent extracts, but also on the residue from the urine of target animals fed the product. Should the data prove positive for carcinogenesis, SOM will apply.

The relatively new field of products from genetically altered organisms will create new problems for the toxicologist. Bioequivalency is only one of the methods for proving safety of a product already on the market, but manufactured under the new technology. New products will also be developed which will required new thought in designing meaningful studies to prove both safety and efficacy.

IX. PRESENTATION OF DATA

The toxicologist also has a role in the presentation of the data to the regulatory agency. The final report of any study must be clear, concise, and lead the reviewer through the study in a logical, scientifically valid manner. The study must have been monitored during its in-life phase, and it must be presented in a format acceptable to the particular agency requiring it. For example, the Center for Drugs and Biologics of FDA issued a "Guideline for the Format and Content of the Summary for New Drug and Antibiotic Applications" in February 1987 which describes the format for the Summary section of the investigational new drug or new drug application, and is partly the responsibility of the toxicologist to prepare. EPA has issued its PR 86-5 Notice on the format for submitting a study to that agency. Failure to follow the guidelines results in delay in the agency evaluation. In fact, EPA will not accept a study which is out of compliance with its guidelines.

X. CONCLUSION

The responsibilities of the toxicologist within the development team for a new drug are tremendous. To meet the challenge, training in basic and applied science is only a beginning; experience in management, regulatory affairs, and research planning are essential. Certainly, the toxicologist must be supported by an enlightened management. Scientific knowledge is continually expanding, and new knowledge requires new thinking on how best to apply the new concepts to the problems of safety evaluation. At stake is the health and welfare of our people and our food supply.

REFERENCES

1. **Gralla, E. J.,** Ed., *Scientific Considerations in Monitoring and Evaluating Toxicological Research,* Hemisphere Publishing, Washington, D.C., 1981.
2. **Douall, J., Klaassen, C. D., and Amdur, M. O.,** Eds., *Cassarett and Douall's Toxicology,* 2nd ed., Macmillan, New York, 1980.
3. **Loomis, T. A.,** *Essentials of Toxicology,* 2nd ed., Lea & Febiger, Philadelphia, 1974.
4. **Goldstein, A., Aranow, L., and Kalman, S. M.,** *Principles of Drug Action,* John Wiley & Sons, New York, 1974.
5. **Paget, G. E.,** Ed., *Methods in Toxicology,* F. A. Davis, Philadelphia, 1970.
6. **La Du, B. N., Mandel, H. G., and Way, E. L.,** Eds., *Fundamentals of Drug Metabolism and Drug Disposition,* Williams & Wilkins, Baltimore, 1971.
7. **Melman, M. A., Shapiro, R. E., and Blumenthal, H.,** Eds., *Advances in Modern Toxicology,* Vol. 1, Hemisphere Publishing, Washington, D.C., 1976.
8. **Beyer, K. H.,** *Discovery, Development and Delivery of New Drugs,* SP Medical & Scientific Books, New York, 1978.
9. **Beyer, K. H.,** From theory to therapy: today and tomorrow, *Proc. West. Pharmacol. Soc.,* 8, 68, 1965.
10. **Fogleman, R. W.,** Toxicology and its role in regulatory practice, in *Toxicology and Occupational Medicine,* Vol. 4, Deichmann, W. B., Elsevier, Amsterdam, 1979.

Chapter 11

PHARMACEUTICAL PRODUCT DEVELOPMENT FROM CONCEPT TO MARKET

Allen J. Polon

TABLE OF CONTENTS

I. INTRODUCTION

Before describing the details of pharmaceutical development, it is important to define the coordinating manager's position. This person is responsible for the coordination of all people and activities required to move a project from its development phase to the marketplace. In the majority of cases, I have observed that this position brings with it tremendous responsibilities with very little authority. Therefore, the manager responsible for coordinating the hundreds (even thousands) of tasks required to develop a new product must have certain attributes, such as the wisdom of King Solomon, the patience of Job, the strength of Hercules, the endurance of a marathon runner, and the ability to not confuse motion with progress.

The successful manager can effect the proper interaction of many departments involved by using good coordination and management techniques. The ultimate goal is to bring a product from the development stage to the market as efficiently as possible at the lowest feasible cost.

For the purpose of this discussion, R & D includes the departments of Product Development, Analytical Services, Pharmacology, Toxicology, Biopharmaceutics, Regulatory, and Medical. The Marketing/Sales Division includes Marketing, Market Planning, Sales, Purchasing, Marketing Research, Manufacturing, Packaging, Pharmaceutical Accounting, New Product Planning and Development, and Advertising/Promotions. The main topics to be discussed are the coordination of pharmaceutical development activities for R & D, product planning and development, and market planning. Specific subjects include clinical material manufacture, package selection, packaging, product specifications for marketing, price estimation for products, profit/cost analysis, draft label and labeling, and coordination between R & D and all departments involved in manufacturing, marketing, sales, and purchasing.

The emphasis in this chapter is on the coordination of the activities. However, select activities are explained in greater detail to aid the manager in avoiding certain pitfalls and overcoming problems.

Before any manager can be effective, corporate management must define the market areas and the types of products they want to pursue. Also, it is requisite for management to understand the expertise and capabilities of R & D. Therefore, open discussions and cross pollination between R & D and corporate management is important for management to have a better understanding of the strengths and potential of R & D for specific areas of new-product development. As a result of this communication, R & D should be requested to place its efforts in areas of its expertise that will bring the company the quickest and greatest return on its investment.

II. MONITORING AND COORDINATING ACTIVITIES

Why are monitoring and coordinating activities necessary? Why can't the department managers simply know what their incremental part of the project is and accomplish the work without being concerned with the input from or output to the other departments involved? In some situations, this has been done, but the result is not usually efficient or economical. For example, how can the purchasing department act without input from the development group, marketing, sales, marketing research, etc.? If one examines the input required by each department from other areas, it soon becomes obvious that interdepartmental and interdivisional relationships are a prerequisite to the proper development and marketing of a product.

It is the responsibility of the coordinating manager to develop an effective network of communication, instill an esprit de corps within the project team, and encourage input and interaction from all members of the team.

A. THE RESEARCH AND DEVELOPMENT TEAM

In the following discussion, assume that the product to be developed is a new chemical entity.

This case describes the development procedures to be followed to develop an Investigational New Drug application (IND) and New Drug Application (NDA) as required by the FDA. However, the coordinating functions for development and marketing can be applied to all types of products, both prescription and over the counter.

Coordination of the R & D functions may be managed by the same individual who will be responsible for coordinating the marketing/sales development. However, in many larger companies these jobs are done by two or more managers responsible for activities within their respective divisions. It is extremely important for these managers to work closely together and keep each other informed of the status and advancement of the project.

B. SELECTING THE PRE-IND ACTIVITIES TEAM

The pre-IND phase requires careful coordination and follow-up by the R & D team to save time and dollars. The initial team should include representatives from the departments of Chemistry, Pharmacology, Toxicology, Metabolic Chemistry, Biopharmaceutics, Pharmacy Research, and Analytical Research. As the project progresses, the coordinating manager invites members of other departments to join the team. For example, the Medical Department and Regulatory Affairs Department will join the group, whereas the Pharmacology Department may leave. Simply remember that flexibility is important. To be effective the team must consist of representatives from those departments required to accomplish the task.

A drug developed in-house undergoes a great amount of early development prior to a project request for product development of a market image. Using Figure 1, follow the early stages of development (pre-IND). After the discovery of a new chemical entity, pharmacological testing (primary screening) is used to determine the activity of the drug. This is done in a manner that will give the Medical Department some insight of what to expect at particular dosage levels in humans. The drug is also tested for its toxic effects in animals. This establishes the safety margin between effective and toxic dose levels.

In conjunction with the above, the metabolic chemists develop an assay for the active ingredient to determine the metabolic route of the drug in animals. This will indicate how much of and in what manner the drug is being metabolized and excreted.

The analytical chemists develop an assay for the drug in order to identify the purity of the raw material and the percent content in a dosage form. During this period, the Pharmacy Development Department may do some preliminary formulation work to determine the "workability" of the compound and its stability in certain forms.

With the great amount of work that goes into the pre-IND phase of a project, is it any wonder that R & D has so much information and input to offer when the product conceptualization phase is initiated by the Marketing/Sales Division? Be sure to include the people in R & D when the "new product" is being developed by Marketing.

When the project reaches the level of development that indicates to R & D management that a potential product exists, a complete report is prepared for review by corporate management. Be certain that it contains an "understandable" summary of the data and all information necessary for the reviewers to give the project proper evaluation. Include in the report such subjects as patent information, the history and background of the project, a definition of the pharmacological activity, the medical area in which the drug would be used, a summary of the completed toxicology, a description of competitive products, and time cost estimates for full development. Explain the advantages and/or disadvantages of the subject product relative to the presently marketed products. To illustrate the work required and the sequence of events that will take place, a good program evaluation and review technique (PERT), precedent network (flow of events) or bar chart is extremely helpful in addition to the written report. An example of a major precedent network is seen in Figure 1. Note the number of activities that can be accomplished in parallel. With this type of information, the executive can make a "go/no go" decision to investigate the potential marketability and profitability of the potential product.

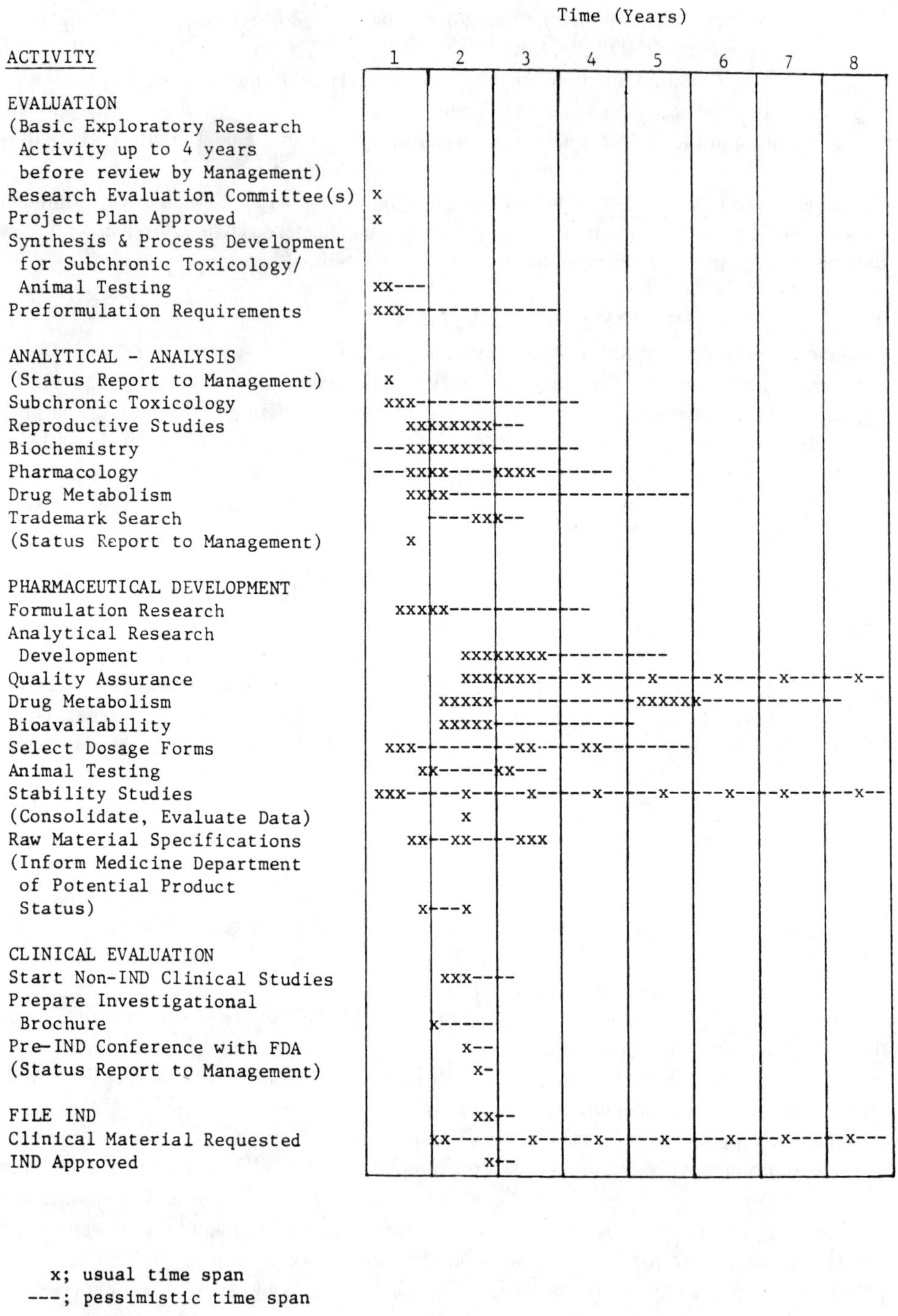

```
                                                      Time (Years)

ACTIVITY                                 1    2    3    4    5    6    7    8

EVALUATION
(Basic Exploratory Research
 Activity up to 4 years
 before review by Management)
Research Evaluation Committee(s)         x
Project Plan Approved                    x
Synthesis & Process Development
 for Subchronic Toxicology/
 Animal Testing                          xx---
Preformulation Requirements              xxx--------------

ANALYTICAL - ANALYSIS
(Status Report to Management)            x
Subchronic Toxicology                    xxx----------------
Reproductive Studies                      xxxxxxxxx---
Biochemistry                             ---xxxxxxxx--------
Pharmacology                             ---xxxx----xxxx-------
Drug Metabolism                           xxxx-----------------------
Trademark Search                            ----xxx--
(Status Report to Management)            x

PHARMACEUTICAL DEVELOPMENT
Formulation Research                      xxxxx-----------
Analytical Research
 Development                                 xxxxxxxx-----------
Quality Assurance                            xxxxxxx---x----x----x----x-----x--
Drug Metabolism                              xxxxx-----------xxxxx------------
Bioavailability                              xxxxx-------------
Select Dosage Forms                      xxx-------xx---xx------
Animal Testing                            xx-----xx---
Stability Studies                        xxx---x----x---x---x----x---x-----x--
(Consolidate, Evaluate Data)                 x
Raw Material Specifications              xx--xx---xxx
(Inform Medicine Department
 of Potential Product
 Status)                                 x---x

CLINICAL EVALUATION
Start Non-IND Clinical Studies              xxx---
Prepare Investigational
 Brochure                                x-----
Pre-IND Conference with FDA              x--
(Status Report to Management)            x-

FILE IND                                  xx--
Clinical Material Requested              xx------x---x----x--x----x---x---
IND Approved                             x--
```

    x; usual time span
    ---; pessimistic time span

FIGURE 1. Activity correlation and time span for typical full-term development project.

C. SELECTING THE MARKETING PRODUCT DEVELOPMENT TEAM

If corporate management (chairman of the board, president, executive vice-president, senior vice-presidents, etc.) approves a "go" decision based on the R & D report, then the next step is to have the Marketing/Sales Division prepare a request for product development.

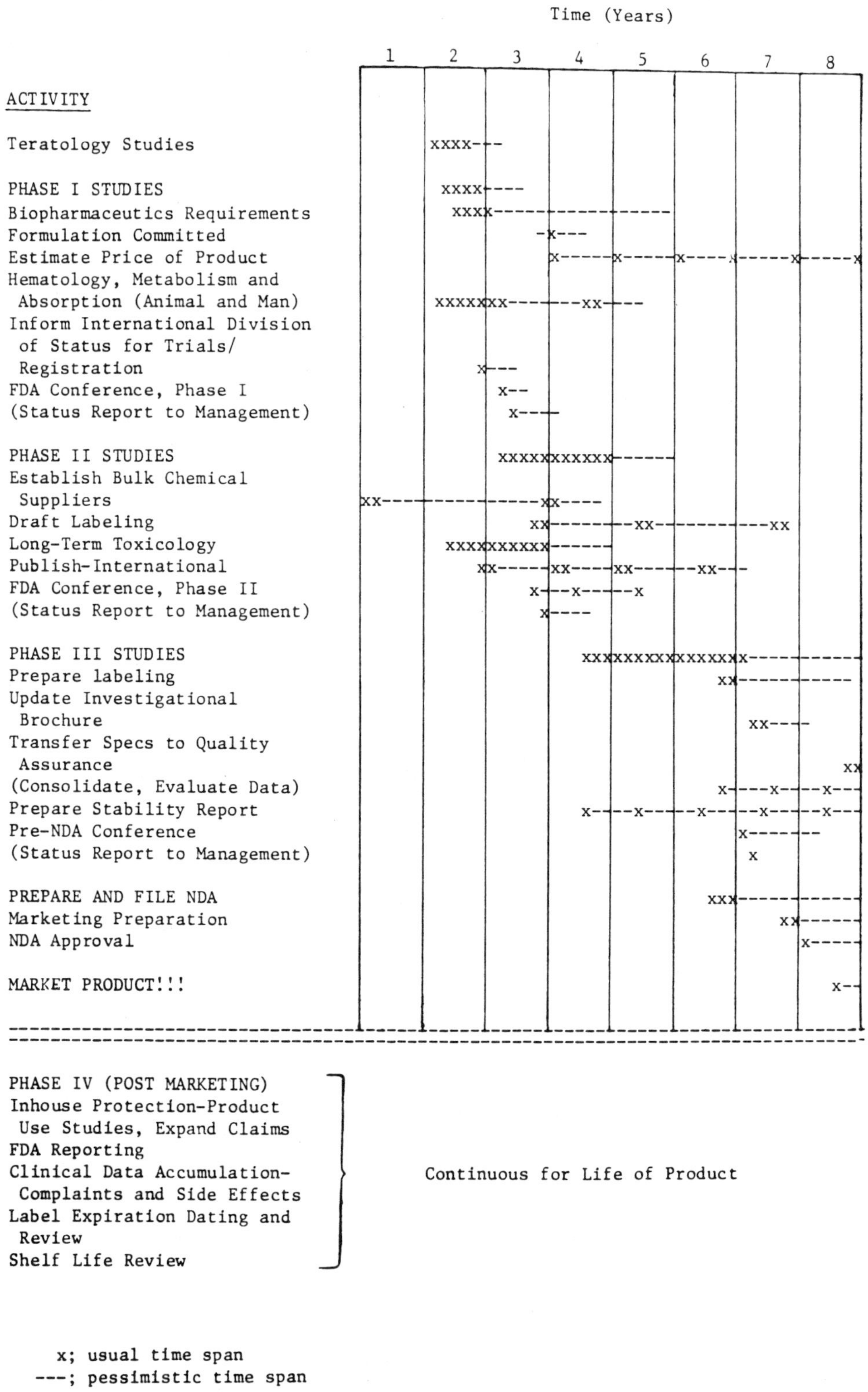

```
                                                Time (Years)

                                1    2    3    4    5    6    7    8

ACTIVITY

Teratology Studies                   xxxx-+-

PHASE I STUDIES                      xxxx+----
Biopharmaceutics Requirements        xxxx-----+-----+-----
Formulation Committed                          -x---
Estimate Price of Product                      x-----x-----x----x-----x-----x
Hematology, Metabolism and
  Absorption (Animal and Man)        xxxxxxx--------xx-+---
Inform International Division
  of Status for Trials/
  Registration                        x---
FDA Conference, Phase I                x--
(Status Report to Management)          x---+

PHASE II STUDIES                       xxxxxxxxxxx------
Establish Bulk Chemical
  Suppliers                     xx----+---------+---xx----
Draft Labeling                                 xx-+----+--xx-------+----xx
Long-Term Toxicology                 xxxxxxxxxx------
Publish-International                  xx-----xx----xx------xx--+
FDA Conference, Phase II                      x-+--x----+--x
(Status Report to Management)                 x----

PHASE III STUDIES                             xxxxxxxxxxxxxxxxx----+------
Prepare labeling                                                xx----+------
Update Investigational
  Brochure                                                         xx---+
Transfer Specs to Quality
  Assurance                                                              xx
(Consolidate, Evaluate Data)                              x-+---x-+--x---
Prepare Stability Report                       x-+--x-+--x---+-x--+-x---
Pre-NDA Conference                                              x-----+--
(Status Report to Management)                                   x

PREPARE AND FILE NDA                                            xxx------+------
Marketing Preparation                                              xx------
NDA Approval                                                       x-----

MARKET PRODUCT!!!                                                       x-+
```

PHASE IV (POST MARKETING)
Inhouse Protection-Product
  Use Studies, Expand Claims
FDA Reporting
Clinical Data Accumulation-   Continuous for Life of Product
  Complaints and Side Effects
Label Expiration Dating and
  Review
Shelf Life Review

    x; usual time span
  ---; pessimistic time span

FIGURE 1 (continued).

With the assistance of the proper departments, establish the market size, sales potential, profit/cost analysis, dosage forms to be developed, and product parameters, such as types of packaging to be used, colors and flavors to be used, size tablet or capsule desired, etc. If the company has an international division, then give them the opportunity to assess the product and express their level of interest and sales potential.

This is the optimal time to determine which departments will be included in the development, how they will be coordinated as a team, the contribution required from each, the period of time they will need to complete their functions, and developmental overlap of activities. In the same manner as a project team was developed in the early stages for R & D, assemble a team for product planning and development within the Marketing/Sales Division. This group will meet periodically as needed with specific members of the R & D Team (such as Product Development) to update each other and exchange ideas and information as the product is developed.

One of the coordinating managers from R & D or Marketing should be made responsible for calling meetings on a regular basis and chairing these meetings between R & D and Marketing.

III. PLANNING A NEW PRODUCT

In many large companies, there exists a Product Planning Group or New Product Department which is responsible for the coordination and development of new products for the Marketing/ Sales Division. However, in some companies, this function may be incorporated into a department such as Marketing. In either case, this department must coordinate the inter- and intradivisional functions for the project. Their main goal is to move the project from R & D to the market by communicating, reporting, and interacting with all sections involved.

A. ACCOMPLISHING THE TASK

Various means have been used to accomplish project planning and product planning and development. The key issue is to develop a system that is uncomplicated, easily understood, and leads to expediency. In order to develop the proper charts, project requests, and reports, it is important to have a complete understanding of the functions of each department and how they interrelate with the other departments in the development and marketing of a product. Lack of this knowledge can be one of the most significant problems encountered by a coordinating manager. It will lead to delays, failures, and disasters. Additionally, without this knowledge it is impossible to be an effective leader for your team.

An overview of the project can be seen using a PERT chart or similar management tool. In addition to a chart describing the activities of the division responsible for marketing the product, there could be a separate one for all R & D functions. The R & D activity chart is shown in Figure 1. A typical network chart for coordinating the Marketing/Sales Division can be seen in Figure 2. These two divisions will overlap at several points, and this can be made obvious in the charts. For detailed jobs within a department, develop a micro or minor chart to ensure proper flow when a project must pass through several sections within that department. Leave nothing to chance.

When a product concept is received by a manager in the Product Planning Department, that person should study in detail all aspects of the particular drug category. Only then will the manager be prepared to request the correct input from other departments, e.g., Marketing, Sales, Purchasing, Product Development, etc., and coordinate it once it is received. These activities are evident in Figure 2.

Due to uncontrollable circumstances one is sometimes "under the gun" to rush the planning and development of a product. However, to rush through this initial planning phase will often lead to a project fraught with built-in problems that may have been avoided if enough time and energy had been spent in the planning stage. It is your responsibility to plan the project well! Request input from all departments and a generous amount of time, money, and energy will be saved in the long run. Only with complete and proper input can a project be planned correctly.

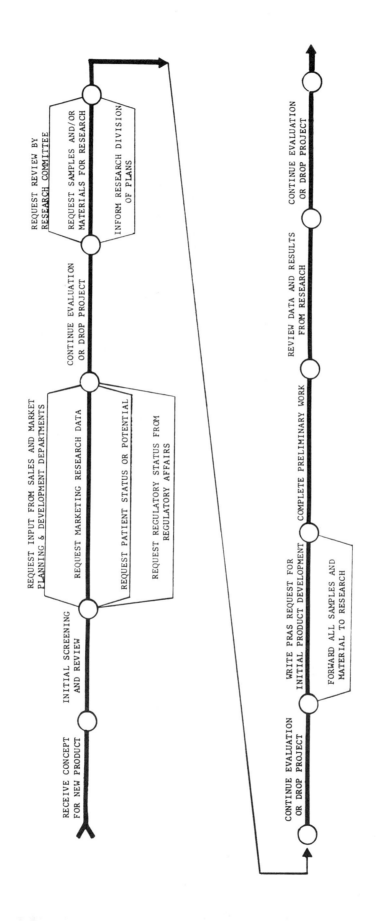

FIGURE 2. Pharmaceutical development of a new product.

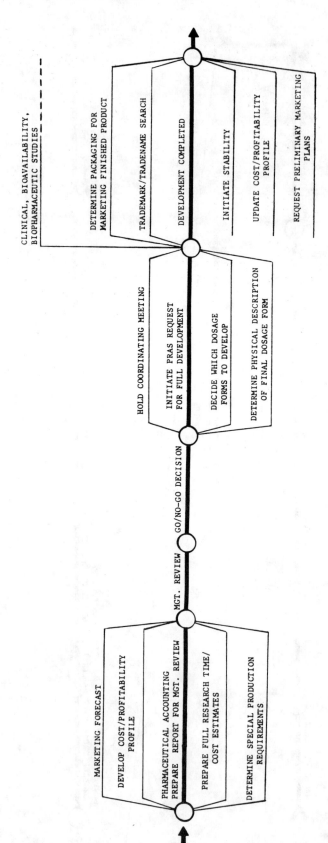

CLINICAL, BIOAVAILABILITY,
BIOPHARMACEUTIC STUDIES

DETERMINE PACKAGING FOR
MARKETING FINISHED PRODUCT

TRADEMARK/TRADENAME SEARCH

DEVELOPMENT COMPLETED

INITIATE STABILITY

UPDATE COST/PROFITABILITY
PROFILE

REQUEST PRELIMINARY MARKETING
PLANS

HOLD COORDINATING MEETING

INITIATE PRAS REQUEST
FOR FULL DEVELOPMENT

DECIDE WHICH DOSAGE
FORMS TO DEVELOP

DETERMINE PHYSICAL DESCRIPTION
OF FINAL DOSAGE FORM

MGT. REVIEW GO/NO-GO DECISION

MARKETING FORECAST

DEVELOP COST/PROFITABILITY
PROFILE

PHARMACEUTICAL ACCOUNTING
PREPARE REPORT FOR MGT. REVIEW

PREPARE FULL RESEARCH TIME/
COST ESTIMATES

DETERMINE SPECIAL PRODUCTION
REQUIREMENTS

FIGURE 2B.

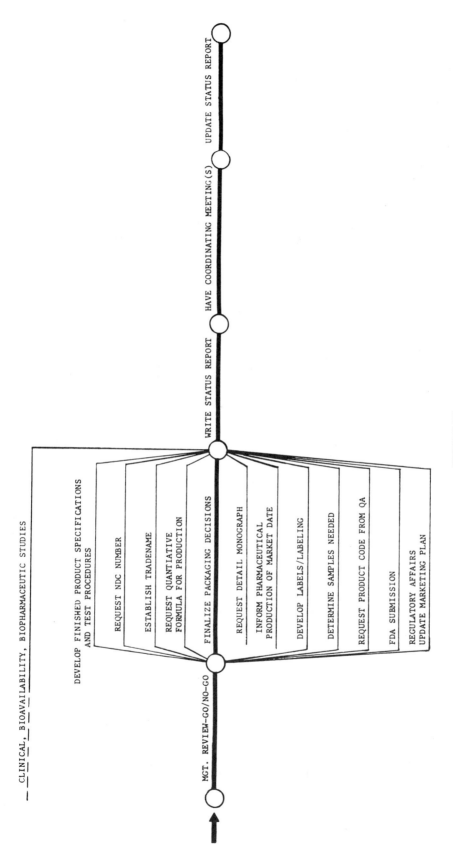

FIGURE 2C.

B. DEVELOPING PRODUCT PARAMETERS

Obviously, it is not desirable to request new products with parameters that are literally impossible to meet. As ridiculous as this may sound, there exists the possibility of this happening in an organization that lacks communication. Several activities should be accomplished before the product development is initiated. First, establish the marketing parameters for the new product by soliciting requests, suggestions, questions, and all other input from the Marketing/Sales Division. Second, act as liaison to be certain the Marketing/Sales input is received by the individuals in the R & D Division who are responsible for the product development. Third, be certain that R & D considers the project to be feasible.

It is important that R & D people have a chance for idea exchanges with the Marketing/Sales Division. They are aware of dosage form concepts from the scientific literature and state of the art, which marketing and sales personnel may not be. They may have suggestions that are synergistic or in concert with market plans. In many companies, the R & D division has in its employ pharmacists and physicians who have practiced their profession and can give insight regarding the sentiments and reactions of their fellow professionals still in practice. Take advantage of this source of knowledge and information.

Fourth, before the development work is initiated, examine a profit/cost analysis. Without a profit margin that meets criteria of the company, a project request should never by initiated. A profit/cost analysis requires a coordinated effort of purchasing, R & D, marketing, marketing research, and sales forecasting. Consider all factors regarding the finished product:

1. R & D can only estimate their development costs, but with time and experience, the figures should be close enough for management's needs; also, a preliminary quantitative product formula is required to determine product costs.
2. Product Planning and Marketing should select several types of packaging and package sizes to be considered. The cost of packaging can then be determined.
3. The sales and shipping departments determine shipping requirements and costs.
4. The place and cost for manufacturing and packaging should be determined.
5. Marketing research and sales forecasts can be used to establish guidelines for material requirements; from this information raw material costs can be forecast.
6. A sales forecast is not only important in making the first "go/no go" decision, it is a necessity. Royalty payments, if involved, can be considered as a direct cost.
7. The projected selling price is derived based on several factors including the company's required percentage profit and market parameters.

With this information, the Accounting Department can determine the profit based on discounts to wholesalers, percentage mark-ups, wholesalers' and retailers' costs, and competitors' prices. Once the cost/profit profile and the forecast are studied, a "go or no go" decision is recommended to management based on expected sales and profit (see Figure 2). Having eliminated much of the guesswork, an informative and accurate project request, setting forth product parameters based on facts, can be written.

Because of the importance of the above planning phase, it is necessary to examine and define certain points more closely.

The dosage form of a product is of the utmost importance; especially to Sales, Marketing, and R & D. Decisions such as whether a solid oral dosage form is to be a tablet or capsule or whether a liquid is a syrup or suspension are dictated by two factors. The first is the physical characteristics of the drug, which, for various reasons, may dictate the dosage form. For example, vitamins are usually either capsules or coated (film or sugar) tablets. A plain, compressed vitamin tablet may be undesirable due to its instability, taste, and odor. Certain drugs may not lend themselves to tablet compression and therefore may be a better candidate for a capsule. However, the reverse can also be true. A hygroscopic material is more stable as

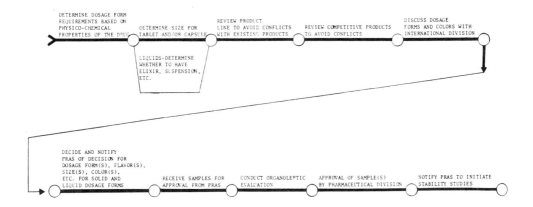

FIGURE 3. Activities for selecting dosage forms.

a film-coated tablet than as a capsule. In summary, the product must be a form and formulation that can be manufactured easily. Forcing the development of a particular tablet or capsule only for its image may end up being a nemesis for the manufacturing people and in the long run cause problems for the final marketed product.

Secondly, the marketing and sales groups will want to have input regarding size, taste, color, etc. For psychological or competitive reasons, a capsule may be preferred to a tablet or vice-versa. The product must be distinguishable from other products of your company as well as competitive ones. Therefore, a particular size or shape or color may not be available because of a conflict with a presently marketed product, and another selection must be made.

'If the product is to be marketed in countries other than the U.S., then consideration should be given to using excipients that are universally acceptable. Input from the international division can help limit the number of formulations required to market the product worldwide. To facilitate the coordination and selection of the dosage forms, develop a flow chart of activities (see Figure 3).

Packaging selection (see Figure 2) for a product is dependent upon manufacturing capabilities, competitor product packaging, supply, costs, preferences of the marketing and sales departments, and package engineering abilities and capabilities. Use the same coordinating effort for this activity as was discussed above for dosage form selection. Once the package is agreed upon, the final recommendation for its market use depends upon the stability of the product in that particular package. If there is any question regarding the suitability of a specific package selection, then insist on back-up package selections and studies to ensure that marketing of the product is not delayed due to instability or other problems related to the package.

Only after compiling all of the information and facts that have been discussed above can a proper project request be written. The request should contain specific details regarding the desired dosage form(s) and packaging.

C. OVERSEEING CRITICAL AREAS

To this point the activities required by R & D and Marketing/Sales to write a project request have been reviewed. Next is an examination of the R & D activities that take place following receipt of the project request and culminating with an NDA submission. This will be followed by a discussion of marketing/sales activities during the same period (NDA development).

Once it is written, the request can be received by one or more of several departments within R & D. If R & D has a program coordination department, then this is the most likely place for the receipt of the request. However, depending upon the system, the request may be sent to Pharmacy Development, office of the vice president of R & D, Regulatory Affairs, or one of several other departments.

After the request for development is received, review the sequence of events that are required for the expanded development and begin coordinating them. Develop proper channels in R & D to prevent the project from sliding or "slipping through the cracks". Never assume that things are happening. Be certain who is doing what, when, and where. Always remember the motto "It's not done til' it's done!"

Continuously monitor the events, update status reports, and meet with the team members individually and as a group on a regularly scheduled basis. Be prepared to inform management at any moment of the details regarding any project:

1. Priorities of projects in the system
2. Stages of development
3. Expenses to date
4. Estimated cost to completion
5. Time elapsed
6. Estimated time to completion
7. Potential problems anticipated
8. Problems encountered
9. Recommended solutions to problems encountered and anticipated.

IV. MANAGING DEVELOPMENT OF THE PRODUCT

A. PHARMACY DEVELOPMENT

Pharmacy Development will initiate development of a dosage form that matches the specifications set forth by the Marketing/Sales Division (see Figure 1). The product must be made in a manner that can be reproduced on a much larger scale in the manufacturing area. As can be seen in Figure 4, to develop a tablet, the formulator selects the proper excipients that will allow the material to be compressable, disintegrate in gastric juice, dissolute and become bioavailable, be packageable (not friable), be esthetically appealing, remain chemically stable, be small enough to swallow or taste good enough to chew, etc. If this is to be an extended action tablet, the problems become far more complicated and the science more sophisticated. If a film or sugar coating is required, the formulator must determine such things as solvent systems, film density and thickness, drying temperatures, pan speed, and exhaust volume.

To develop a capsule, the formulator selects excipients that will allow the material to flow, compact, disintegrate, dissolute, and remain stable. If the product is to be long acting or time release, the process of developing the active material particles or matrix becomes a primary concern.

Formulating stable liquids can be very difficult. Many chemicals in a liquid medium are far less stable than in a solid form. This includes suspensions, syrups, elixirs, and injectables. Therefore, the R & D staff must develop a product that is not only esthetically appealing with a pleasant taste, but also is stable in a medium that lends itself to instability in many cases. The formulator carefully selects the proper excipients, e.g., antioxidants, a chelating agent, sweeteners, flavors, colors, and preservatives. The optimum pH, viscosity, and clarity must be established. A container and cap must be selected that will maintain product stability while not leaking or cap locking.

There are other dosage forms that may be requested, e.g., ointments, suppositories, powders, and granules; however, there is no need to delve into the trials and tribulations of the formulator in each instance. Let it suffice to say that one should have considerable respect for Pharmacy Research. One cannot simply put a request in and immediately receive a product to meet the criteria. Development of a product is the result of the proper balance of science, personal skills, knowledge of the scientific area, and state of the art.

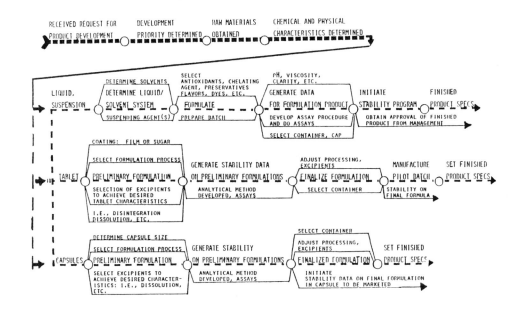

FIGURE 4. Development of a liquid, tablet, or capsule.

During the development phase, the project manager is the main thread of communication and understanding between management and those doing the work. Be aware of any problems or difficulties experienced by departments working on the project in order to update the time/cost estimates, reevaluate priorities, and keep management informed.

Once Pharmacy Research has developed the product and it meets the parameters of the project request, send product samples to Marketing/Sales management for evaluation and approval of the physical characteristics. Only with management approval should R & D feel comfortable with the product they developed.

B. ANALYTICAL CHEMISTRY AND THE STABILITY PROGRAM

Now that Pharmacy Development has produced a dosage form containing many excipients, it is the task of the analytical chemist to assay the mixture and determine the amount of active ingredient in each dosage unit. The excipients may cause complications by interfering with the assay used for the drug by itself. Until an assay method is available, the stability assays will be delayed. This can be the source of a costly and time-delaying problem. If it is, then reschedule the project accordingly and inform management of the problem and the steps being taken to resolve the situation. An updated chart and status report should be issued to reflect any changes.

Following the preliminary formulation and subsequent development of the assay, a short stability study can be conducted to assure everyone the product is stable. The product can be stored at various and extreme temperatures to produce stability data in a relatively short period of time that will be representative of the long-term shelf life of the product. However, to study a product at temperatures that are too high can give results directly related to elevated temperatures, but with no application to an Arrhenius plot (curve used to determine stability of a product in years based on short-term data at elevated temperatures).

Working together, Pharmacy Research and Analytical Services are responsible for initiating the stability program using the package(s) selected for marketing the product. A pilot batch is manufactured by the development group and assayed by the analytical section to ensure that the procedures that worked for lab-size batches will work for scale-up batches.

Parallel to the above activities, the dosage form is tested in animals to determine the bioavailability of the drug. In addition, the pharmacy lab should run *in vitro* studies to determine the release of the drug in artificial gastric juice. Long-acting or slow-release products are placed in gastric juice first and then in artificial intestinal juice to simulate the manner in which a product actually passes through an *in vivo* system.

C. PREPARING FOR CLINICAL TESTING

The Regulatory Affairs Department can assemble the IND using the information and data available from the Departments of Pharmacology, Toxicology, Metabolism and Bioavailability, Analytical Research and Development, Pharmacy Research and Development, and Clinical Research. During the 30-day waiting period following the submission of the IND, development work can continue; e.g., secondary (back-up) formulas completed and stability studies initiated, development of raw material test procedures and specifications initiated, pilot batches made, clinical materials made ready for distribution, etc.

When the IND is submitted to the FDA, the Clinical Research and Clinical Material Supply departments become active in concert. The Medical Department will have investigators selected and protocols written for Phase I clinical pharmacology studies. Therefore, the quantity of clinical material requirements for Phase I should be known and a clinical material request initiated as soon as possible.

Manufacturing and processing clinical materials for several sections of the Medical Department can be a complicated task. Examine the situation in detail and develop a system that allows enough lead time for the Clinical Materials Section to complete the job properly and have the drug in the physician's hands when required.

If the schedule for the project is to be maintained, there are certain pitfalls to be avoided regarding supply of clinical materials. Have the section heads agree upon a predetermined time allotment for manufacturing, packaging, labeling, and shipping the material. Be certain that everyone involved understands the necessity for interdepartmental communications if requests are to be met and supplies readied at the proper time. This function demands constant monitoring.

The Clinical Material Section will prefer to package and label a product *after* the product is approved by Analytical Services, since everything would be for naught if the product does not pass the assay and must be remade. All packages would require destroying because the alternatives are so very costly. Not only would the product be discarded, but the cost of containers, labels, and labor would also be lost. Obviously, this would be an extremely wasteful and costly event.

Several factors combined will determine the schedule for clinical material supply. The Clinical Materials Section has limited personnel that respond to many requests from the Medical Department simultaneously. By receiving proper advance notice, active drug, excipients, and packaging components can be ordered and labels can be produced. Consider also the shipping time for receipt of raw materials and distribution of finished product. Several things can hinder shipment: Christmas, New Years, Thanksgiving, weekends, winter snow, summer vacations, etc. Altering schedules (including those for new orders coming into the department and old orders already there) may be necessary if the assay for a product is too low or too high and a batch remake is required.

One of the worst sins befalling a clinical study is a delay due to poor planning of clinical material inventory. Develop an inventory reporting system to keep the Medical Department informed of product inventory levels. When additional medication is required, it should be available immediately. If two or more sections of the Medical Department are ordering drugs from the same batch, notify the sections through the reporting system (computer, handwritten, or oral). When levels become low, but before depletion occurs, be certain new clinical material requests are made. If a supply problem occurs despite proper planning, be ready to evaluate priorities and recommend to management any changes that will alleviate the problem without causing others.

While the three phases of clinical studies are being conducted, there are several other R & D functions to be completed (see Figure 1). The final dosage form is established, the stability program initiated, and enough data collected to determine a reasonable expiration date for the product to be marketed. In conjunction with the formulation commitment, determine whether or not special manufacturing equipment will be required. Notify the proper personnel in the Production Department and request that they make provisions for these needs. Examples of equipment that may require ordering are punches and dies, mixers, blenders, tablet presses, drying equipment, packaging machinery, etc. One or more sources of supply for the bulk raw materials is established by the Purchasing Department with the assistance of R & D if necessary. In certain instances, there may be only one supplier. In this case, to guarantee the supply of raw material requirements, consider a contract for minimum and/or maximum requirements.

The toxicology studies completed prior to the IND submission are acute and subacute. Now the chronic or long-term toxicology and teratology studies are initiated (see Figure 1). The chronic studies will be used to demonstrate the long-term effects of the drug on animals and the teratology studies will be used to determine any genetic effect on future generations caused by the drug. These data are required for the NDA submission. "Red flags" in either case can mean the demise of the project. It must be proven that the drug is relatively a nontoxic agent with beneficial pharmacological and physiological properties when taken for specific medical problems; in short, safe and effective.

Monitor the ongoing activities continuously and distribute periodic status reports plus updated activity charts to keep everyone informed. In addition, notify management of all changes that may affect the decision to continue the project. Good decisions can be made only if the executives are kept well informed and properly advised. For example, a change in FDA point of view for a particular category of drugs or a change in the over-the-counter monograph may alter company plans for marketing a particular product. Other types of changes of which management should be made aware are a scientific breakthrough (change in the state of the art) or the marketing of a new product by a competitor.

Following each of the three phases of clinical studies, the data are reviewed and summarized by the Medical Department with the assistance of statisticians. The required departments present to the FDA the results of the work completed and the plans and protocols for that which is proposed. As the Phase III clinical studies come to a close and the toxicology studies are completed, the product specifications and analytical procedures are made ready for the NDA submission and transfer to Quality Assurance.

The data and information from all studies should be consolidated and a pre-NDA submission conference arranged with the FDA for the purpose of establishing the intent of the company and to be certain that the FDA requirements are fulfilled before making the final NDA submission. This will conclude the *concentrated* effort spent by R & D beginning with the synthesis of a chemical entity and ending with a NDA for a drug product. However, participation of R & D is far from finished. There is a need to continue stability studies, investigate new medical activities of the drug, conduct Phase IV clinical studies, assist Quality Assurance and production as required, develop new dosage forms to expand the product line, etc.

V. PLANNING FOR THE MARKET

Now the discussion turns to the activities of the Marketing/Sales Division following the project request. These activities will be reviewed and the overlap and interface with the R & D division examined. Emphasis is placed on planning the sequence of events and the paralleling of activities as shown in Figure 2. A quick review of information acquired and/or activities completed prior to writing the project request will be helpful before discussing product planning and development from a Marketing/Sales viewpoint:

1.   Market data/marketing research
2.   Consumer input
3.   Sales forecast
4.   Cost/profit profile
5.   R & D time/cost estimates for development
6.   Special production requirements
7.   Dosage forms desired for marketing

When the product is prepared for stability studies, all departments in Marketing/Sales should be in agreement on packaging. A desire by anyone to change the packaging following initiation of stability should be discussed with all involved departments. Changes can nullify all of the stability data that could be used to support the expiration dating. This increases the direct in-house cost, plus for every month of market time delayed due to insufficient stability data, the company loses approximately $1/12$ of a year's sales for that product, patent protection time, and perhaps, market time without competition.

A. SELECTING THE TRADE NAME

Initiate the selection of a trade name during the early stages of the project. It is a creative and time-consuming job that may span a large part of development time. A list of suggested trade names for a new product can be compiled in several ways. A specific department can make the list, select the name, and do the search, or it can be a contributory effort by everyone in the company with one department acting as the coordinating and responsible party. Special meetings can be held to discuss the pros and cons for various names. This may be a synergistic means of arriving at the best possible trade name. Another method is to retain an outside company to select the name of the product.

It is necessary to establish the trade name before the label/labeling can be written. Labels are written by a specific department with input from Regulatory Affairs, the Medical Department, and the Legal Department. The labeling (e.g., package insert) is written by the Medical Department with input from Regulatory Affairs if necessary. Both labels and labeling should be routed to the departments responsible for approval before final printing, e.g., Legal, Medical, Regulatory Affairs, Marketing, etc.

B. INITIATING THE MARKET PLAN

A preliminary market plan from the Marketing Department can be used for future planning by the production area, Purchasing department, Shipping department, Sales and Advertising departments, and for more accurate sales forecasting. The market plan should be updated and reissued as the market changes and in-house plans approach reality.

C. COORDINATING AND MANAGING THE FINAL DEVELOPMENT

The finished product specifications and test procedures are transferred from Analytical Services to Quality Assurance in conjunction with NDA approval prior to manufacturing the product. The two sections should work closely together in assuring that the product will meet the specifications and tests as established by Analytical Services and that Quality Assurance understands the procedures and can duplicate the methodology and results.

Have the quantitative formula for the product transferred to Production and be certain the Purchasing Department has all materials in-house before Production is ready to begin manufac-turing. To assure a smooth transfer of technology, product development personnel should work with the production personnel on pilot batches and the first two or three production runs.

When equipment and materials required for manufacturing and packaging are ordered, consideration should be given to the time remaining before the expected NDA approval and the time required for receipt of new equipment and materials. Never pre-empt by ordering equipment that is costly and may sit idle for months, or perhaps years. This requires input from Regulatory Affairs, Medical, Purchasing, Manufacturing, Marketing, Sales, and perhaps others.

The sales force will require product information. Request the detail brochure and physician information from the Medical Department. If a situation arises that will prevent the printing and distribution of this material at the proper time, then consider outside assistance from experts in the particular medical area. The detail information may be difficult to write depending on the depth of knowledge and level of education of the sales representatives reading it. In many companies, there are professional people in Marketing/Sales management positions who work with the sales force. Any guidance or assistance that can be offered to the medical writer by professional people (physicians, pharmacists, chemists, biologists, etc.) working with the sales force should be helpful and, if offered in the right spirit, appreciated.

VI. SUMMARY

Constantly monitor all activities to keep the project on schedule. Keep all lines of communication open between departments and divisions and be certain that the charts are followed and the schedule met. Be alert to potential problems and act as liaison and goodwill ambassador when necessary. During the period between the initiation of clinical studies and the NDA approval, the activities necessary to bring the product to the market-ready stage are completed.

When the final FDA approval letter for the NDA is received, everything should be "push-button" ready. If a good system for coordinating and monitoring the project has been developed and adhered to, then the company will successfully market a new product shortly after receipt of the approval letter, and everyone will bask in the glory.

Chapter 12

NOTICE OF CLAIMED INVESTIGATIONAL EXEMPTION FOR A NEW DRUG

Joyce Williams

TABLE OF CONTENTS

I. INTRODUCTION

Preparing to initiate clinical studies with a promising new drug is a significant stage in the drug development process. By now, there has already been a significant investment in identifying an active pharmacologic compound, developing a stable formulation, and conducting the basic pharmacological and toxicological tests. Safety in animal models has been established to a degree that the pharmaceutical firm feels that there are sufficient data to begin testing in humans.

At this point, an Investigational New Drug Application (IND), the first formal submission of data concerning this potential new therapy, must be filed with the Food and Drug Administration (FDA). This chapter will discuss the preparation and filing of this document and the required follow-up reporting during the clinical development phase.

The extent of information in an IND will depend upon the newness of the drug, whether or not it has been previously studied, possible risks to patients, and the developmental phase of the drug. The IND sponsor must consider all these parameters in determining the amount and type of information needed in the IND to permit the start of clinical trials.

Since this is an important step in the drug development process, considerable planning and preparation should preceed the filing of the IND to avoid any delay in advancing to the clinical testing phase. For the firm to submit a complete, well-planned IND, the Regulatory Affairs staff or regulatory consultant should be involved early in the development program so that all FDA requirements can be anticipated and prepared for in advance.

The IND is not approved by the FDA; rather the sponsor must wait 30 days following the filing of the application, and if not contacted by the FDA to the contrary, then the clinical studies may begin. At the end of this 30-day period, the IND is said to become effective. Instead, if during the initial 30-day period, the FDA has safety concerns regarding initiating the studies, it will issue a clinical hold. This is a notification that a clinical study may not be started or continued if already in progress. Trials in humans may not begin until the sponsor has resolved those safety concerns and the clinical hold has been lifted.

For Phase I studies, a clinical hold will be imposed only if there are concerns regarding the safety of the study subjects; however, in Phase II or III studies, the FDA may also place a clinical hold on a study that is so deficient in design that the study would not be able to establish safety and effectiveness. A clinical hold may be imposed by telephone, other means of rapid communication, or in writing and will identify the studies to which the hold applies and briefly state the reason for the hold. Within 30 days after the hold is instituted, the FDA will explain in writing, if not done so previously, the basis for the hold. If all studies remain on hold for more than 1 year, the FDA may place the IND on inactive status. If the FDA determines that an investigation presents an immediate and substantial danger to subjects, the FDA may immediately terminate the IND by written notice at any time.

II. EXEMPTION TO CONDUCT CLINICAL STUDIES

An IND is an application for an exemption from the premarketing approval requirements of Section 505 or 507 of the Federal Food, Drug and Cosmetic Act or the licensing provisions of the Public Health Service Act. The Food, Drug and Cosmetic Act requires that no new drug can be marketed until its safety and efficacy has been established. In order to obtain the data from clinical studies required to prove that these two standards have been met, the sponsoring firm must be given an exemption so that the investigational drug may be legally shipped in interstate commerce to the clinical investigators.

The IND provisions were originally legislated in 1962 under the Kefauver-Harris Amendments to the Food, Drug and Cosmetic Act and, for the first time, required proof of efficacy. Effective on June 17, 1987,[1] the FDA revised its regulations (21 CFR, Part 312) for the format of an IND. These new regulations are known as the "IND Rewrite" and sought to focus the earlier stages of the IND process on patient safety while allowing the sponsor more freedom to revise the design of studies at this stage. Only later, in the more advanced stages of the clinical research, would the FDA also be concerned that the clinical study design would lead to a demonstration of efficacy. This is the first time that the FDA has attempted to adopt different standards for the various stages of clinical research. These regulations also formally instituted a clinical hold procedure and defined when it can be imposed.

The IND Rewrite encourages consultations between industry and the FDA regarding the plan and design for clinical studies. These meetings are intended to facilitate designing the major clinical studies in such a way that they will support marketing approval if the test results are favorable. This change in emphasis is aimed at encouraging innovation while still assuring patient safety and, thus, hasten the overall drug development process and make it more efficient.

III. FORMAT AND PREPARATION

INDs should be formatted following the sections enumerated in Form FDA 1571. The FDA feels that this format will result in well-organized applications and facilitate FDA review. An original and two copies of the IND should be submitted. The FDA has issued several guidelines pertinent to the content and assembly of INDs and New Drug Applications (NDAs)[2] and they should be carefully followed regarding the format and assembly of the application. While several of the guidelines will be helpful in formatting some of the technical sections of the IND, they were developed primarily for preparing NDAs so the level of detail suggested by the guideline for an NDA may not always be available at this stage of the development. In fact, the IND Rewrite underlines the point that the type and amount of chemistry and toxicology data to be filed depends on the scope of the proposed clinical studies for the next year.

Planning for the documentation and submission of an IND should be started well in advance of the time planned for initiation of clinical studies. Responsibilities for each of the reports or sections comprising the IND should be identified early and the content of each section should be discussed in detail so that all departments agree on the data that will be needed. A schedule for completion of all reports and the preparation, review, and tentative filing date of the IND should be prepared. Once the key people are in agreement that there are sufficient data to support beginning clinical studies, preparation of the IND can begin.

Accuracy and completeness of all the information in an IND is important to avoid clinical holds or delays in FDA review. For this reason, attention should be given to checking and cross-checking all information. The document needs to be well organized and complete so that the FDA reviewers can understand the company rationale in establishing the safety of the drug.

It is helpful to include a cover letter with the IND. This letter should briefly describe the new drug, summarize the key information presented, and state the type of clinical study initially proposed.

A. FORM FDA 1571

Form FDA 1571 must be completed, signed, and included in the original IND and all amendments and reports. This form was extensively revised and reissued in 1987 in conjunction with the IND Rewrite. All appropriate sections of this form must be completed. By signing this form the sponsor agrees to wait 30 days, or longer if a clinical hold is imposed, before initiating clinical studies, that all studies will be reviewed and approved by a qualified Institutional Review Board (IRB), and that all other applicable regulations will be followed in the conduct of the clinical studies. If the sponsor does not reside in the U.S., the form must be countersigned by an attorney, agent, or other authorized official who resides in the U.S.

The current FDA 1571 also requires identification of the person who will monitor the clinical study, the person(s) responsible for review and evaluation of the information provided relevant to the safety of the drug, and, if any of the sponsor's obligations have been transferred to a contract research organization, identification of the organization and the obligations transferred. These provisions were added with the IND Rewrite.

B. TABLE OF CONTENTS

The table of contents should include the page and volume number for all major sections and subsections to the degree that it would be helpful to the FDA reviewer to locate information. In addition to the comprehensive table of contents, in lengthy applications it is also useful to include more detailed tables of contents in each individual section.

C. INTRODUCTORY STATEMENT

This is a brief statement including the name of the drug product and drug substance (active ingredient), the pharmacological class of the drug, the structural formula of the drug substance (if known), the formulation of the drug product (dosage form), the route of administration, and the objectives and duration of the clinical investigation.

If there is any previous human experience (worldwide) with the drug, it must be briefly summarized here. Specific information relative to the proposed clinical investigation should be described.

Likewise, if the drug has ever been withdrawn from testing or marketing in any country for safety or efficacy reasons, this must be explained. The country (or countries) where the drug was withdrawn must be listed as well as the reasons for withdrawal.

D. GENERAL INVESTIGATIONAL PLAN

In this section, the FDA is interested in having the sponsor briefly describe the clinical plan for this drug for the next year. The following information should be included:

1. Rationale for the drug or research study
2. Indication to be studied
3. The general approach to be used to evaluate the drug
4. The types of clinical trials to be conducted in the first year following submission of the IND
5. Estimated number of patients to be studied
6. Identification of serious or severe risks anticipated based on previous human or animal studies in this or related drugs

If the sponsor, at the time of submitting the IND, has not yet determined the full first-year clinical plan, that should be stated. In that case, only the protocol which has been defined need be described in this section.

This overview can usually be stated in two or three pages. Clinical plans beyond the first year should not be included. The sponsor may make changes in this investigational plan at any time without notifying the FDA.

E. INVESTIGATOR'S BROCHURE

All pertinent information known about the drug must be furnished by the sponsor to all clinical investigators in a document known as the investigator's brochure. As the investigations proceed, this brochure will be periodically updated to report new findings, particularly with respect to adverse effects. The investigator's brochure will eventually form the basis of the package insert for the product.

Initially, the investigator's brochure will contain the following information:

1. A brief description of the drug substance (active ingredient), including the structural formula and the formulation of the drug product (dosage form)
2. A summary of the pharmacological and toxicological effects in animals and, if any data exist, in humans
3. A summary of the pharmacokinetics and biological disposition of the drug in animals and in humans, if any data exist
4. A summary of safety and effectiveness information from prior clinical studies, if any
5. A description of possible risks and side effects based on prior experience with this or related drugs and a description of precautions or special monitoring

F. PROTOCOL

This section of the application includes the clinical protocol(s) and information concerning the clinical investigator, the clinical facilities, and the IRB. The initial submission of the IND only needs to include the protocol for the first study planned if others are not yet available.

The traditional phases of the clinical study program will be explained in greater detail later in other chapters, but a brief delineation of the phases here will be helpful in understanding FDA expectations and review of the protocols to be submitted. Phase I studies determine pharmacology, drug metabolism, and dose response with limited numbers of healthy subjects or patients with the target disease. Phase II studies are the first well-controlled trials to evaluate effectiveness and safety, particularly common short-term side effects and risks of the drug. Phase III studies are a further expansion of the controlled trials to investigate effectiveness, to establish the proper dosing regimen, and to provide additional safety data to establish the overall risk-benefit ratio.

Phase I protocols may be less detailed and more flexible than Phase II and III protocols. A Phase I protocol will provide an outline of the study including an estimate of the number of patients to be studied, a description of safety exclusions, and a description of the dosing plan including duration, dose, or method to be used in determining the dose. It should detail only those elements of the study that are critical to safety, such as monitoring vital signs and blood chemistries. Phase I design modifications not affecting critical safety assessments should be submitted in the annual report.

For phases II and III, detailed protocols are required describing all aspects of the study. If it is anticipated that a protocol change might be required, alternatives can be designed into the study initially, wherever possible.

A protocol should include the following elements:

1. A statement of the objectives and purpose of the study
2. The name and address and a statement of the qualifications of each investigator, the name

of each subinvestigator working under the supervision of the investigator, the name and address of the research facilities to be used, and the name and address of each IRB
3.   The criteria for patient selection and for exclusion of patients and an estimate of the number of patients to be studied
4.   A description of the study design including the control group, if any, and a description of methods to minimize bias on the part of subjects, investigators, and analysts
5.   The method for determining the dose to be administered, the planned maximum dosage, and the duration of individual patient exposure to the drug
6.   A description of the observations and measurements to be made
7.   A description of the clinical procedures, laboratory tests, or other measures to monitor the effects of the drug and to minimize risk

G. CHEMISTRY, MANUFACTURING, AND CONTROL DATA

At the stage at which an IND is first filed, the structure of the drug substance may not be completely defined or the formulation of the dosage form may still be subject to change. The FDA does not expect that the full extent of chemistry, manufacturing, and controls information required in an NDA will be available this early in the development process, but there must be sufficient information to define the entity to be studied and to assure that the dosage form will be stable for the duration of the clinical study. The amount of information needed will vary with the phase of the investigation, the proposed duration of the investigation, the dosage form, and the amount of other information available.

1. Drug Substance

To prepare this subsection, the FDA's "Guideline for Submitting Supporting Documentation in Drug Applications for the Manufacture of Drug Substances" should be consulted. Pages 49 to 55 of the guideline specifically pertain to chemical entities in INDs and further describe the differences in the information required for the different phases of the clinical investigation. If the drug substance is being purchased from another firm, the sponsor can reference the manufacturer's Drug Master File, particularly for the synthesis information required in this section.

a. Physical and Chemical Characteristics

For Phases I and II, the physical and chemical characteristics need to be described as appropriate to profile the drug substance. If it is an asymmetric molecule, the potential stereoisomers should be separated and characterized. Specifications and tests to control the ratios of any isomer admixtures must be established. It is important to know which of the stereoisomers have pharmacological or toxicological properties and which are being clinically tested.

b. Manufacture of the New Drug Substance

The name and address of the manufacturer of the drug substance must be given. The synthesis, isolation and/or extraction, and purification of the drug substance must be explained. This should include a flow chart of the procedure listing reagents and intermediates and should be accompanied by a written description of the procedure. If there are any patents or published articles which elucidate the preparation, copies should be included. After the initial filing of the IND, major changes in the pathway or scale of the synthesis will require an amendment or update in the next annual report.

As the IND studies progress to Phase III testing, the manufacturing procedure should approach the detail required in an NDA. If there have been significant changes in the synthesis, it should be clear which process was used in the manufacture of each lot of clinical material.

c. Analytical Methods

This subsection must include limits and methods to assure the identity, strength, quality, and purity of the drug substance. Analytical methods for the early phases of the clinical studies need to include at least one specific identity test, a test for at least one impurity, and an assay. Ideally, the impurity method should be a chromatography test. At this point it may be difficult to establish tight specification limits and it is accepted that these limits may be revised and refined as more information becomes known about the drug substance.

Elucidation of the reference standard should be documented as much as is possible at this time. Testing of the reference standard is expected to be more extensive than for the drug substance itself.

By the initiation of Phase III studies, the test methods and specifications should be more completely developed. All significant impurities must be isolated and identified by appropriate test methodology and specification limits set at the lowest achievable levels. Any additional information relating to stereoisomers and their possible effects should be provided. Studies of any solid-state forms should be completed and specifications developed. The relevance of the solid-state form to the bioavailability of the dosage form should have also been studied.

d. Stability

Information is needed to support the stability of the drug substance during the toxicological studies and the planned clinical trials.

2. Drug Product

As in the previous subsection, the FDA's "Guideline for Submitting Documentation for the Manufacture of and Controls for Drug Products" (pages 12 to 17 apply to investigational formulations), the "Guideline for Submitting Documentation for Packaging for Human Drugs and Biologics" (specifically page 17), and the "Guideline for Submitting Documentation for the Stability of Human Drugs and Biologics" (pages 38 to 40 cover INDs) should be utilized to develop this portion of the application.

After the initial submission, information amendments should be submitted when the formula or scale of production of the clinical material changes. Production scale-up changes are critical because they can affect key chemical or physical properties of the drug, including content uniformity, hardness, moisture content, or dissolution. Differences in these properties may lead to changes in drug bioavailability and thus be of clinical significance.

a. Components

All components of the dosage form should be listed, including processing materials, whether or not they appear in the finished product. Each component should be identified by its established name or chemical name along with a designation of its grade (e.g., American Chemical Society [ACS], U.S. Pharmacopoeia [USP]).

Alternative components may be provided for, but must be justified. Major changes in the formulation must be explained in an amendment to the IND.

b. Composition

This is a quantitative statement of the drug composition. Ranges for certain ingredients may be provided as necessary. A representative batch formula for the manufacture of the investigational drug needs to be provided and it must include all ingredients whether or not they appear in the finished dosage form. Formulation numbers should be used to identify each different formulation studied.

All presentations of the composition should be on the basis of 100% potency. Any excesses over the label declaration should be designated with the percent excess shown. Overages in the batch formula other than for manufacturing losses must be explained.

c. Specifications and Analytical Methods for Inactive Components

Specifications and test methods must be provided for all inactive components whether or not they appear in the finished product.

d. Manufacturer

The name and location of each facility involved in the manufacture or controls of the drug product must be listed. This includes any of the following which may apply:

1. Manufacturer of the drug product
2. Contract packager or labeler
3. Contract quality control laboratories
4. Suppliers of inactive components of the drug product

e. Methods of Manufacturing and Packaging

The production and packaging operations should be described in detail appropriate to the phase of testing.

In Phases I and II, the packaging should assure adequate protection of the drug, and stability studies with this packaging should be initiated. By the end of Phase III, the IND should contain complete information regarding the packaging of the drug including the proposed market package and the relevent stability and compatibility data.

To protect the subjects of clinical studies, investigational materials should be manufactured in conformance with current good manufacturing practices (GMPs). Adverse reactions, toxicity effects, or physiological activity of the drug may vary, resulting from potency variations or contaminants. Lack of product uniformity because of manufacturing variations could affect the clinical studies. For specific information on meeting GMP requirements for clinical trial supplies, the sponsor can refer to the FDA's "Draft Guideline on the Preparation of Investigational New Drug Products".

f. Specifications and Analytical Methods

Assurance of the identity, strength, quality, and purity of the drug product must be provided. At this point in the developmental process, the specifications and test methods will probably not be as well developed as they will be later, but, by the end of Phase III testing, they should be of the level of detail required in an NDA.

For Phases I and II, an assay method including adequate acceptance specifications for testing the new drug substance in the dosage form is needed. The assay should include a reference standard with data to support its integrity. Limits may be wider at this stage than they will be later. Unless the assay is also a specific identity test, a separate identity test must be submitted. For solid oral dosage forms, chemical and physical tests to characterize the dosage form should include uniformity of dosage unit and a dissolution profile in an appropriate medium. For injectable products, a sterility test, a measurement of particulates, and a pyrogenicity test should be part of this testing.

Information supporting the specificity, linearity, precision, and accuracy is needed for any specific quantitative methods.

By the time of Phase III testing, a full description of the identity tests, assay methods, and specifications must be available as well as any other tests necessary for the specific dosage form. For solid oral dosage forms, an *in vitro* dissolution rate test and specifications should be included. Information supporting the reference standard should be as complete as that required for the NDA.

g. Stability

For Phase I testing, stability information can be limited to that needed to demonstrate that the clinical product would be stable for the duration of the investigation. Stability studies on the investigational formulations should be well underway by the end of Phase II. Stability tests in these first two phases will evaluate the stability of the investigational formulations used in the clinical trials and to obtain additional information for development of a final formulation (e.g., compatibility studies that show interactions between the drug substance and other components).

The stability program for Phase III testing will test the formulation intended for commercial production in the market package, determine the expiration dating of the product, and study any degradation products. It is desirable to complete and file the data to support the proposed expiration dating period during the Phase III testing.

3. Placebo

This section applies if a placebo is proposed for the clinical testing and should include a brief general description of the composition, manufacture, and control of the placebo. Precautions taken to ensure the absence of the new drug substance from the placebo should be described. Similarities between the placebo and the active dosage form as far as physical characteristics and packaging should also be explained.

This information is needed to establish that the blinded nature of the clinical study will not be compromised by differences between the study drug and the placebo in such parameters as odor, taste, texture, or other physical characteristic.

4. Labeling

A copy of all labels and labeling to be given to the investigators must be provided. These may be provided in draft form. The immediate package label must bear the statement, "Caution: New Drug — Limited by Federal law to investigational use".

5. Environmental Assessment

Certain agency actions require consideration of the environmental implications of that action and they, thus, require that the sponsor prepare an environmental assessment. Submission and review of an IND is one of those actions. Therefore, the IND must include an environmental assessment under 21 CFR 25.31 which describes formats for preparing the environmental assessment or a claim for a categorical exclusion under 21 CFR 25.24.

H. PHARMACOLOGY AND TOXICOLOGY DATA

This section covers the information about the pharmacological and toxicological studies of the drug which form the basis upon which the sponsor has determined that it is reasonably safe to initiate the proposed clinical studies. The kind, duration, and scope of these tests will vary with the duration and nature of the proposed clinical investigations. This information must include the identification and qualifications of the individuals who evaluated the results of these studies and concluded that it is safe to begin the proposed investigations and a statement of where the investigations were conducted and where the records are available for inspection. As the sponsor proceeds through the clinical testing program, it is expected that information amendments will be submitted to the IND with additional pertinent safety information. The format of the individual reports and general organization should follow the FDA's "Guideline for the Format and Content of the Nonclinical Pharmacology/Toxicology Section of an Application". Submission of raw data in this section is not required, but the test results must be filed in sufficient detail to permit adequate scientific review by the FDA. In most cases, data tabulations will be adequate for review and should include all observations, pathology findings, and laboratory measurements that relate to an evaluation of the safety of the drug.

1. Pharmacology and Drug Disposition

The pharmacological effects and mechanism of action of the drug in animals, and information, if known, on the absorption, distribution, metabolism, and excretion of the drug should be reported. The order of presentation of these results should follow the guidelines.

2. Toxicology

This subsection should begin with an integrated summary of the toxicological effects of the drug in animals and *in vitro*. These studies will vary depending upon the nature of the drug and the phase of the investigation and may include some or all of the following: results of acute, subacute, and chronic toxicity tests, tests of the drug's effects on reproduction and the developing fetus, any special toxicity test related to the particular mode of administration of the drug or conditions of use (e.g., inhalation, dermal, or ocular toxicology), and any *in vitro* toxicity studies. For each key toxicology study that supports the safety of the proposed clinical investigation, a full tabulation of data must be provided.

Acute toxicity studies should include the following information:

1. Pretest conditioning and age of animals, dosing procedures, vehicles, and dosage volumes for each study
2. Types and severity of toxic signs and their onset and progression, or reversal in relationship to dosage and time after dosing for each species
3. Lethal-dose data tabulated for interstudy and/or interspecies comparison, including total numbers dosed and mortality incidence with time of death for each sex at each dose
4. Order of species and routes of administration as specified in the guidelines

Subchronic and chronic studies should be listed and briefly described in a table. Studies should be grouped by species, in order of increasing duration and/or route of administration in the order recommended in the guideline. Detailed study reports should be grouped by species as organized in the table. Important findings should be summarized with any relationships to dose and duration of treatment emphasized. Specific report formats are described in the guideline.

Any special toxicity studies for a particular formulation or route of administration should be tabulated for *in vivo* studies to show group comparison and time-related or progressive effects within each group and for *in vitro* studies to show the type of test, dose range in increasing order, and effects related to dose.

3. Good Laboratory Practices

Each study subject to the good laboratory practice regulations under 21 CFR 58 must include a statement that the study was conducted in compliance with those regulations, or, if not conducted in compliance, a brief statement of the reason for the noncompliance.

I. PREVIOUS HUMAN EXPERIENCE

Previous human experience with the drug, if any, known to the sponsor should be summarized. Detailed information relevant to the safety of the proposed investigation should be presented. If there were controlled trials, detailed information on those trials relevant to an assessment of drug effectiveness for the proposed investigation should be provided. Published articles should be attached if directly related to the proposed clinical trial or included in a bibliography if less directly relevant.

If the drug has been marketed in other countries, a list should be provided of the countries in which it is marketed and in which it has been withdrawn from marketing, if any, for safety or effectiveness reasons.

J. ADDITIONAL INFORMATION

In some applications certain other information may be needed. If the drug is a psychotropic compound or has abuse potential, clinical and animal studies on drug dependence and abuse potential will be required. For radioactive drugs, human or animal data to calculate the radiation-absorbed dose to the whole body and critical human organs is needed as part of Phase I.

IV. MEETINGS WITH THE FDA

To improve communications and resolve questions, the FDA encourages meetings with sponsors and recommends them at prescribed intervals for certain INDs.

End-of-Phase II meetings can be helpful in planning later studies. The purpose of this meeting is to determine the safety of proceeding to Phase III, to evaluate the Phase III protocols and the investigational plan, and to identify any other studies needed for marketing approval.

End-of-Phase II meetings are mainly intended for INDs of new molecular entities or major new uses of marketed drugs, but any IND sponsor may request such a meeting. At least 1 month in advance of the meeting, the sponsor should provide the FDA with background information on the Phase III plan, summaries of Phases I and II studies, plans for any additional nonclinical studies, and draft labeling, if available. Written minutes of the meeting will serve as a record of agreements between the sponsor and the FDA.

Also formalized in the regulations is the pre-NDA meeting, which will be addressed in a later chapter. In some cases, the drug developer may want to have a pre-IND meeting with the FDA if there are questions regarding design of appropriate preclinical or Phase I studies.

V. AMENDMENTS

With the IND Rewrite, amendments are divided into two types, protocol and information amendments. All significant changes to the IND must be filed as amendments.

A. PROTOCOL AMENDMENTS

Following submission of the original application, any additional protocols or modifications to a submitted protocol must be filed as protocol amendments. To implement changes to an existing protocol or to add a new protocol, it must be submitted to the FDA for its review and must be approved by a qualified IRB. Submission to the FDA and approval by the IRB may occur in any order.

For protocol changes in Phase I, only those which significantly affect the safety of subjects must be submitted. In Phases II or III, a change that significantly affects the safety of subjects, the scope of the investigation, or the scientific quality of the study must be submitted. Examples of the type of changes which must be submitted are

1. An increase in drug dosage or duration of exposure of subjects to the drug or a significant increase in the number of subjects
2. A significant change in the protocol design, e.g., addition or deletion of a control group
3. Addition of a new test or procedure to improve monitoring for, or reduce the risk of, adverse effects, or dropping a test which was monitoring safety

A protocol amendment is also needed to add a new investigator to a previously submitted protocol. For treatment protocols, new investigators are only required to be added in the annual report. Protocol amendments for new investigators must be filed within 30 days of adding the investigator, and they may be grouped together.

The protocol amendment must be prominently marked as a protocol amendment and the specific change noted, i.e., Protocol Amendment: New Investigator. The original IND submission is to be numbered "000" and all amendments and safety reports thereafter are serially numbered in chronological order.

For new protocols, the amendment must include a copy of the new protocol and a brief description of the most clinically significant differences between it and previous protocols. For protocol changes, a brief description of the change and a reference by date and amendment number to the original protocol should be given. Amendments for new investigators must contain the investigator's name, his qualifications to conduct the study, reference by date and amendment number to the protocol to which the investigator is being added, the names of any subinvestigators, the name and address of the research facility, and the name and address of the IRB. Protocol amendments to eliminate an immediate hazard to patients may be implemented immediately and the FDA informed later.

B. INFORMATION AMENDMENTS

Information amendments will be filed to add or change information in the IND that is not within the scope of a protocol amendment, a safety report, or an annual report. This information may include new toxicology, chemistry, or other technical information, or a report that a clinical study is being discontinued.

As with the protocol amendment, the information amendment must be prominently marked to identify its contents (e.g., Information Amendment: Chemistry, Manufacturing, and Controls) and serially numbered with the other amendments. Information to be included in the amendment is a statement of the nature and purpose of the amendment and an organized presentation of the data. Information amendments may also be grouped and submitted in 30-day intervals.

VI. SAFETY REPORTS

An IND sponsor is responsible for reviewing all relevant safety information from all sources worldwide of clinical studies, animal investigations, commercial marketing, scientific literature, and unpublished scientific reports. Two types of safety reports are required: written reports and telephone reports.

A written safety report must be sent to the FDA and all participating investigators of any adverse experience associated with the drug that is both serious and unexpected. An unexpected reaction is one that is not listed in the current investigator's brochure. The written safety report must be submitted within 10 days of initially receiving the information and should be prominently marked "IND Safety Report". Each report shall identify all previously filed reports involving a similar adverse experience and shall analyze the significance of this adverse effect in relation to the others. Written safety reports are to be numbered serially along with amendments.

Telephone reports to the FDA are required for any unexpected fatal or life-threatening experience associated with the use of the drug in clinical studies under the IND. These telephone reports must be made within 3 days of receiving the information. This is intended as an early warning system for the most serious adverse reactions and allows discussions between the FDA and the sponsor regarding whether or not any changes are needed in the study design.

VII. ANNUAL REPORTS

Within 60 days of the anniversary of the date that the IND became effective, the sponsor must annually submit a brief report of the progress of the investigation to cover the following information:

A. Individual study information comprising a brief summary of the status of each study in progress and each study completed during the previous year and including:

 1. The title of the study, its purpose, a brief statement identifying the patient population, and a statement as to whether or not the study is completed
 2. The total number of subjects initially planned for inclusion in the study, the number entered into the study to date, the number whose participation in the study was completed as planned, and the number who dropped out of the study for any reason
 3. If the study has been completed, or if interim results are known, a brief description of any available study results

B. Summary information obtained during clinical and nonclinical investigations of the previous year including:

1. A narrative or tabular summary showing the most frequent and most serious adverse experiences by body system
2. A summary of all IND safety reports submitted during the past year
3. A list of subjects who died during participation in the investigation with the cause of death for each subject
4. A list of subjects who dropped out during the course of the investigation in association with any adverse experience, whether or not thought to be drug related
5   A brief description of what, if anything, was obtained that is pertinent to an understanding of the actions of the drug, including such information as dose-response data, controlled trial information, and bioavailability data
6. A list of the preclinical studies completed or in progress during the past year and a summary of the major preclinical findings
7. A summary of any significant manufacturing or microbiological changes made during the past year

C. A description of the general investigational plan for the coming year to replace that submitted the previous year
D. If the investigator's brochure has been revised, an explanation of the revisions and a copy of the revised brochure
E. A description of any significant Phase I protocol modifications made during the previous year and not previously reported in a protocol amendment
F. A brief summary of any foreign marketing developments with the drug during the past year, such as approval or withdrawal of marketing in any country
G. If desired by the sponsor, a log of any outstanding business regarding the IND for which the sponsor requests a reply or meeting with the FDA

VIII. DRUG CLASSIFICATION SYSTEM

All new drugs filed with the FDA are given a classification that characterizes its chemical type and the expected therapeutic gain to be provided by that drug. Specific classifications are usually assigned during the IND stage and carry through the NDA review, although they may change during this time based on new information.

Chemical types receive a number classification:

- Type 1 — New molecular entity. The active moiety is not yet marketed in the U.S. either as a single entity or as part of a combination product.
- Type 2 — New salt. The active moiety is marketed in the U.S., but the particular salt or ester has not been marketed.
- Type 3 — New formulation. The compound is marketed in the U.S., but the particular dosage form or formulation is not.
- Type 4 — New combination. The drug product contains two or more compounds which have not previously been marketed together in the U.S.
- Type 5 — Already marketed drug product. The product duplicates a drug product already marketed in the U.S. by another firm.
- Type 6 — Already marketed drug product by the same firm. This designation is used primarily for new indications for marketed drugs.

Therapeutic potential types are classified by number:

- Type A — Important therapeutic gain. The drug would provide effective therapy or diagnosis for a disease not adequately treated or diagnosed by any marketed drug, or would provide improved treatment of a disease through improved effectiveness or safety.

- Type B — Modest therapeutic gain. The drug has a modest, but real, potential advantage over other available marketed drugs (such as greater patient convenience, elimination of an annoying adverse effect, the potential for a large cost reduction, a less frequent dosage schedule, or usefulness in a specific disease subpopulation).
- Type C — Little or no therapeutic gain. The drug duplicates in medical importance and therapeutic usage a drug already marketed.
- Type D — Special situation. The drug has decreased safety or effectiveness compared to a marketed drug, but has a compensating advantage (e.g., it treats patients who do not respond to the marketed drug).
- Type E — Drug Efficacy Study Implementation/Over the Counter (DESI/OTC) claim. The IND/NDA was filed to support a "less than effective" claim under DESI or OTC review.
- Type M — The drug is already marketed in a foreign country.
- Type P — The packaging or container is a very important feature.
- Type R — The drug is subject to specific unique conditions of approval listed in an approvable/approval letter for an NDA.
- Type S — The application is sensitive because of wide publicity, congressional interest, etc.
- Type T — There is an important problem in toxicity with the drug.
- Type U — The drug is likely to be used in children.

None of the chemical designations are mutually exclusive and, therefore, more than one can be assigned as appropriate. For the therapeutic potential designations, types A to E are mutually exclusive, but the remainder are not. Each drug will be assigned both a number and a letter designation.

These designations are utilized by the FDA to prioritize the handling and review of applications, with those containing new molecular entities and important therapeutic gains receiving higher priority than those drugs representing less therapeutic advantage. This is intended to help focus FDA activities to speed the review and approval of the more promising, breakthrough drugs. More recently, the FDA developed a special designation for drugs to treat acquired immune deficiency syndrome (AIDS). These drugs are now designated "1-AA", which is the top priority for review.

IX. TREATMENT IND

In an attempt to make certain experimental drugs for treating life-threatening diseases more broadly available prior to marketing approval, the FDA permits Treatment INDs to meet this need. This regulation (21 CFR 312.34) formalized a procedure that had already been allowed for many years in other INDs.

Criteria that must be met for a drug to qualify for a Treatment IND are

1. The drug is intended to treat a serious or immediately life-threatening disease.
2. There is no comparable or satisfactory alternative to treat that stage of the disease in the intended population.
3. The drug is under investigation in a controlled clinical trial under an IND in effect for the trial or all clinical trials have been completed and these trials have shown evidence of effectiveness.
4. The sponsor of the controlled clinical trial is actively pursuing marketing approval of the investigational drug with due diligence.

The sponsor and investigators must comply with all safeguards of the regular IND process, specifically including informed consent (21 CFR 50), which is not subject to FDA waiver and IRB review and approval (21 CFR 56) of all protocols.

The sponsor must still conform with all applicable portions of the IND regulations (21 CFR 312), especially including distribution of the drug through qualified experts (qualified licensed medical practitioners or treating physicians) who must comply with 21 CFR Parts 50, 56, and 312, maintenance of adequate manufacturing facilities with GMP compliance, and submission of IND safety reports. Unlike other INDs, the FDA will here more closely review the company's GMP records and may even request an inspection of the manufacturing facility.

These regulations also allow for charging the patients for the investigational drug. This provision should be helpful to smaller companies, many of whom are emerging biotechnology firms. Charging for the drug would only be granted upon a showing of why charging is needed for the sponsor to undertake or continue the clinical trial. There must be adequate enrollment in the ongoing clinical investigations under the authorized IND. The sale does not constitute commercial marketing of a new drug for which an NDA has not been approved and the drug must not be commercially promoted or advertised. The sponsor of the drug must also be actively pursuing marketing approval with due diligence. The sponsor may not charge a price greater than that necessary to recover cost of manufacture, research, development, and handling of the investigational drug.

A Treatment IND must meet all of the same requirements as a regular IND. If the sponsor wants to charge for the investigational drug, the sponsor must notify the FDA in writing prior to commencing charges. A sponsor of a clinical investigation who intends to sponsor a treatment use for the drug shall submit a treatment protocol containing the following elements:

1. The intended use of the drug
2. An explanation of the rationale for use of the drug
3. A brief description of the criteria for patient selection
4. The method of administration of the drug and a statement of the dosage
5. A description of the clinical procedures, laboratory tests, or other measures to monitor the effects of the drug and to minimize risk

X. EXPEDITED DEVELOPMENT OF DRUGS FOR LIFE-THREATENING ILLNESSES

To respond to concerns that there needed to be a faster approval process for drugs to treat desperately ill patients, particularly those with AIDS, the FDA issued special regulations[3] (21 CFR 312.80-312.88) in 1988 describing procedures for expediting the approval of these types of products. These regulations do not establish a new regulatory mechanism, but rather provide for the review and approval of a new drug at an earlier stage in the clinical testing program.

The major features of this expedited development program include:

1. Early consultation with the FDA both at the pre-IND stage and at the end of Phase I should result in agreement on a testing plan that can allow for the approval of a product after the completion of Phase II testing.
2. Utilization of Treatment INDs will permit wider use of the drug between the completion and analysis of Phase II testing and marketing approval.
3. Risk-benefit analysis will be utilized by the FDA to access the approvability of the marketing application based upon the seriousness of the disease being treated.
4. Phase IV studies will be employed to learn additional information about the risks, benefits, and optimal use of the drug. These will be postmarketing studies and might include investigation of different doses or patient populations.

5. Focused FDA regulatory research (e.g., development of manufacturing standards and assays for vaccine or biotechnology products) may be undertaken in certain circumstances.
6. Active monitoring of conduct and evaluation of clinical trials may be undertaken by the FDA to assure that the studies are proceeding on schedule.
7. Safeguards for patient safety inherent in other FDA regulations will all still apply for the testing of drugs being developed under this process.

A key to expediting the process is earlier and more frequent consultation with the FDA to reach early agreement on the design of studies needed for approval of the drug. This will be especially helpful during the preclinical and Phase I clinical studies.

XI. CONCLUSION

The IND Rewrite, Treatment INDs, and Expedited Development of Drugs for Life-Threatening Illnesses regulations all are attempts by the FDA to improve and accelerate the drug development process. A general consensus, spurred by the AIDS crisis, is forming to explore additional mechanisms to speed and improve this process, thereby shortening the time required to develop the preclinical and clinical data needed for new drug approval.

The IND or clinical investigation stage of the drug development process is a critical step in getting a new product to market, since, if the preclinical or clinical studies are not properly designed, marketing approval will never be granted. Likewise, it would also be a mistake to expend efforts on filing the original IND, but not continue to keep it updated with current information from the development process. The IND and its amendments and reports are an ongoing description of the progress during this phase of the experimentation.

REFERENCES

1. *Fed. Regist.,* Vol. 52, No. 53, March 19, 1987, 8798 — 8847.
2. Department of Health and Human Services, Food and Drug Administration, Center for Drug Evaluation and Research
    a. Guideline for the Format and Content of the Chemistry, Manufacturing, and Controls Section of an Application, February 1987.
    b. Guideline for Submitting Documentation for the Manufacture of and Controls for Drug Products, February 1987.
    c. Guideline for Submitting Documentation for the Stability of Human Drugs and Biologics, February 1987.
    d. Guideline for Submitting Documentation for Packaging for Human Drugs and Biologics, February 1987.
    e. Guideline for Submitting Supporting Documentation in Drug Applications for the Manufacture of Drug Substances, February 1987.
    f. Guideline for the Format and Content of the Nonclinical Pharmacology/Toxicology Section of an Application, February 1987.
    g. Draft guideline on the Preparation of Investigational New Drug Products, February 1988.
3. *Fed. Regist.,* Vol. 53, No. 204, October 21, 1988, 41516 — 41524.

Chapter 13

BIOPHARMACEUTIC AND PHARMACOKINETIC STUDIES

John H. Wood

TABLE OF CONTENTS

I. INTRODUCTION

Often the development of background biopharmaceutic and pharmacokinetic data for a new drug is looked upon as part of the necessary obstacles that must be overcome in the Notice of Claimed Investigational Exemption for a New Drug (IND) and later the New Drug Application (NDA) process. Rather, this process should be looked upon as an opportunity, if properly utilized, to develop a body of information that should support the ongoing clinical studies of the IND Phase III process. In addition, if unexpected results develop in population subsets during Phase III or in any post-NDA Phase IV or surveillance studies, properly executed IND studies may provide adequate information to contain the problem.

To this end, it is not intended in this chapter to provide any review of basic concepts in biopharmaceutics or pharmacokinetics. These are quite adequately covered in the existing literature, and any repetition would be redundant. Rather it is the object here to emphasize where required information may be best obtained during the investigation and how it may contribute to support a quality drug introduction.

Too frequently, pharmacokinetic investigation is delayed as long as possible in the clinical studies in order to minimize expenditures if the investigational drug study is prematurely terminated. When done, it is generally as a pure kinetic study rather than as an essential component in the development of the ongoing studies.

Even if only minimal animal drug disposition data are developed before the initiation of Phase I clinical studies, these data should develop rapidly during the clinical studies to serve as a guide for the human investigation of drug fate.

Often the acronym ADME is used to cover the range of what is needed both in animals and in man. The four letters of ADME are the first letters of absorption, distribution, metabolism, and excretion. Until recently, inability to perform suitable drug assays at the low concentrations frequently found for the therapeutic range, particularly for free unbound drug, served as a legitimate excuse to preclude the development of adequate data on many new drugs. Too often, because of expiring patents, there is little incentive to adequately restudy the older drugs. Today, as these drugs go generic, no company has a financial incentive to conduct other than required bioavailability studies.

Indeed, the bioavailability data filed with the FDA under requirements of Abbreviated New Drug Applications (ANDAs) and NDAs must constitute a virtual gold mine of clinically relevant, but legally inaccessible data permitting further evaluation of these drugs. More important, implicit within all these data, even for recent NDA filings, is a measure of the inherent intersubject and even possibly intrasubject variability. This type of information is rarely available in the open published literature, and certainly is virtually never developed for the published literature in a manner useful or applicable to clinicians who are not familiar with the statistical nuances of the presented data.

Today, as pharmacokinetics is being utilized to an increasing degree in the clinical setting, we will have a greater demand for such information in a form readily suited to clinical application. If, for a given drug, the population forms a tight statistical distribution of values for all parameters of the ADME blanket, this drug may be rigidly described in its desired dosing range and expected results, and is not likely to require therapeutic drug level monitoring unless the therapeutic to toxicologic index is extremely close. However, a drug with an extremely wide range of parameters across the population is likely to cause reporting of frequent adverse reactions as well as therapeutic failures. Indeed, if the prevalence is too high, a drug recall might be the extreme solution. It is for this reason that this author believes that it is in the best interests of the manufacturer to fully develop the ADME blanket beyond the minimal requirements for the acceptance of an NDA in order to minimize clinical misadventures with the general utilization of the drug. Today a caveat requiring therapeutic monitoring of plasma levels of a new drug, in spite of marketing objections, is likely to be welcomed by the newer breed of physicians and clinical pharmacists. Much more important, however, is the fact that adverse publicity is much less likely to ever develop, reflecting back as equating with a good drug and a quality company.

II. ANIMAL STUDIES

A. PRECLINICAL
1. Choice of Test Animal Species and Mode of Administration
a. General

Initially, animal studies are intended only to provide the necessary pharmacological and toxicological observations to determine that the entity being investigated is indeed a potential drug of exploitable value. Once that decision has been made, animal disposition studies need to be initiated. These will develop as the study of the chemical continues, until a complete profile is developed. However, a minimal knowledge is essential before use in man can be justified.

Classically, pharmacological testing in conscious animals is restricted to three modes of administration: oral, i.p., and i.v. Rarely is the i.m. or the s.c. route utilized except for specific applications, while the percutaneous is applicable only for dermal preparations and for dermal toxicology.

However, for use in man the oral route dominates, except for a few special situations for which the i.v. route is required. The i.p. route is of no general significance. Similarly, the i.m. route is normally of clinical importance only when solubility prevents an i.v. dose, when more pain results from i.v. than i.m. injection, when delayed release is desired, or when medical convenience indicates it for rapid absorption. The dermal routes, percutaneous or s.c., represent special situations which do not fit the general study mode. They, along with ocular administration and various types of suppositories and inserts, require specialized treatments.

The general state of knowledge of drug metabolism development today permits reasonable guesses to be made of possible or probable metabolic pathways for clearance of a drug after administration. If it is concluded that the drug is unlikely to have appreciable clearance without prior metabolism, extensive analytical method development will eventually be required. If the drug is already sufficiently polar that appreciable renal excretion of unchanged drug is probable, then initial analytical requirements for study are simplified.

b. Bioavailability Requirements for Any ADME Study

Too often in initial ADME studies, minimal concern is placed on the potential completeness of absorption, in contrast to final recovery in the excretion. However, if absorption is not complete, conclusions from animal studies for extrapolation to man are suspect. Obviously, the i.v. route, if possible, is the ideal goal as a reference standard against which to initially judge all other routes. If essentially no fecal drug loss occurs in this route, but fecal loss does occur with oral administration, this fecal loss is a measure of absorption failure. If the molecular weight and geometry of the drug is such that biliary excretion will be significant, evaluation of oral dosage may become difficult.

The use of small animals generally necessitates some form of lavage administration for oral dosing. If suspending agents are used to provide a suitable drug suspension, these agents may have coated some drug particles with a virtually insoluble layer, thus minimizing timely release of drug. Moreover, the additional fluid volume utilized may provide too rapid a gastric transit to assure a reasonable opportunity for absorption. Hence, unless the drug is soluble at the desired concentration levels for study, data from smaller animals may be somewhat suspect.

Within classic pharmacology, the big animal has tended to mean the dog. The dog will generally accept oral dosage forms equivalent in shape and size to those intended for humans. Hence the oral dosage can be backed by laboratory *in vitro* data implying probability of *in vivo* availability. Also the size of the dog permits reasonable blood sampling for initial pharmacokinetics. If necessary, a urinary catheter may be inserted with minimal difficulty into the bladder so as to assure a clean, separate catch of urine and of feces. Because of alleged similarities to human metabolism, the minipig is becoming more common. However, this cannot be considered an animal of convenience.

Any analytical work-up of samples is a significant financial cost that makes it desirable for the study to be as valid as practical. The quality of the test materials at any stage should be unambiguous. Input from formulations specialists as consultants should be sought at this stage to assure later credibility.

c. Use of Radioactive Drug

In general, any initial distribution or metabolism studies in animals will be greatly facilitated by the availability of drug appropriately labeled with one or more radioactive elements. In the preparation of such labeled compounds, it is desirable that the label be in a portion of the molecule not subject to loss by any probable metabolic detoxication mechanisms. In those cases in which the drug fragments into two major entities, it may become necessary to trace both portions by having a label in each. It should be emphasized that the chemical purity of the labeled compound is essential. Initial use of the label is to permit the isolation of fractions containing one or more metabolites. Any label fractions characteristic of metabolism of labeled drug impurities, but not of the drug itself, lead only to an excessive and expensive burden on the chemists involved in the metabolite elucidation.

The actual specific activity of the administered labeled drug (that is a measure of the relative number of radioactive atoms in the total drug used) may depend on limitations from the synthetic steps used as well as the amount of cold carrier drug required.

Generally, with radioactive drug it is not expedient to do any dose-dependency studies. Instead, a rather high, but clearly sublethal drug dosage is administered. In this way sufficient drug becomes available, wherever label is found, to provide material for chemical identification.

Obvious initial observations include time course blood samples to the extent permitted by the physical size of the test animal, as well as total urine and fecal accumulation by time intervals. These should be as frequent as practical. If time studies are performed with both blood and excretia, a preliminary kinetic evaluation of half-life and volume of distribution is possible. Considering the cost involved in synthesizing a labeled drug and maintaining animal facilities in compliance with good laboratory practice, the additional cost of timed samples and their counting for preliminary kinetics are virtually nil.

When total excretion radioactivity does not balance the activity given the animal, rigorous autopsy studies are essential to determine the organs or sites of drug retention. It is then incumbent on the investigators to further evaluate the rate of elimination or clearance of this retained activity both by longer-term urine and fecal collection, and by periodic sacrifice of animals to directly evaluate disappearance from the site(s) of retention.

Separately, it is desirable to sacrifice a few animals during the period of distribution and clearance in order to determine whether or not any transitory sites of drug accumulation exist. This should be done even though the drug is determined to be readily cleared completely.

Until the chemical isolation and identification of all radioactive excretion fractions using the best of chromatographic separation techniques, we cannot begin to develop the appropriate analytical techniques to quantitate the drug and its metabolites separately in body tissues and fluids. Thus the kinetic observations made by total radioactivity alone may always represent additional components beyond the parent drug and therefore provide guidance only.

d. Metabolic Fate of the Drug

Although logical and expected metabolic clearance mechanisms may be predicted on structural considerations, the elucidation of the metabolic pathways must first be achieved by appropriate chemical identification studies. Next, quantitative analytical methods for unambiguous determination of parent unchanged drug and major metabolites in primary body fluids must be developed. Frequently, this quantitative aspect is delayed until Phase III clinical studies are initiated. This may be viewed as cost effective if Phase II and initial Phase III studies are less than optimal. However, availability of analytical methodology may indicate lack of human absorption or unanticipated metabolism to have produced the chemical failure. Thus, if the parent compound was, in fact, a prodrug metabolized to an active drug, it is conceivable that man might not make that metabolite in adequate amounts.

Recognition of the metabolite identity and a determination of its activity might lead in such a situation to a successful drug instead of to another clinical failure. Obviously, the economic aspects of "what if" are difficult or impossible to evaluate to justify fuller initial work-ups. With new, unique compounds, this potential to overlook the real drug could be greater than in more traditionally structured molecules.

Even though quantitative analytical methods may not be immediately available, the radioactive drug administration and metabolite identification does permit a determination of the primary modes of drug clearance and of fraction by each route. Generally, basic metabolic fate in rats and in dogs is desirable before any human studies are initiated. The addition of information from either rabbits or guinea pigs is not likely to be of great additional value.

If the initial human studies contemplate the use of radioactive drug because the analytical methodology does not exist, it is of particular importance to assure from the animal studies that no accumulation in humans is likely to occur, and that the metabolic pathways utilized by the animal models are likely to be adequate in humans.

Thus, although examples may be well known in which animal metabolic fate was not adequately determined prior to human test use, these clearly should be justifiable exceptions rather than the rule. Any delay means that any form of success in Phase II and Phase III studies could mean an urgent need for catch-up in animal and human metabolism and subsequent kinetic studies.

e. Metabolism and Route of Administration

Just as it is impossible, *a priori*, to state that a specific animal species will provide the most satisfactory data for comparison with man, conflicting information is accumulating as to the route of administration and its effect on drug metabolism. It is clearly evident that in man, so-called "first pass" effects during absorption may occur either in the gastrointestinal lumen and in the mesenteric system walls or in the hepatic enzyme mass. Very limited data exist to relate any first pass effects in animals to those in man. Indeed, very few data are available to distinguish first pass effects in animals from general excretion metabolism from steady-state load.

It is unfortunate that virtually no general studies have been undertaken in animals to determine the extent to which the animal systems may even be used to supplement human studies. By analogy to the human, the use of i.p. administration in animals is looked upon with suspicion as a mode of administration for metabolism and kinetic studies. Presumably the fluid return is by a mixture of plasma capillaries and lymph recovery. It would seem reasonable that general absorption metabolism might be expected to be intermediate between that obtained by the classic oral and i.v. routes. Hence, it should still be looked upon as an acceptable mode provided the bioavailability is adequate.

Indeed, the growing use of support procedures for the renally impaired such as continuous ambulatory peritoneal dialysis as an alternative to the kidney dialysis machines will make it imperative for more detailed studies of drug absorption and of clearance by the peritoneal route. Presently, most peritoneal absorption studies relate to antibiotics used when infections occur. Absorption of highly polar molecules does seem to be reasonably rapid. If i.p. administration can be determined to reduce first pass metabolic destruction of a drug, it may be that such patients could appreciably reduce essential drug intake by adding these drugs to the residual fluid left in the cavity after dialysis.

f. Pharmacokinetics

Even though analytical procedures suitable to quantitate metabolite levels with time may not be available when human work is initiated, in general, some analytic determination of apparent free drug levels with time should generally have been obtained in animals. The term "apparent free drug" is used in recognition that initially the determination may not be specific to the drug alone, but may analyze one or more metabolites as contributing to the apparent drug content.

This same analytical procedure should be adequate to determine at least qualitatively whether the drug is highly bound to human serum proteins or to the red cells by *in vitro* addition studies.

B. STUDIES CONCURRENT WITH THE CLINICAL TRIALS
1. Metabolism
a. Short-Term Studies

As the clinical studies proceed, it becomes increasingly important that any ambiguities or uncertainties existing from the preclinical studies be rapidly resolved. In particular, the analytical methodology for unchanged drug and any circulating metabolites should become available. The methodology and its sensitivity should be adequate to clearly determine the metabolic rates in the animal species chosen for test.

Concurrently, human data should be developing in parallel. It becomes desirable to identify one or more animal species in which the metabolic fate is similar to that in man. Too often, unfortunately, this is a goal which is not attainable. In that case it is acceptable to utilize two species that between them do display all the pathways utilized by man, but do not exhibit additional metabolites not found in man.

There is an important restriction regarding this last limitation that is essential to consider. If this additional pathway is one that is suspected in other drugs to be involved in the development of adverse effects, particularly damage to tissues or organs, that animal model might reveal a mechanism for a low-incidence adverse reaction in man. This is particularly relevant for subjects who are clinically overdosed or who may have abnormal metabolic patterns (to be discussed later). However, adverse animal responses later attributed to a metabolic path not found significant in man may result in the discontinuing of the development of a drug of value.

With a choice of the more suitable animal species, linear dose-response effects in metabolic patterns should be carefully examined (see also the later section on kinetics). Any shift in the relative ratios of the metabolites as a function of dose is a clear indication of dose-dependent kinetics. In some situations the metabolite ratio shift may be a more sensitive and positive criterion of this than direct kinetic studies. If two metabolites are independently being formed from the parent drug, then the relative amounts of each metabolite should be in the ratio of their first order rate constants of formation. Thus, if drug D is forming two metabolites A and B, then

$$\frac{dA}{dt} = k_A D \tag{1}$$

and also

$$\frac{dB}{dt} = k_B D \tag{2}$$

where k_A and k_B are the metabolic formation, first-order rate constants. Then it will follow that for complete collection

$$\frac{A}{B} = \frac{k_A}{k_B} \tag{3}$$

Because of the sampling times chosen or required, the evaluation of the rate constants may have more experimental error than the direct determination of total metabolites.

This approach is equally valuable for recognizing possible saturable symptoms of renal clearance, either active or passive excretion or resorption. The greatest sensitivity results if comparisons are also made for reasonable time intervals rather than just for totals. Then the actual transitory effect of load is enhanced. For this reason, steady-state-type observations, using 24-h collections in the multiple dosing mode, have obvious advantages.

Ideally, the same animals will be used for the steadily increasing dose in order to permit each animal to be evaluated separately for dose dependency rather than pooling observations across many different animals. Generally, much more work will be required if many different animals are used and the results averaged. Too often a massive array of data is assumed to be superior and preferable to careful, detailed studies of a limited number of test animals or humans. Quantity should never substitute for quality in experimental design.

Continuously increasing dosage studies may be confounded by enzyme inductive actions. This must be clearly determined in the long-term tests.

b. Long-Term Tests

Normally, the long-term animal studies are identified as being associated with long-term chronic toxicity studies. These studies can and should also serve as a vehicle to provide data in metabolic and kinetic studies.

Thus, if metabolite ratios are established at the initiation of the chronic study by the use of total 24-h urine and feces collection and are repeated periodically, these can clearly establish whether or not autoinduction of enzyme function does occur, and if so, in what time frame. The results of such an observation are clearly of clinical relevance, either as a warning or as a reassurance.

Of even more importance for the long-term clinical safety of the drug would be any indication that formation of any metabolite was being impaired. The toxicological implications of such an observation should be examined at that time even though no other animal tests might warrant such a study.

After a suitable period of chronic use, administration of a few doses of radiolabeled drug in a limited number of animals is desirable, even though the thought of such an approach might horrify the toxicologist. The purpose is to determine whether or not chronic usage may have stimulated metabolic clearance modes not observed in the initial metabolic work-up.

2. Pharmacokinetics
a. When Needed

Once clinical studies have been initiated in man, it is difficult to rationalize extensive further single-dose pharmacokinetics in animals, except for studies not ethically permissible or desirable in man.

In that regard the animal model permits forcing saturation of clearance, resorption, and metabolic systems. Unfortunately, we do not have a ready means of projecting whole-body animal Michaelis-Menten kinetic parameters to equivalent ones in man. However, high steady-state levels, for which nonlinear kinetics are evident, permit the evaluation of whether or not concomitant administration of other drugs will change clearance kinetics. A systematic study of probable concurrent medications in this manner is more desirable than the observation of an interaction in a patient as a result of an unanticipated difficulty. This type of anticipatory screening examination is unfortunately not as common as it should be today. Screening in such studies would include pharmacokinetic changes resulting from binding displacement with highly bound drugs as well as for classic competitive metabolism.

Once the general metabolic fate and binding characteristics of a new drug have been determined, a checklist of probable drug interaction candidates can be easily developed. It is not, and never should be, necessary or desirable that such a list be exhaustive. Rather, here we should develop information for prototypes. Following that, reasonable persons should be able to recognize when unlisted alternatives can be expected to exhibit similar behavior, and hence the possibility of occurrence in the patient should be anticipated.

Another aspect of the high-dose studies, paralleling the metabolism studies discussed earlier, is whether or not, in the test species being studied for chronic toxicity, any dose-dependent kinetics are observable and whether or not these observations are paralleled in man. It is particularly important to determine what kinetic pattern exists at toxic levels. If the kinetics are not significantly shifted at high to toxic doses and the half-life is reasonable, overdosed patients would be best given supportive therapy only, rather than attempting dialysis, etc., for removal of drug already absorbed. Information regarding management of overdoses is not generally developed in IND investigation unless an accident occurs. There is no reason for the animal pharmacokinetic studies not to address this point to the extent possible so that supportive information is available in an emergency.

b. Chronic Administration Studies

As we discussed under the metabolism heading, the test animals maintained for chronic toxicity studies should be utilized to assure whether or not enzyme induction or some form of inhibition may not occur with time. Even rats may yield several small blood samples at intervals without jeopardizing their health or status as long-term test animals. Two samples could reflect maximum and minimum levels during dosing intervals. This might be done initially at 10-d intervals with the intervals increasing with the total elapsed time. Larger animals, such as the dog, permit additional samples so as to evaluate the area under the curve (AUC) between doses and the beta (β) decay elimination pattern. The constancy of the pattern of change resulting from such observations could be as an important element in the chronic toxicity study as many of the currently relevant parameters.

III. HUMAN STUDIES

A. PHASE I INVESTIGATION
1. Purpose

Phase I studies represent the first use of the drug in man. Except for certain special situations such as for many cancer and AIDS drugs where no truly safe dose can be anticipated, these studies are performed in normal healthy voluntccrs. The purpose is to establish a dose-response tolerance relationship, limited by the onset of unacceptable adverse effects. Two modes of dosing are general. The first is an increasing single dose either daily or every alternate day. The other involves multiple dosing at each level prior to increase. Presently, the choice of mode, initial dose level, and interval for increase are considered to be primarily clinical decisions based upon prior animal toxicology. Obviously, if no prior pharmacokinetics is performed, there can be no projection from the animal as to how this might best guide in this initial human screen.

Once this tolerance and safety screen is complete, the studies advance into efficacy and tolerance in patients. The only other times in which normals will be again used is in formalized kinetics and bioavailability investigations (to be discussed under a later subheading). However, legally, all studies performed in normal subjects are properly Phase I studies even if conducted late in the IND process.

2. Other Derivable Information

However the initial Phase I study is conducted, it provides a source of the critical data difficult to ethically develop at a later date. It is probable that never again will dosage levels ever be deliberately pushed to as high a level in normals as at this point. Later studies for bioavailability assessment and pure pharmacokinetics should terminate before reaching levels capable of inducing any major adverse observations.

It is therefore essential that meaningful blood and urine samples be collected during this study even if appropriate analytical methodology for their evaluation is not yet available. These samples, in most cases, can be adequately preserved frozen. The number and size of blood samples obviously must be balanced by the other demands for blood dictated by the toxicological safety screening during the course of the Phase I study. Ideally, this study is performed in a minimal lapsed time frame of a few weeks so that the sample size and frequency becomes significant. However, there is no practical limitation on urine collection. Indeed, because these studies should be conducted under tight control, complete monitoring and collection of urine and of feces is readily obtained.

Optimally, samples should be obtained at least at the assumed peak time of blood concentration and at suitable intervals during the decline phase. These timings should not interfere with the time course of the Phase I study proper, but should require all dosing to be rigidly conforming to reproducible pharmacokinetic intervals for all subjects in test. Urine collections should be subdivided into practical time intervals, suitable for pharmacokinetic evaluation. Aliquots and composites should be carefully prepared by volume. Too often it is assumed that if a 24-h urine collection is needed for a specific clinical test, appropriate aliquots and composites for kinetic evaluation cannot be obtained. Too many research and clinical studies are faulted by this absurd concept. There is no test used today that requires that the total urine collection be available; only a representative aliquot sufficient for the analytical needs is required.

Even in outpatient studies all urine samples should be collected separately. Preferably, these are immediately measured for volume, and a suitably sized aliquot retained. Time of urination, volume, and aliquot serial number designation are recorded on a patient diary page. If measurement is not practical the whole sample is retained in a urine bag and frozen. A technician then subsequently thaws the sample, thoroughly homogenizes it, measures it, and retains the aliquot. Suitably sized composites are prepared later by the laboratory personnel using variable-volume pipettes. Ideally, simple decimal multiples are used. Thus a 325-ml original sample might contribute 325 µl or 3.25 ml to a composite as would be judged desirable for the total volume required. In this way suitable 12-, 24-, or 48-h composites can be prepared and still permit retaining each individual sample, if needed, for pharmacokinetic work-up.

Obviously, very large aliquots may need to be retained for composites suitable for metabolite identification studies. However, it is unlikely that if the majority of the urine is retained for metabolite composites, all other composites and aliquots for safety tests and for pharmacokinetics can affect the recovery studies in any way. It is essential that, for economy of effort, these initial studies be used for evaluation of the metabolism in man in order to permit initiation of meaningful chronic animal studies as early as possible if continued study and development of the drug is elected.

At least as important as the wide dose range pharmacokinetic information available in this way is the separate utilization of the information to determine whether the blood level response to dose is relatively uniform or highly variable between test subjects, and thus whether the onset of adverse reactions is more related to blood levels attained or to dosage when these two factors are not tightly associated. Similarly, we obtain immediately a measure of the homogeneity of the test population as to clearance parameters. Admittedly, there is a limit as to the statistical chances for recognition of aberrant values in a very limited size of population, but certainly if there are population differences that are common, these will be seen.

Of increasing importance today is the recognition that varying types of nonlinear dose response are possible, both as they relate to apparent effective absorption with plateauing of resultant plasma levels and in saturation of excretory processes with dramatic increasing of plateau levels. The ascending-dose studies of Phase I and later of Phase II should determine this and the degree to which it may be clinically significant. It is inexcusable that such an observation wait until late in the Phase III clinical trials, or worse until general marketing use of the drug occurs.

3. Later Studies for Pharmacokinetics
a. Radiolabeled Drug

Even if unambiguous analytical methods for drug and the metabolites found in animals are available before initiation of clinical studies, sampling from the ascending-dose study may not permit a complete material balance. For a single-dose administration, it is desirable that this be assured as early as possible in a separate study using a couple of subjects. The use of a radiolabeled dose for this purpose can be very valuable, especially if the analytical techniques do not permit complete quantitation for the whole dose even in animals. In this way it is possible to be assured that no new metabolic pathway occurs in man that had not previously been recognized in the animal models.

If reasonable progress has not yet been made in the analytical development, then the use of radioactive material is essential in order to provide clearance estimates for man, and also information for the fuller animal studies.

It should be recognized, however, that use of radiolabeled drug in man must be clearly justified if there is any tendency in animals for long-term drug accumulation. In particular, potential sites or organs of concentration should be carefully reviewed by the health physicist in the light of the available animal information regarding levels and their duration.

Occasionally, attempts are made to assess dosage bioavailability utilizing incorporated radioactivity. Such trials should be examined with skepticism, since frequently the dosage unit used is analogous to, but not exactly identical with a normal dosage.

b. Bioavailability Studies

Initial bioavailability assurance for Phase I and Phase II studies can be best assumed if the solubility of the drug permits its administration by solution. If solubility does not permit this, then a fine suspension is normally the next most desirable dosage for test and later reference for more commercially normal forms.

It must be recognized that as the clinical studies proceed, investigation of alternate salts, possibly different esters, etc., may appear desirable. These cannot be substituted into clinical studies without *in vivo* characterization by a Phase I investigation to document their equivalence, greater reproducibility, etc. depending on the reason for their choice. A series of clinical studies, each using different types of dosages, can create confusion and apprehension among those reviewing the studies. For this reason it is urgent to optimize the dosage form as early as possible in the clinical studies. This again emphasizes the need to develop all the supporting analytical methodology as soon as practical during the study of the drug chemical. In this regard it should be noted that the use of the ultimate reference standard, the investigative i.v. dose, requires a greater level of animal safety data acceptable to the FDA than does the investigative oral administration.

From time to time the question is raised as to why a new drug oral dosage form must have optimal bioavailability rather than merely controlled uniformity of release level. There are two principle reasons for this. Most important, a lack of full reproducible bioavailability parallels increasing potential for subject variability, and hence less reproducibility in response. Also there is a problem with which the drug innovator may not identify. As generic drugs develop, severe problems occur when the generics show appreciably better bioavailability than the innovator upon which the clinical experience was based. Generally, then, a solution is not interchangeable with a tablet, and problems in special situations occur if a patient temporarily cannot swallow tablets. For these reasons the optimal dosage form is required by the FDA, and its quality should be based upon an unambiguous reference standard such as oral solution or i.v. dose whenever possible.

Formal documenting of the bioavailability of the test dosage form against the reference should be conducted with a standard bioavailability protocol. This requires adequate panel size to assure the appropriate level of statistical confidence, and the use of a crossover design. It is important when extensive Phase III clinical studies have been completed, or even just initiated, that any change in dosage form be fully documented for equivalence or superiority in order not to raise questions later as to the validity of these results for clinical dose response.

There can be perturbing factors to the use of a solution as a bioavailability standard. There have been several studies in the literature which could be interpreted to imply that a drug administered in a small volume of fluid may have a greater bioavailability than if a larger volume was used. This is in spite of the common acceptance of drug absorption occurring along most of the gastrointestinal tract. Hence it is possible that, for some drugs at least, higher fluid volume washes drug past the more active absorption areas. Data exist to indicate this is certainly possible for digoxin, digitoxin, and tetracycline. However, only differences of less than 15% occur in such cases.

Of extreme importance in bioavailability assessment of dosage forms is the pattern first pass effects may produce. The amount of free, unchanged drug reaching the general circulation will depend upon the absorption flux. In general, slower absorption will yield more first pass metabolism and less bioavailability, while increasing dosage size tends to increase the percentage of unchanged drug reaching the circulation. Also, bioavailability tends to increase for first pass drugs when they are taken with food. For such drugs absorption may be complete as determined by total urine output even though effective bioavailability is very clearly related to dosage absorption parameters. Because the degree of first pass metabolism tends to be less reproducible for test subjects, a higher variability is to be expected for these drugs in contrast to the observations for those that are essentially completely absorbed unchanged.

The actual evaluation of bioavailability or of bioequivalence can be properly performed only in conjunction with the simultaneous evaluation of pharmacokinetic parameters which will be discussed in the next section. However it should be emphasized that the bioavailability, F, of a dosage relative to that of a reference is given by

$$F = \frac{(AUC)_{Test}}{(AUC)_{Reference}} \tag{4}$$

where AUC is the total area under the plasma unchanged drug concentration time curve for a single dose for the test and reference dosage forms as indicated.

In addition, for dosing to a steady-state plasma concentration, it is required in linear pharmacokinetics that the total AUC for a single dose must equal the AUC between doses. If, however, there is found to be nonlinear kinetics, the bioavailability assessment becomes more difficult mathematically. Reference to standard texts will provide the necessary mathematical treatment.

Bioequivalence requires, in addition to equivalent values of AUC, that the time profile of concentration be identical within the appropriate statistical confidence bounds.

Thus, although separate in title, bioavailability and elementary kinetics can be mutually dependent parameters.

c. Kinetic Studies

As indicated earlier, the use of radioisotopes without chemical resolution to measure the decrease of drug in general circulation may lead to erroneous conclusions if appreciable circulating levels of drug metabolites are present, because these are assumed to be drug. Thus, in the extreme, all unchanged drug may have disappeared from general circulation, but appreciable metabolite may still be present. Therefore, the half-life observed from the blood level radioactive decay curve will be the maximum possible for the drug, but in reality could be appreciably shorter.

It is for this reason that definitive assays are needed as early as possible. It may be if the drug half-life was short, but that of one metabolite prolonged, that multiple dosing to obtain a satisfactory blood level of drug could provide excessive metabolite buildup. It is not sufficient merely to assay for original drug in the plasma.

From oral dosages it is generally difficult to evaluate distributive rate constants unless distribution is very slow. However, from the plasma concentrations Cp resulting from the single-dose oral administration the following parameters can be directly determined: Time, t_{max}, for maximum concentration, C_{max}, to occur; elimination half-life $t_{1/2}$; and area under the curve to infinity AUC. In addition, the values of the parameters from Equation 5

$$Cp = A\left(e^{-Kt} - e^{-K_a t}\right) \tag{5}$$

where A is a constant given by

$$A = \frac{Fk_a D}{V_d(k_a - K)} \tag{6}$$

K and k_a are the rate constants for elimination and absorption, respectively, D the dose with fraction F bioavailable, and Vd the volume of distribution, may be evaluated.

In this form K and $t_{1/2}$ are related by Equation 7

$$K = \frac{0.693}{t_{1/2}} \tag{7}$$

With this equation, it is possible to fit the data and derive the parameters manually from graphs. More frequently, however, computer fitting of the data is employed.

The apparent overall rate constant for clearance is better known as the beta (β) constant. We can evaluate an apparent volume of distribution from the area data by Equation 8.

$$V_d\beta = \frac{FD}{(AUC)(\beta)} \tag{8}$$

The volume so determined is often referred to as the Beta Volume.

Similarly, the overall body clearance (Cl) of drug is given by

$$Cl = (\beta)(V_d\beta) \tag{9}$$

$$= \frac{FD}{AUC}$$

It will be the parameters $V_d\beta$, β, AUC, and Cl that are most critical to compare between normal subjects and disease patients of the subsequent clinical studies.

Although this simple one-compartment open model is an oversimplification of the real situation, it is remarkably adequate for most clinical studies. Occasionally, when the distribution phase becomes apparent, either because of very rapid absorption or of slow distribution, then an additional exponential is required for Equation 5, which now becomes

$$Cp = Ae^{-\alpha t} + Be^{-\beta t} + Ce^{-\gamma t} \tag{10}$$

The constants involved here, A, B, C, α, β and γ may be related back to the parameters of the open two-compartment distributive model. However, reference to a standard text should be made. This is not normally an efficient or accurate method for parameter evaluation.

These distributive parameters are more reliably determined by following plasma concentrations subsequent to an i.v. dose when that is possible.

As repeatedly discussed earlier, it is essential to evaluate the linearity or proportionality of the dose to plasma concentration. If any nonlinearity occurs, it will follow that all parameters such as β, V_d, AUC, and Cl, will become dose or concentration dependent. If these departures from linearity are significant this will make dose adjustment and maintenance more difficult during clinical studies. In particular, the samples obtained during the ascending-dose study for drug tolerance become invaluable at this time.

There are some investigators who prefer or who routinely develop Moment Parameters in addition to the more classic ones. At the present time it is not clear that useful information can be developed by Moment Theory that is otherwise unavailable. The reader is referred to current textbooks and literature for further information in this regard.

In examining the dose-tolerance data it is important to construct a plot of adverse reaction incidence and severity as a function of plasma concentration occurs with dose, to determine whether or not the adverse reactions do become more noticeable in parallel with departures from linearity. This response curve should be compared with one similarly developed for patients in Phase II.

As mentioned earlier, the studies on normals are Phase I regardless of the time frame in which they are performed. As Phase II studies are completed, it becomes desirable to assure that the single-dose kinetics are predictive of the multiple-dose administration. If the linearity in single-dose studies has been clearly established or the degree of departure clearly evaluated, multiple dosing should provide no surprises. If the Phase II studies are anomalous in this regard, a careful reevaluation of the kinetics becomes obligatory.

B. PHASE II INVESTIGATION
1. Purpose
These studies are intended to determine, by ascending doses, the multiple-dose drug level required for a therapeutic response. Today the FDA is becoming increasingly concerned with a clear recognition of the lower levels for adequate therapeutic response in order to minimize the incidence of adverse reactions in susceptible patients.

Since alternate normal medication is being withheld from the subject, it is desirable that an effective dose be found by relatively rapidly increasing the dosage within the parameters determined by the Phase I study. As an effective tolerated dose range is found, the studies will increase to evaluate steady-state maintenance levels. Normally, patients in Phase II studies will not be exposed to the highest drug level reached for more than 2 weeks. However, it is possible for Phase II patients to carry over into Phase III studies for longer terms.

2. Other Derivable Information
a. Similarity of Parameters to Those of Normal Subjects
As patients are placed on the test protocol it is desirable to obtain blood and urine samples to determine whether or not the basic pharmacokinetic parameters for patients are equivalent to those observed in normals. As in the Phase I studies, the ascending-dosage regimen utilized at this stage provides unique sampling opportunities not normally available at a later point in time. Obviously, samples drawn in such a follow-through would probably never be analyzed if the chemical does not prove to be therapeutic. However, if it becomes evident that Phase III studies will be initiated, then these samples become important.

If the time course of the drug levels in patients appears entirely similar to that developed in normals, and if the levels from multiple dosing are as expected from single-dose studies, the need for any extensive pharmacokinetic studies in patients is minimized.

If, however, any of the pharmacokinetic parameters differ significantly between normals and patients, it is essential to define the differences clearly and to determine their cause and implications for clinical use. This will require appropriate studies in patients to be performed in a manner most acceptable for the disease state(s) involved.

b. Dose Response and Drug Level

Plasma levels obtained during the ascending doses permit a determination of therapeutic response as a function of drug concentration. Also, as with Phase I studies, the incidence of adverse reactions with concentration should also be noted. Monitoring of levels at steady state permits a preliminary determination of whether or not any metabolic induction may occur, thus reducing the plasma concentration to somewhat less than expected from single-dose values alone.

c. Pharmacodynamics

Today, the time course of pharmacologic effects resulting from drug administration is being actively studied both in normals and in patients. This response measure is generally followed for those clinically related parameters most amenable to quantitation. However, optimally the response of every observable parameter, clinically desirable or adverse, should be followed with time in dose-response studies. Obviously some drugs, as for example cardioactive, are easier to study in this manner than others.

Clearly establishing differences in pharmacodynamic response as a function of the time course of plasma drug concentration has not yet been adequately documented for a variety of drugs. However, we should expect that a major increase in the development of these data in the future and the concurrent development of modeling concepts that will handle these observations.

The development of these parameters and their modeling belongs in the Phase I and Phase II area of the IND.

C. PHASE III INVESTIGATIONS

In general, unless indicated by the Phase II studies, it is unlikely that patients in Phase III studies will be utilized for routine biopharmaceutic pharmacokinetic evaluations. However, as Phase III progresses, patients with more than one disease condition will enter the study. The potential of other medications to affect or be affected by the test drug should then be examined carefully. No absolute guidelines can be set for this, but potential based upon level of drug binding, of common metabolic pathways, or of known enzyme induction potential should guide the screening evaluation.

As the type of patient population is expanded, the nature of other disease states may dramatically affect the use of the drug. The better the pharmacokinetic and metabolic disposition of the drug has been developed, the greater the assurance that no surprises will arise during the extension of the drug use to the general population.

D. SOME ASPECTS OF DATA EVALUATION
1. Modeling of Pharmacokinetic Data

A variety of very sophisticated computer programs exist to determine the best mathematical fit of pharmacokinetic model parameters to the observed data. These programs, by minimizing the deviations between the observed and calculated model values, also imply which is the best model. Mathematically, these fits have clearly computed confidence bounds, but these bounds tend to become ignored. Only the knowledgeable kineticist recognizes that the permissible bounds on his calculated model parameters are often shockingly large. Frequently, however, data from crossover studies are presented for each dosage form as if the subject distribution parameters are indeed different for each dosage studied, and sufficient significant figures are used that this would appear to be self-evident. Because computed confidence bounds seem to be, in fact, unrealistically wide, they tend to be ignored entirely. The assumptions of randomness for a set of consecutive time points may possibly overweigh the model constraints that oblige each point to follow the preceding one smoothly. It is possible that adjacent points cannot each have the variance that they display as independent points. Although the parameters calculated for each administration do vary, the resultant model calculated values are generally more in agreement than would be expected from the calculated confidence bounds. Indeed, applied clinical pharmacokinetics dose calculations depend on this constancy.

It should also be recognized that the "best" calculated model is the best fit of an assumed model to the real data. It does not assure that the model does, in fact, have a real physiologically identifiable counterpart. Rather, the body as a whole reduces to the model, but specific organs or tissues, if they could be isolated, behave quite differently.

In this regard, a careful examination of much blood level-time data, especially if the values are obtained at frequent intervals, clearly exhibits undulations superimposed on the best smooth curve. These data are clearly the resultant of cycling of drug, with or without circadial rhythm superimposed. Routine fitting to standard models cannot handle these, and consequently the significance and reality of these undulations are ignored.

The exact fitting of data by very complex mathematical expressions requires parameters that cannot be related even for individual subjects when several sets of data are available. The author feels that no useful predictive generalizations can follow from such model-independent fittings.

Only an adequate physiologic model can be expected to be capable of matching complex variations such as undulations. The challenge is to develop a reduced physiologic model which adequately predicts observed phenomena, hence providing a recognition of the processes involved, without rendering it too complex to be usable. Only such models are likely to be of value in pharmacodynamic response modeling because only they can be related to concepts of receptor effects.

2. Michaelis-Menten Kinetic Data

Computer modeling of plasma concentration dosage time curves does permit the research evaluation of Michaelis-Menten parameters. Such a procedure is, however, impractical to use in a patient. Similarly, dose- and body load-dependent kinetic urine metabolite levels are not a convenient procedure for patients. Consequently, unless we are dealing with unique situations such as phenytoin, where the saturable pathway is the dominant mode of clearance, there is presently no suitable procedure for treating dosage adjustments due to saturation kinetics of important, but not dominant, clearance pathway for drugs. We do need new mathematical techniques for evaluation of data to permit some level of pragmatic dosage adjustment for drugs in which some level of saturable control of kinetics occurs.

Thus, we have dozens of drug combinations for which we clearly recognize and accept that competitive metabolism occurs. Yet many will not accept the consequent concept that competition can only occur while some level of saturation is present!

At the present time there are few, if any, clearly defined metabolic systems for which we do not have at least one drug known to exhibit saturable metabolism either within the therapeutic dose range or in some degree of toxic overload. The present regulatory state of anticipatory precaution may make the issuance of a drug approval for a drug primarily cleared by a single saturable pathway difficult or impossible. However, if our kinetic studies are well done, we may find that such a restriction could become the rule rather than the exception. This cannot be a rationalization of why such kinetic studies should not be complete. The scene will be visited in routine dosing without knowledge. Such occurrences result in frequent adverse reports which either jeopardize acceptance of the drug or result in the extreme in the eventual recall of the drug from the market. It is for this reason that we do need to develop new computation techniques leading to nomograms that could ease dosage calculations for general practitioner acceptance. This need is real.

Of greatest concern, once potentially saturable metabolic routes are recognized, is the role of coadministered other drugs. By virtue of the magnitude of their doses and their intrinsic enzyme activities, these may dominate clearance by mass-action thermodynamic requirements. Coadministration of large quantities of common medications such as aspirin, acetaminophen, or vitamin C may markedly dominate metabolic paths needed for the active drug under investigation.

The saturability of renal pathways is now beginning to become recognized as an area inducing significant kinetic effects. Tubular secretion and resorption are both significant pathways in drug clearance. Both are capable of competitive inhibition with significant clearance changes. This is a growing area of active research.

3. Characterization of Populations

There is the tendency to consider that the pharmacokinetic parameters for a population exhibit a reasonably normal distribution of values. The central value becomes the accepted value used for calculating dosages to be used for the general population. This holds if the therapeutic index is reasonable. Only if persons from one tail of the distribution exhibit signs of overdosing while those at the other extreme are underdosed, does it become necessary to realize that dosage adjustments are needed as a clinical judgment. When the population distribution is very wide, then the frequency of these occurrences makes this a recognizable situation warranting prescribing precautions. Many of our oxidatively metabolized drugs exhibit such wide distributions and yet have been capable of routine use without plasma concentration monitoring. Today, most such wide distributions in pharmacokinetic parameters are recognized to be two adjacent distributions, sufficiently close that they overlap and require special mathematical examination to separate them into their separate entities. Indeed, in the case of clear genetic allele inheritance, such as acetylation, we recognize the existence of trimodal distributions. In single ethnic population groups one mode, either the fastest or the slowest, often tends to disappear and be manifested only as a long tail to the next major mode.

When the population of a mode drops below 10%, the clear recognition of the mode becomes obscured and it is recognized only as a tail. This is characteristic of the debrisioquine-type drugs, where a small fraction of a Caucasian or Black population cannot metabolically clear the drug. Many of these newer drugs have been unacceptable in the U.S. because of the danger to a small population subset not otherwise readily identifiable. Whether or not we will eventually recognize clear genetic phenotype distributions for oxidative metabolism comparable to the commonly accepted acetylation types for isoniazid, hydrazaline, procainamide, and the sulfa drugs remains to be seen. However, the evidence is beginning to tend in that direction.

Rather than saying that we should not have certain drugs because we cannot safely handle their dosing, it is necessary to develop as markers reasonably innocuous drugs that can readily be determined analytically in blood or urine. These markers will serve as prototypes for these metabolic pathways of importance. With such a development, we may find it possible to rapidly screen an individual patient for how available a specific metabolic path is, and thus know a safe dosage to initiate.

When data are presented in the form of the range, average, and standard deviation for half-lives or other pharmacokinetic parameters, we cannot readily recognize whether the distribution is continuous or exhibits nodes. Future drug studies should clearly characterize the distribution of pharmacokinetic parameters in order to permit a clear recognition of the range of values involved.

Nevertheless, it is now evident that many Phase I and all Phase II metabolic reactions are quite variable in capacity across wide population distributions. The safer drugs will therefore be those for which several metabolic paths are available. Competition for path by other necessary coadministered drugs or the genetic limitation of a major path will not lead to dangerous drug accumulations before recognition. Admittedly, this means use of a suggested initial dose followed by a successive buildup as needed as the general rule for the initiation of therapy. However, there is no inherent pharmacokinetic trap likely to induce adverse reactions in a population subset when this is the approach taken.

As pharmacodynamic effects are more fully evaluated, similar concepts in population subsets for sensitivity to drugs may logically be expected. Pharmacogenetics has two major thrusts, the effect of the host on the clearance of the drug and the effect of the drug on the host. Indeed, then, in our modern parlance these two genetic manifestations are exhibited in pharmacokinetics and in pharmacodynamics.

IV. CONCLUSIONS

Data development for new drugs must be provided in the manner desired by the FDA to obtain approval. However, the groups developing these data should review this material for publication of the pharmacokinetic implications in the clinical literature in a mode communicative to the practitioner. Too often, if available, it is available only in sophisticated treatments suitable for full appreciation only by others of equivalent knowledge. The meaningful complete distribution of information is an obligation of the drug innovator.

Chapter 14

MANAGING AND CONDUCTING PHASE I AND PHASE II CLINICAL STUDIES

John A. Owen, Jr.

TABLE OF CONTENTS

I. INTRODUCTION

The decision to proceed to Phase I testing — the first introduction of a new chemical entity into a human being — is certainly a watershed in drug development. It is never a simple decision, but rather balances the obvious commitments of time, work, and money, plus the risks of failure, against the possible gains in terms of therapeutic advantage. The new product may be stronger, safer, cheaper, or simply more convenient to use. But if the previous basic research has been comprehensive and productive, if the clinical need exists, and if consultants concur, the decision to proceed can be made with some degree of confidence that a product with demonstrable clinical usefulness will eventually emerge.

II. GOALS OF PHASE I TESTING

Once made, the decision must be implemented by the preparation of a protocol, involving essentially normal subjects. The initial goals of the protocol are (1) to measure the pharmacological impact of the drug, (2) to determine the pharmacokinetic behavior of the drug, and (3) to detect any untoward effects. A more detailed discussion of these considerations is found in Chapter 13.[1-6]

To achieve these goals, the sponsor must go back to the animal data to review exactly which organ systems have shown a response to the drug, so as to pick out which human systems need to be monitored. Every bit of animal data contributes significantly at this point, including manufacturers' unpublished data as well as anything that may have already appeared in the literature. It is often desirable to review the information available on older comparable products, even though they may overlap only partially the characteristics of the new drug in question. It is equally important to show how the new drug differs from, as well as resembles, older, more thoroughly studied compounds. Review of the Phase I studies on these latter drugs often provides useful suggestions as to how to study the new drug. Of course the sponsor is always torn between the temptation to make these studies completely comprehensive and the realistic necessity to keep them within practicable limits.

III. CONSIDERATIONS IN DESIGN OF PROTOCOL

It is not difficult to arrange for the testing of human physiological parameters that are altered by drugs which affect normal function, e.g., a diuretic is easily tested in normal subjects by measuring the volume of urine secreted, its sodium content, and changes in renal clearance. These findings can then be easily extrapolated to later Phase II and Phase III studies of edematous patients who would benefit from a diuretic. The problem is considerably more difficult when the drug is designed to treat a disease state, such as cancer or infection, and its impact can only be measured in terms of amelioration of the disease. In such cases there can be no discernible therapeutic effect in normal subjects; the primary goals of such Phase I studies are in the pharmacokinetic area, and in the documentation of adverse effects, particularly in relation to blood levels. Finally, there are some drugs that fall into an intermediate area, i.e., able to relieve certain symptoms that might be experimentally produced. An example of this might be the titration of an analgesic effect, in which subjects are exposed to painful stimuli, their perceptions of which may be attenuated or blocked by the drug.

In all these studies, it is desirable to use assessment measures which are comparable to those used in the previous animal studies and at the same time are not too dissimilar from those which may be used clinically in the evaluation of disease and in the response of that disease to appropriate treatment. It is also desirable that, insofar as it is possible, these be relatively nonstressful, noninvasive, and of low risk so that they may be repeated several times during the course of treatment for comparison with baseline findings.

The pharmacokinetic information to be derived from Phase I trials is extremely important to everyone involved, but especially to the manufacturer. Therefore, these experiments should be as carefully designed and thoroughly reviewed as any other aspect of the testing (see Table 1). It is essential first to measure the rate of disappearance of the drug after i.v. injection, in order to determine the apparent volume of distribution and the plasma half-life or half-lives, depending on how many compartments occupy the theoretical model. Assessment of urinary and/or fecal excretion, with an analysis of the various metabolites of the drug, is also necessary in order to be able to anticipate potential problems of administration in patients with liver or renal disease. If the drug is available in an oral preparation, it is important to measure the bioavailability of a single dose, and the cumulative effect of interval dosing, so as to establish the dosage frequency necessary to produce therapeutic drug levels. For many drugs it will be necessary to measure both the peak and the trough of the blood levels following a single oral dose, in both the fasting and fed states. Using a multiple range of doses, it should be possible to establish a dose-response curve; this can then be compared with dose-response curves of comparable drugs already in clinical use. It is also important to know the degree of protein binding in plasma, so as to be able to predict possible drug interactions with other agents which might compete for binding sites and displace free drug from carrier protein for greater effect at tissue sites.[7]

Adverse effects are mostly subjective, except for the frequent skin rashes which, though obvious, are usually nonspecific. Every attempt should be made to correlate adverse effects with plasma levels when they are available. Repeated laboratory screening is essential in any Phase I study, and this should include complete blood counts, urinalysis, and usual laboratory chemistries, particularly including liver enzymes, uric acid, measures of renal function, etc. If the drug resembles a family of drugs which frequently produces characteristic adverse effects such as ototoxicity, special testing routines (e.g., audiometry) should be set up to monitor any changes occurring during or after use of the drug.

Any experiment, particularly a clinical trial, should be designed so as to provide sufficient and appropriate data for the statistical analyses which best suit the investigators' hypotheses. This requirement raises several important issues about data and methods which should be incorporated into the design of the experiment.

First, the data must be in sufficient quantity to answer the questions posed by the hypotheses, as well as the empirical results. In other words, the size of the subject groups must be sufficiently large so as to have the chance of showing the results one expects (the power of the design), and that chance must hold up when the results are actually examined after the experiment has been run.

Second, the data must have been obtained from subjects which are appropriate to the hypothetical relationship being examined. The population of normal subjects must be sufficiently homogeneous so as to give consistent outcomes (or, if more broad scale implication for the results is desired, heterogeneous normal populations must have potential differences in response factored into the calculation of experimental power).

Third, the statistical methods must properly fit the hypotheses. This is a much more complex issue than points one and two, and, for most experiments and investigators, implies that a biostatistician be involved in the design from the very beginning. A huge variety of statistical methods exist, only a few of which will be appropriate to any individual experiment. An experienced biostatistician will not only assist in the selection of analysis methods, but will also help in identifying design issues which may enhance the probable success of the trial. If the sponsor of the project will be conducting the analysis, the investigator should ask the sponsor's statistical unit for help. They will probably be anxious to get involved early in the project, rather than to face unresolved problems which may turn up after the study has actually been completed.

IV. CONSIDERATIONS OF THE PRINCIPAL INVESTIGATOR

Once the complete protocol for Phase I testing has been established by the sponsor, the next step is to find an investigator to carry out the study. Since well-trained clinical pharmacologists

TABLE 1
Essential Pharmacokinetic Data in Drug Testing

1. Oral availability (%)
2. Urinary excretion (%) — identification of metabolites
3. Plasma protein binding (%)
4. Clearance (ml/min/kg body weight)
5. Volume of distribution (l/kg body weight)
6. Plasma half-life (h)
7. Peak plasma concentration (C_{max})
8. Time to peak (T_{max})
9. Area under the curve (AUC 0 to 12 h, 0 to 24 h, and 0 to 0<)
10. Effective concentrations — may not be available
11. Toxic concentrations — may or may not be available

are always in short supply, this may be no easy task. In general, an investigator is more apt to become interested in such testing if he has a clinical interest in the general class of drugs represented, if he has had previous experience in Phase I testing of any drugs, and (most of all) if he has ever done Phase I studies before for the current sponsor. This shared experience and this prior understanding can save much time and facilitate the early establishment of a good working relationship. Usually, the investigator has a long-term affiliation with the institution where the studies are to be done, which renders the processing of the necessary paperwork less time consuming and expedites the handling of the grant funds. It goes without saying that for best results the investigator, as well as the sponsor and the institutional authorities where the testing will be done, must all be enthusiastically committed to carrying this study through to completion.

The clinical pharmacologist usually approaches his task by studying in great care the detailed protocol which is now available from the sponsor. He is mentally comparing this study with others that he has done, in terms of any unfamiliar features or other possible problem areas. At this time a monitor from the sponsoring company will usually meet with him and discuss the protocol in detail, after which both parties may wish to make some procedural adjustments, either for simplification or to provide additional data which is now seen to be desirable. In general, the clinical pharmacologist is well advised to resist the temptation to make the study more complicated than it already is, since in actuality, it is usually much more time consuming than his most extreme estimates anyway. Some of his concerns are summarized in Table 2.

A. SUBJECT POPULATION

Of major concern to the clinical pharmacologist is the population of normal subjects available to him for testing. He must have a clear understanding as to any restrictions in terms of age, body build, race, sex, previous and current disease history, or drug ingestion, etc. The risk of drug effects on the fetus must be clearly understood and obviated by requiring occlusive birth control methods or proven sterility as precondition for participation by females in the child-bearing age. The investigator will want to know whether or not it is possible to study several small groups of subjects in sequence or whether or not all subjects must be enrolled and started on treatment at the same time. The latter is more difficult, because it requires much more preplanned cooperation on the part of other physicians and ancillary personnel. It is also important to have a shared understanding in advance about subjects who drop out. Should the investigator enroll an extra 20% as a margin of safety, enroll new subjects to fill in the gaps as they occur, or leave them unfilled?

B. FACILITIES

Another question that is of equal concern to the investigator is whether or not his facilities

TABLE 2
Essentials in Planning a Phase I Trial

1.   Subject population
2.   Facilities
     a.   Area for study; hospitalization
     b.   Collaboration
     c.   Laboratory facilities
3.   Time commitments
4.   Ancillary personnel
5.   Budget
6.   Administrative approval
7.   Institutional Review Board (IRB) approval

are adequate for the investigation that is planned. He must have available space to receive the supply of drugs, must keep them under satisfactory storage conditions, must maintain an accurate inventory, and must use appropriate techniques for assessment of the presumed pharmacological effects. If these studies are to be continued longer than a few hours, it will be necessary to house the subjects overnight; this is best done in a clinical research unit or similar setting in a teaching hospital. Undoubtedly, other personnel will be involved in some of the basic evaluation such as interpretations of the X-rays, electrocardiograms, pulmonary function tests, etc., and their agreement to participate must be obtained in advance. It must be decided where the necessary laboratory studies are to be done, particularly those involving plasma samples for blood level determinations. If these are to be shipped back to the sponsoring company, there must be a clear-cut mechanism established for packing, refrigerating, and shipping of these samples to avoid deterioration. Thus, in summary, the clinical pharmacologist is like a builder who must make sure that his bulldozers, brick masons, carpenters, electricians, plumbers, painters, roofers, and plasterers are all ready and willing to go, in proper sequence, before undertaking to build a house.

C. TIME COMMITMENTS

Another essential part of the planning is a realistic appraisal of the time required to complete the studies, and of the time available to the clinical pharmacologist to devote to them. This will depend a great deal on what facilities are available and how many patients can be handled at a time. Normal subjects must have some inducement in order to participate in such studies, and this may be easier at some times of the year than others. Adult students, for example, often find it attractive to participate for pay in clinical trials while on holiday from their school work. On the other hand, this may be a time when the ancillary help is in short supply and the facilities are inadequate to handle the load of human material planned for the test. The investigator himself must budget his own time and look ahead to times of greater and lesser commitment to other enterprises.

D. ANCILLARY PERSONNEL

It is impossible to be specific about the number of ancillary personnel available, but there are a number of functions which are invaluable to a satisfactory completion of the whole task. There is always a good deal of secretarial work involved and records must be up-to-date, precise, and properly filed. Other professional assistance in the form of clinical pharmacologists or general physicians, specially trained nurses, the essential laboratory technicians, and others must be available and willing to devote the time required for the study. A highly desirable addition to the team would be the part-time services of an experienced pharmacist, who would take pains to make sure that all of the experimental drug is stored, dispensed, and accounted for by techniques of strict inventory control. These last activities are often of little interest to the clinical pharmacologist, but of urgent necessity to the sponsor, who must eventually satisfy the FDA that all materials have been shipped, received, stored, dispensed, and recorded faithfully and without error.

E. BUDGET

Finally, the sponsor and the clinical pharmacologist working together must arrive at a budget that is realistic. While it is unlikely that any clinical pharmacologist ever becomes rich just performing clinical drug testing, it is undeniably true that it is a seller's market as far as his services are concerned. The needs of the sponsor to find experts to test the drug are usually greater than the need of the investigator to fill huge empty spaces on his schedule by participating in the Phase I trial. Still, it is usually the intellectual curiosity of the latter, rather than monetary gain, that enlists his support. The budget must be worked out so as to provide for all the necessities of the experimentation, plus a professional fee for the time and effort expended by the principal investigators. It must also be arranged so as to enable payment of the "subcontractors" in a way that is efficient and acceptable to all. The institution will also require that overhead be included, which is accepted as a necessary aspect of the entire program of drug development in any research-oriented drug company.

F. ADMINISTRATIVE APPROVAL

Once the budget has been agreed on, the investigator must submit the necessary documentation of his qualifications to the drug company and to the FDA. Finally, the contract or grant agreement must be approved by the local institutional authorities and by the sponsoring drug company. Then as soon as the investigator has received his final protocol, recordkeeping material, and supplies of the drug, he is now in a position to begin his research. Somewhere along the line, though, one other hurdle must be overcome. The protocol must be thoroughly reviewed and cleared by the Institutional Review Board (IRB) at the institution where the work is to be done.

V. THE INSTITUTIONAL REVIEW BOARD

The IRB has gradually evolved from its official beginning back in 1966, to the point where it has become a critical administrative element in all institutions in which human research is being done. In essence, the Department of Health and Human Service (HHS) and/or the FDA have delegated to local IRBs the authority to examine and analyze the protocol of any research proposal involving human subjects, to ensure that such research correctly balances the potential benefits against the risks to which the subjects will be exposed, and finally, to specify exactly what information must be presented to the subject before he or she can be said to have given informed consent.[11,12]

This is an interesting stepwise delegation of authority. An adverse decision by an IRB may be appealed by an investigator, and that decision may be reversed at the higher levels within his own institution. The board, on the other hand, has the right to appeal to the Secretary of HHS if it determines that, despite interdiction, unauthorized research continues to be conducted with a clear threat to human health and life. HHS and the FDA, in turn, may intervene to enforce, or even to reverse, decisions already made by the IRB. It must be noted that such drastic steps as the last two mechanisms are rarely brought into play.

On the whole, the IRB functions well insofar as it is composed of dedicated, conscientious members who are willing to spend a great deal of time reviewing the research plans of others, and who are able to transmit a sense of their concern for the human rights of subjects as well as an understanding of the pressures on the investigators.

Usually the board is composed of individuals who are appointed by the parent institution, and every attempt is made to balance the various disciplines represented and to include lay members

TABLE 3
Concerns of the Institutional Review Board (IRB)

1. Is everything clearly in understandable lay language?
2. Is the preclinical data base sufficiently comprehensive?
3. Are subjects appropriately screened?
4. Are risks accurately and fully described?
5. Are benefits realistically estimated?
6. Does the pregnancy clause receive sufficient emphasis?
7. Are subjects assured of privacy and confidentiality?
8. Are the recompense and liability conditions clearly and expressly stated?
9. Is the subject's freedom to withdraw or refuse expressly preserved?
10. Are the rights of minors or incompetents protected by signatures of parents or guardians?
11. Does each subject receive a copy of the consent form with the name and telephone number of someone on the investigational team?
12. How much is research vs. routine clinical?
13. Someone to call re research subject's rights.

with no specific scientific experience. It is highly desirable to have on the board members representing the clergy, the legal profession, consumer groups, minority groups, or others who have their own perspective on the ethics of informed consent.

Most institutions find that it is simpler to give a blanket jurisdiction to the IRB to consider any and all research, whether it be supported by a federal or local governmental agency, a commercial firm, a private source, or whether it represents an unsponsored pilot study. The mechanics of approval require that the investigator submit a fairly detailed protocol of what he proposes to do and a carefully composed consent form which conveys to the subjects in lay language the actual details of the human research, the risks and benefits, the assurance of monetary reward and liability compensation, and the information regarding the ability to contact the investigators at any time and to withdraw from the investigation at any time without prejudice. The consent form should also include considerable information about a new drug whenever this is the subject of the study. In addition, it is essential to have the Notice of Claimed Investigational Exemption of a New Drug (IND) number of any investigational drugs or of Claimed Investigational Exemption of a New Device (IDE) number for investigational devices. Furthermore, most institutions will require a letter of indemnification from the sponsor which will set forth the limits to which the sponsor will support the investigators and reimburse the subjects in the event of any untoward or adverse reactions (*vide infra*).

The major thrust of board deliberations is the format and wording of the consent form, since, in general, the overall research design is not strictly within its purview. There are many concerns and considerations to be covered in informed consent, no matter how routine or unusual the actual research. Hence, as an aid to the investigator, some boards offer a model to be followed as closely as possible. An example is provided in the Addendum.[13]

The IRB must consider each proposal with these and other questions in mind (Table 3). After thorough discussion, a favorable decision is usually forthcoming, but is often contingent upon certain modifications of the consent form. This is conveyed to the investigator, and when all is revised and correct, a letter or form (HHS-596) authorizing the investigator to begin his research is issued. However, the function of the board does not stop at that point. The investigator is required to contact the board immediately if any unexpected adverse effects or disasters occur in the course of the study, and to report periodically on the progress of his study until it has been completed.

The board has the authority to defer granting approval to investigation, and also to request its suspension or termination if circumstances indicate that the risks of continuation would be prohibitive. In such an extreme situation, the parent institutional authorities and sponsor are informed immediately and must be prepared either to back up the board decision or else to intervene actively to bring about a resolution of the disagreement. Finally, as a last resort, the board may always communicate directly with the HHS in order to alert the federal government to the problems of investigations which otherwise cannot be resolved. HHS in turn may, at this point, suspend payment to the institution, not only of the funding for this particular project, but of all federal funding of any sort, until such a time as it is felt that all human investigation is in compliance with federal guidelines.

The literature in this area is growing rapidly. In addition to federal guidelines (which are continually under revision), there is a growing volume of state and local guidelines[14] and regulations regarding human investigation, in addition to those which may have been established by the institution itself.

In recent years both HHS and the FDA have been preparing separate sets of guidelines for human investigation and for the operation of IRBs. There have been differences in philosophy and in wording between these two regulations, and many efforts have been made at high levels to bring the two versions closer together. It is this continuing effort to resolve differences which has perhaps delayed so long the final appearance of these regulations in their most permanent form. It is quite possible, of course, that some further crisis in human experimentation, such as the thalidomide disaster, may sponsor a renewed spurt of activity and even more restrictive revision of the regulations. It seems highly unlikely that any event or nonevent would ever stimulate further attempts to revise these regulations to make them more lenient, wishful thinking to the contrary notwithstanding. It therefore behooves every investigator, as well as every sponsor, and particularly every IRB, to become thoroughly familiar with the wording and intent behind the federal regulations when they have finally become effective. Periodically, the structure and operations of the IRB are monitored by means of an on-site audit by an inspector from the FDA.

VI. MANAGEMENT OF THE PHASE I CLINICAL TRIAL

The previous discussion has focused on the planning of the Phase I trial in considerable detail, which does not leave much to say about the actual conduct of the trial. If it has been planned well, it will go well.

In brief, the investigator needs now only to make himself obsessive-compulsive about following every detail of his protocol and he will secure the information he is seeking. The problems that he encounters once the trial has begun will fall into four categories.

Disappearing time — The first subject to go through the clinical trial will take considerably more time than was anticipated. The problem will soon solve itself as practice makes perfect, as the investigator learns to get all things in readiness before actually beginning each trial, as technical difficulties are mastered, etc. However, he also finds that the overall time projected for the completion of the entire study is slipping by faster than he thought. Tempo is of the essence; once the investigator gets behind schedule on a study, his efficiency seems to suffer and enthusiasm cools. Again, planning is the answer: subjects and time must be lined up in advance so that no unforeseen delays will upset the schedule unduly.

Disappearing subjects — A change of mind, unexpected emergencies, waning interest, illness, etc., will invariably affect some members of the proposed study population. Hence it is always desirable to recruit a greater number than actually required and to keep in frequent contact with them all, to ensure that a prepared and suitable subject is always available for study.

Disappearing drug — In a perfect trial, every ampule, every milliliter, every tablet should be accounted for. The receipt, inventory, storage, and reinventory of unused supplies are tedious but essential tasks. Not only is this aspect a requirement of the FDA, but it is one of those trifles which make perfection. In a perfect trial, there is no disappearance of the drug.

Disappearing data — Here, too, the perfect study is one with every bit of data in place — a condition which is rarely met. Broken, clotted, or insufficient blood samples, missed observations, shipments lost in the mail or in the lab are all par for the course. Sometimes if a particular laboratory study is absolutely crucial, it is well worthwhile obtaining duplicate samples on everyone, every time, to be sure that no missing values will ruin the study. How damaging such deficiencies are will depend on the experimental design and statistical analysis and whether or not it is possible to recruit additional subjects later on.

In summary, a successful clinical trial requires three qualities in the investigator: planning, perfectionism, and overall determination to carry through the study, organize and analyze the data, and report his findings. If these are present, the task will not prove to be too difficult. It may appear that the difficulties have been exaggerated, but, if so, the purpose has been to enable the reader to avoid them in future Phase I clinical trials of his own.

VII. THE PHASE II CLINICAL TRIAL

With the successful completion of Phase I testing, it is essential to move on the planning for Phase II trials. Here the objectives and stratagems are quite different. Whereas in Phase I testing the primary question concerns the pharmacologic effect of the drug in normal subjects, in Phase II we are studying its therapeutic impact on human disease in terms of how well it reverses the pathophysiology and/or relieves the symptoms of illness.

One of the watershed papers in clinical pharmacology is the well-known study of Mahon and Daniel, which established for all time the four cornerstones of a meaningful clinical trial: suitable controls, random assignment to treatment, removal of observer bias, and appropriate statistical analysis.[15] Sooner or later every clinical trial, especially every Phase II clinical trial, must be measured against those criteria. Failure to measure up will not only cast doubt on the scientific validity of the study, but will further delay and prolong the decision by the FDA on the final New Drug Application.

Since a general discussion of statistical analysis was summarized earlier in this chapter, we will here confine our attention to the decisions which seek to satisfy the first three requirements of Mahon and Daniel.[15] In many significant ways the planning of Phase II trials involves considerations largely, if not wholly, absent from Phase I testing, such as:

1. Choice of the target illness.
2. Characterization of patients who might be subjects.
3. Choice of controls: longitudinal, parallel, or crossover?
4. Choice of parameters to assess drug effect and of criteria of success or failure.
5. Selection of appropriate dosage forms.
6. Use of placebos.
7. Randomization in assignment to treatment?
8. Observer blinding.
9. Decisions as to length of study, criteria for drop out, post-trial follow-up, etc.
10. Ethical issues of Phase II trials.

A. THE TARGET ILLNESS

Some drugs must of necessity have extremely restricted clinical indications, e.g., synthetic vasopressin is appropriately studied only in subjects with true diabetes insipidus. On the other hand, a new nonsteroidal anti-inflammatory agent can be tested as a therapeutic agent in rheumatoid arthritis, osteoarthritis, ankylosing spondylitis, gout, acute skeletal muscle pain, minor postoperative pain, simple tension headache, etc. In general, the decision as to which disease to study depends on the availability of suitable patients, the past experience with comparable drugs, the potential market value of a new agent for any given specific disease, as well as on the previously demonstrated pharmacology of the drug.

B. CHARACTERIZATION OF PATIENT SUBJECTS

It is advantageous to utilize established and relatively objective criteria for the diagnosis of the disease under study, as this makes it clear which patients may or may not be considered potential subjects of study. The crucial question is whether or not the process of selection can be described in such a way as to immediately satisfy an objective expert that these are indeed appropriate examples of the disease for which the new therapeutic agent would be useful.

C. SELECTION OF CONTROLS

In Phase I testing each subject may serve as his own control, but this is usually not appropriate in Phase II. If the disease progress is relatively transient, e.g., tension headache, spontaneous improvement may confound interpretation of drug effects, necessitating a parallel control group receiving placebos. If the course is chronic and progressive, it is good to compare the new drug with an active agent of accepted therapeutic value; even better is a comparison of placebo vs. both standard treatment and the new drug, provided that active treatment can be withdrawn for a significant period without great harm to the patient. Perhaps the most ironclad comparison of all is the parallel crossover study with "washout" periods on placebo preceding and following each period of drug administration, i.e., Group 1: placebo, standard drug, placebo, new drug, placebo and Group 2: placebo, new drug, placebo, standard drug, placebo.

Of all the decisions in experimental design of Phase II trials, none is more important than the selection of suitable controls, and in making that decision there is no substitute for a firsthand knowledge of the natural history of the disease.

D. PARAMETERS AND CRITERIA

Sometimes the consideration of these topics is best approached in reverse, proceeding from the end to the means. Unless a trial produces results which can be analyzed for statistical significance, the entire effort is in vain and probably unethical for that reason. For statistical analysis one must have numbers; therefore, the parameters of study must be susceptible to numerical expression, either quantitative or by classifying subjects as treatment success or failure. It is, of course, equally essential that these parameters represent the fundamental measures of the disease, preferably the actual diagnostic criteria themselves or the customary ways of quantitating severity of disease. If no such parameters are available, it may be necessary to devise a rating scale, basically subjective, but as clearcut as possible in providing a quantitative assessment of the severity of the overall disease process at any given time.

E. SELECTION OF APPROPRIATE DOSAGE FORMS

This is mainly a pharmaceutical problem, but it involves consideration of the dosage forms of standard drug therapy and of the requirements to be fulfilled in preparing the corresponding placebo. In general, it is desirable to make dose size and frequency such as to facilitate compliance, not only during the trial, but in possible future widespread clinical use.

F. USE OF PLACEBO

The need for comparable controls has been discussed earlier, and the decision whether to use placebo and/or standard active drug involves practical as well as ethical questions. Much depends, again, on the natural history of the disease, but now also upon the pharmacokinetics of the drug in question. How long does it persist in the blood or other compartments after the last dose? How long does it take for an untreated patient to relapse to any given level or morbidity? If either or both of these time periods are lengthy, placebo controls become logical, even essential. On the other hand, if therapeutic progress is always slow and precious and relapse rapid and disastrous, ethical considerations must militate against placebos. Sometimes it is possible to compromise, by combining active drug and placebo in a variable ratio in each patient's regimen, reducing the drug content as much and as long as the patient's condition will permit without seriously threatening life or health.

G. RANDOMIZATION

If controls and experimental subjects are to be selected from the same population, there can be little excuse for not using strict randomization techniques in assigning patients to the new drug or to placebo treatment. If the disease varies widely in severity, it may be desirable to stratify the randomization in order to avoid the unlikely possibility of getting most of the milder cases in the new drug group and the more severe ones in the placebo group, or vice versa.

H. OBSERVER BLINDING

It is generally accepted that validity of observations requires that patients should be prevented from knowing whether they are receiving active drug or placebo. This has usually been extended to include also the investigative team, which makes the trial "double-blind". Sometimes the variations in disease or the side effects make it almost impossible for a curious observer not to guess which patient is receiving the active drug. Here some protocols have been able to achieve "triple-blinding", in which one observer evaluates the therapeutic impact of the drug, but avoids examining its side effects or toxicity, while another observer checks for toxic but not therapeutic effects. Thoughtful investigators have recently begun to reexamine the dogma that only double-blind trials are valid, and it must be admitted that in some cases the data generated would appear to be so objective as to be bias-proof. In general, however, it is still advisable to lean over backward in order to remove any possibility of observer bias rather than to risk the lingering doubts that might otherwise be voiced.

I. MISCELLANEOUS CONSIDERATIONS

The length of the study is an important decision, again requiring a profound knowledge of the natural history of the disease and of the rapidity of action of the drug in animal studies. Prolonged studies are expensive, in terms both of financial outlay and of the delay in obtaining definitive answers. In every study, some patients will elect to drop out, and this number will naturally be greater in longer trials or those with greater drug toxicity. It is well to establish in advance some fairly clear criteria which would necessitate dropping the patient from the study, or breaking the code to see whether his continued participation involves unacceptable risks.

When the trial is over, the patient must have, and must know that he has, the option of changing over to the best established drug therapy available. If he has responded well to the test drug, it would be ideal to let him continue on it in a Phase III trial. In any event, these patients must continue to receive special attention and follow-up for 1 to 2 years, to allow evaluation for prolonged or deferred development or toxicity or of therapeutic benefit.

J. MEDICO-LEGAL CONSIDERATIONS

For a number of years, the liability aspects of human investigation were wishfully considered to be mainly theoretical, but as time goes by the medico-legal implications of the investigational risks to subjects have become a difficult problem.

Federal regulations require that informed consent carry a statement about liability which is usually expressed in words like those of the model: "If you should suffer physical injury directly resulting from the research procedures, no financial compensation for such things as lost wages, disability or discomfort is available, but medical treatment that is not covered by your insurance will be provided free of charge at (the institution)." This carefully worded sentence is notable for what it does and does not say.

1. In case of chemotherapy with expected severe side effects, the consent form may list all of these, stress their unavoidability, and insert "unexpected" between "suffer" and "physical".
2. Note that psychic injury, pain, and suffering are excluded, although in actual practice it is sometimes prudent to give way on this point.
3. Since the promise of free treatment applies only to side effects of research procedures,

it becomes extremely important that the Investigational Procedures section of the consent form spell out exactly what is research and what is routine clinical treatment.

4.   Usually neither the investigator nor the subject knows exactly what the latter's insurance will cover and there seems to be a growing reluctance on the part of carriers to cover investigational procedures. The above phraseology is the best we can do.

5.   It is clear that subjects who desire compensation for lost wages, disability, or discomfort have no recourse via the consent form, so must institute legal action to obtain it. Such lawsuits are usually based on the claim of negligence or inadequately informed consent or both.

While the informed consent statement is not primarily written with the intent to provide documentary defense against a lawsuit, there are several areas that will repay careful consideration in preparation.

1.   The need to separate the experimental from the customary has been noted above.

2.   It never hurts to repeat in the consent form the criteria for exclusion of subjects ineligible for investigation. Often those who suffer side effects should never have been in the study to begin with, and claim they were wrongfully included. The interdiction against pregnancy in females should be coupled with the responsibility to report any such suspicions promptly.

3.   The use of placebos and randomization must be described in such a way as to be technically accurate without providing any clues that would destroy the double-blind. This may be difficult or impossible to do, in which case the legal considerations, unfortunately, take precedence.

4.   Side effects to be expected must be described as precisely as possible, e.g., if a possible side effect is hemorrhagic (but not thrombotic) stroke, that specificity should be stated. The requisite prompt action to be taken by subjects and by investigational staff, in the event of a side effect, should also be described generally.

5.   Payment should be itemized and prorated for partial but incomplete completion of a study.

6.   There should be a clear identification of contacts (name and phone number) to be called in case of emergency, and this should be dependably responsive, 24 hours a day, 7 days a week.

To return to the blanket liability statement, if treatment is to be provided at the institution free of charge, who actually pays the bill? In some cases, the institution seeks commercial coverage for research misadventures; for most unsponsored research, it relies on self-insurance. The wording of this is a matter for the sponsor's own legal advisors, but it would seem basic to include:

1.   The name and title of all investigators and of the specific research protocol (updated by any subsequent modifications), plus the location and durations of the study.

2.   A reference to the approved consent form to be used.

3.   A promise that the sponsor will reimburse the institution for such medical treatment, provided (a) eligible subjects only were enrolled, (b) a valid consent was obtained, (c) the protocol was followed exactly, (d) the sponsor was promptly notified of the event, and (e) investigator and institution cooperate fully with the sponsor in providing time and materials for legal defense.

In case of a lawsuit, it is incumbent that sponsor and institution present an unbroken position, that the investigator was acting both at the direction of the sponsor and as one whose research was approved by his institution; the plaintiff's case will inevitably attempt to wedge these apart. Most of these cases result in some settlement, without prejudice, if the loss through disability is clearly indisputable and long-lasting.

This has been a rather detailed discussion of a problem which may surface only once in a thousand clinical trials. To avoid becoming that 0.1%, however, this section is worth rereading.

K. ETHICAL CONSIDERATIONS

The ethical issues of the Phase I trial are fairly straightforward. So long as all known risks are fully presented, and the monetary inducement is satisfactory, it is a viable reasonable contract between consenting adults: *caveat emptor*. But in Phase II trials the patients are in a difficult and often ambiguous position, and the investigator must lean over backwards to protect their rights.

First, the attending physician who wishes to conduct clinical research on his own patients is assuming a double role at considerable risk of conflict of interest. It is clearly to his interest to induce his patients to enter the study and to stay in it despite adversity: no matter how loudly he proclaims their freedom of choice, it is clear what he really wants, and the doctor-patient relationship will usually guarantee that that is what he gets. To avoid this conflict, it is far, far better for the physician to acquire a "research associate" who will actually solicit patients to enter the trial.

Second, a major ethical problem has to do with taking patients off standard therapy to try the new drug. This is not so bad if standard therapy, per se, is not so good, but even so, it is no less unacceptable to destroy faith in the old drug than to raise false hopes in the new drug. The clear goal of all proper trials is to find the best treatment for the individual patient, and to provide assurance that this best treatment, once found, will continue to be available.

Third, use of placebos is always a troublesome issue. The risks of deterioration of the patient's condition due to withdrawal of needed medication must be kept to an absolute minimum, even at the price of having to expand or prolong the study to compensate for the dropouts. And the patient-subject must be clearly informed of these risks and of the techniques to minimize them, of the randomization procedure, and of the preestablished criteria for dropout. The justification for all diagnostic tests must be clearly stated, including those which serve to monitor toxicity.

Fourth, every effort must be made to protect privacy and guarantee confidentiality, to set forth honestly the limits of liability on the part of sponsor and investigator, and to state the terms of compensation or other inducement to the participants.

Finally, the investigator must not only promise, but must enthusiastically deliver, appropriate care to anyone who suffers adverse reactions. And it must be kept up for as long as necessary, nor should the patient ever have cause to feel that he is an embarrassment to the investigator, to be shunted aside, treated in a hasty and perfunctory way, or dismissed without a return appointment. These hangdog tactics are not only callous, but unethical; they constitute an open invitation to legal action.

To a lesser degree this admonition applies also to those who successfully complete the trial without incident. They have lived in an atmosphere of enhanced interest and rapport, but now they have come down to earth. No matter how busy he is with other patients or new trials, the investigator must never seem to forget that he and the subject, "for one shining hour", shared a very special relationship on the cutting edge of scientific research. If this has had an enduring beneficial effect on both their lives, then truly this clinical research has passed the final ethical test.

ADDENDUM
("Model" Consent)

CONSENT TO PARTICIPATE IN A STUDY
(Title of Study)

We invite you (your child,_____,) to participate in a study of _____.
We hope to learn _____. You were (Your child was) selected for this study because
_____.

Investigational Procedures

If you choose (agree to permit your child) to participate in this study, we will
_____.

Risks and Benefits

Research studies often involve some risks. The risks of this study are _____. In addition, it is possible in any experiment that harmful effects which are not now known could occur. Of course, we will take every precaution to watch for and prevent any harmful side effect. If you are pregnant, we want you to tell us and we will not include you in the experiment, because to do so might be harmful to your unborn baby; we also want you to avoid getting pregnant during this study, and expect you to use an effective method of birth control. If you should become pregnant in spite of all precautions, please contact immediately the investigator whose phone number is listed below and he/she will discuss with you the choices available for your consideration.

If you (your child) participate(s) in this study you (your child) may experience _____. We do not guarantee or promise, however, that you (your child) will receive any of these benefits.

Alternative Treatments

Often, the treatment for your (child's) condition would be _____. However, in order to test the effectiveness of our experimental treatment, we must necessarily withhold (delay) customary treatments. If the experimental treatment is not effectively improving your (child's) condition, we will treat you (your child) with _____ (customary treatment).

Other alternatives to participating in this experiment include _____ or simply a decision not to participate.

Privacy of Records

Any information that we learn about you (your child) that can be individually traced to you (your child) will be used responsibly and will be protected against release to unauthorized people. In addition to the members of the health care staff who usually have access to your (child's) file, you (your child's) records are likely to be shown to _____ (e.g., FDA and employees of the sponsor). If you sign this form, you have given us permission to release information to those other people. The results of this study may be published in the medical literature, but no publication will contain any information that will identify you (your child).

Payment

You (your child) will (will not) receive _____ dollars (any payment) for participating in and completing this study.

In the event you (your child) suffer(s) physical injury directly resulting from the research procedures, no financial compensation for such things as lost wages, disability, or discomfort is available, but medical treatment that is not covered by your insurance will be provided free of charge. If you have any questions concerning financial compensation for injuries caused by the experiment, you should talk to _____ at _____.

Conclusion

Neither your decision not to (allow your child to) participate in this study, nor your decision to stop and withdraw from the study after having agreed to participate will hurt your future care at this hospital. Of course, we will tell you anything we learn during the study that may help you decide whether or not to continue participating.

You are making a decision whether or not you (your child) will participate in this study. If you sign this form, you have agreed that you (your child) will participate based upon reading and understanding this form. If you have any questions about the study, please ask _____ before signing.

If you have any questions regarding research subjects' rights, please contact_____, Chairman of the _____, at _____.

You will receive an unsigned copy of this form to keep.

_____

Witness_____   Signature_____

_____

Member of Research Team_____   Signature of Parent or Guardian

                                                   _____

                                                   Date

NOTE: The same version of the consent form should not be used for both adults and children. The bracketed references to children should be omitted from adult forms. The brackets and preceding language should be omitted if the study is confined to children.

REFERENCES

1. **Waife, S. O. and Shapiro, A. S.,** Eds., *Clinical Testing of New Drugs,* Paul B. Hoeber, New York, 1959.
2. **Nodine, J. H. and Siegler, P. E.,** Eds., *Animal and Clinical Pharmacological Techniques in Drug Evaluation,* Year Book Medical Publishers, Chicago, 1964.
3. **Herrick, A. D. and Cattell, Mc. K.,** Eds., *Clinical Testing of New Drugs,* Revere Publishing, New York, 1965.
4. **Feinstein, A. R.,** Clinical epidemiology, in *The Architecture of Clinical Research,* W. B. Saunders, Philadelphia, 1985.
5. **MacMahon, F. G.,** *Principles and Techniques of Human Research and Therapeutics, Selected Topics,* Futura Publishing, Mt. Kisco, NY, 1985.
6. **Meinert, C. L.,** *Clinical Trials, Design, Conduct and Analysis,* Oxford University Press, New York, 1986.
7. **Benet, L. Z., and Sheiner, L. B.,** Design and optimization of dosage regimens: pharmacokinetic data, in *The Pharmacological Basis of Therapeutics,* 6th ed., Gilman, A. G., Goodman, L. S., and Gilman, A., Eds., Macmillan, New York, 1980, 1675.
8. **Cochran, W. G. and Cox, G. M.,** *Experimental Designs,* 2nd ed., John Wiley & Sons, New York, 1957.
9. **Mainland, D. B.,** *Elementary Medical Statistics,* 2nd ed., W. B. Saunders, Philadelphia, 1963.
10. **Siegal, S.,** *Nonparametric Statistics for the Behavioral Sciences,* McGraw-Hill, New York, 1956.
11. **Annas, G. J., Glantz, L. H., and Katz, B. F.,** *Informed Consent to Human Experimentation: The Subject's Dilemma,* Ballinger Publishing, Cambridge, MA, 1977.
12. President's Commission for the Study of Ethical Problems in Medicine and Biomedical and Behavioral Research, *Volume One: Report,* U.S. Government Printing Office, Washington, D.C., 1982.
13. **Prentice, E. D. and Antonson, D. L.,** A protocol review guide to reduce IRB inconsistency, *IRB,* 9, 9, 1987.
14. 45 C.F.R., 46:103 (c) as amended by 43 *Federal Register,* 51, 559, 1978; also 51, 20204, 1986 and 52, 19466, 1987.
15. **Mahon, W. A. and Daniel, E. E.,** A method for the assessment of reports of drug trials, *Can. Med. Assoc. J.,* 90, 565, 1964.

Chapter 15

CONDUCTING PHASE III AND PHASE IV CLINICAL TRIALS

Carlos R. Ayers

TABLE OF CONTENTS

I. INTRODUCTION

A few years back a group of medical doctors were interviewing a small, select number of young aspiring medical students. Their purpose in scrutinizing these young scholars lay in selecting one of the students as the recipient of a memorial scholarship prize. The final question put to the students was this: what do you feel has been the single most outstanding medical advancement in this century? One of the students answered the question by announcing that, in his opinion, the development of antibiotic therapy, specifically penicillin, was not only a great medical advancement, but a major contribution to society as a whole.

This illustration serves to reaffirm popularity of the belief that drug therapy is the cornerstone of treatment for many disease states in peoples all over the world. Therefore, if society is to be justly served, it makes good common sense that drug development be placed in a category abreast of that never ending continuum which is medical progress.

Previous chapters in this book have dealt with the embryonic stages of drug development. Thus far, we have learned that each new drug is conceived in the laboratory — for it is in the laboratory where the chemical formula mapped out on paper is synthesized. The "drug" does not become a pharmacologic entity, however, until its worth has been demonstrated.[1] Pharmaceutical companies design Phase I and Phase II projects which will afford an exquisitely detailed picture of the new compound. Details of pharmacodynamics, human toleration, and preliminary discussions of the overall drug validity are among the overall objectives. Therefore, Phase II is deemed a success only when the specific pharmacologic test agent demonstrates the desired effect in patients without possessing toxic properties which would preclude its use.

A more thorough analysis of Phase II clinical trials is presented in the previous chapter. The author succinctly describes a multitude of parameters inherent to the scope and objectives at this level of investigation. Indeed, the importance of Phase II trials cannot be overstated as it serves to lay a firm foundation for a true appreciation of the intricacies of Phase III and Phase IV studies.

Having achieved this end, we may now embark upon our discussion of conducting Phase III and Phase IV clinical trials.

Phase III and IV constitute the final two steps in drug development. Successful completion of these two phases entitles the pharmaceutical company to seek marketing approval from the FDA. Suffice it to say, then, that extreme care is exercised when conducting the clinical trials in these phases. We shall therefore view each phase separately and later shift our focus to general adminstrative aspects of both Phase III and Phase IV clinical drug protocols.

A. PHASE III

In the development of any given pharmacologic agent, Phase III precedes registration of a new drug application (NDA) with the FDA. Therefore, protocols at this level of investigation are designed to evaluate efficacy and safety in a large number of patients. The protocol must be so constructed as to emphasize the patients' general ability to tolerate the drug. Formulating approaches to overdose, addressing the problems of drug interactions, and addiction qualities are additional items composing the fabric of Phase III trials.

Controlled, as well as uncontrolled, clinical trials are employed in the Phase III stage of drug development. Controlled trials are those in which the test drug is compared to a placebo or another medication. A particularly useful research tool, the controlled trial provides answers to comparative therapeutic questions in a convincing manner, especially when there are only minute differences expected.[2] Uncontrolled trials do not involve any comparison studies and simply entail direct administration of the drug to the patient. This method is a straightforward means of evaluating general patient drug tolerance, efficacy, and dose scheduling under conditions that will closely approximate actual practice.

B. PHASE IV

Successful completion of Phase III clinical trials is accompanied by FDA support of the NDA, and emanating from this are Phase IV clinical trials. Protocols at the Phase IV level of clinical investigation are less rigid in structure in contrast to previous phases. Again, both controlled and uncontrolled trials are used to elucidate further details of drug action and oftentimes investigators are allowed to conduct their own special studies. Special studies are frequently quite helpful in obtaining a wealth of information regarding the specific drug effects of body systems. Investigators often utilize "study drugs" to expand and enhance their own academic research programs. Indeed, it is within this framework that the special study serves a dual purpose; it broadens the scope of the investigator's research and provides the pharmaceutical sponsor with specific answers to questions about the drug, its side effects, mechanism of action, and general worth as a therapeutic agent.

Protocols of the third and fourth phases in drug development are tailored to meet the needs of both the patient and the sponsor. It goes without saying that a protocol design so complex as to preclude both investigator and patient compliance is of little value to either the sponsor or the study patient.

II. STUDY ADMINISTRATION

A. STUDY INITIATION

It becomes appropriate at this point in our discussion to disgress momentarily and consider the question, "Who are the qualified investigators?" Many parameters require thorough analysis in answering this question. The disease entity which the study drug has been designed to treat should be closely aligned with the prospective investigator's area of expertise. For example, it would be inappropriate to select a dermatologist to conduct a clinical trial of a new antihypertensive agent. Due consideration is also afforded the prospective investigator's other duties and whether conducting the clinical trial consitutes a low- or a high-priority goal item. Additionally, will the investigator become intimately involved with the study or will he function simply as a bureaucratic figurehead? Observations need to be made by an experienced clinical practitioner. The patient resources available within the institution is another consideration. Often, considerable effort is required in screening patients to ultimately obtain the total number necessary to complete the study population.

Following the selection of the investigator, several tasks require attention before active patient recruitment begins. While meeting to discuss the study budget, the pharmaceutical representative and the investigator also discuss the specifics of institutional review of the protocol and consider the topic of patient "informed consent". In addition, the pharmaceutical sponsor visits the clinical laboratory to obtain convincing evidence that this facility will perform adequately.

The aforementioned discussion between the drug sponsor and the clinical investigator pertains to the issues of data collection and responsibilities of the recorder. The investigator must be briefed in advance as to the requirements for completing and submitting case report forms to the sponsor's clinical drug monitor. Accurate records are filed in a manner which affords easy retrieval of data. Every protocol provides guidelines for dispensing and cataloging of drugs and these regulations should be carefully delineated by the sponsor at the outset.

Finally, and prior to study initiation, the subject of adverse clinical experiences is examined in great detail. A uniform procedure for the evaluation, treatment, and reporting of adverse experiences is essential in meeting the general protocol objective. Without strict adherence to a standard policy, drug safety cannot be accurately assessed.

B. THE IMPORTANCE OF INFORMED CONSENT

When the patient signs the consent form agreeing to participate in the drug protocol, he is permitting the investigator to perform laboratory tests and treatment as well as to administer the new therapeutic agent to the patient as required by the clinical trial protocol. This act constitutes patient consent, but it may not be inferred that he is giving "informed consent". It becomes necessary, then, to distinguish between "patient consent" and "informed consent".

The term "informed consent" takes the patient a step beyond the ritual of signing a document. An important element of study initiation, obtaining a patient's informed consent, denotes that the investigator or his designee has educated the patient with respect to the manner in which the participant's daily lifestyle will be affected.[3,4] Every step of the protocol is explained to the patient. Layman's terms are preferable to confusing scientific jargon. The investigator must never hesitate to answer all questions the patient asks, thereby creating a general atmosphere of congeniality, mutual trust, and respect. The patient who signs a consent form after he becomes an "informed" patient is often an excellent, cooperative, protocol participant.

C. DEVELOPING A CONSENT FORM

Pharmaceutical companies often supply a sample patient consent form, but, in reality, it is the responsibility of the investigator to compose a consent form which may be easily understood by his patients and acceptable to his institutional review committee.

The best consent form is one which, as previously stated, is written in laymen's language. It is paramount to all concerned that the patient be able to comprehend what he reads. Details of protocol design and procedures are outlined in a orderly fashion. Any experimental procedures should be identified and explained.

Consent forms also include clauses which clearly state that the patient may or may not reap benefits through participation. The possibility of side effects or discomforts demand attention, but the beneficial qualities the medication may possess should be mentioned. A section which explores alternatives to study participation should be included.

Another important point to keep in mind when constructing the consent form is the patient's future care. Communicate to the prospective study patient that he is free to withdraw from the study whenever he chooses without compromising the quality of his future medical care. The consent form also assures the patient that his questions regarding drug side effects, benefits, and general risks will be duly addressed by the members of the research team.

No consent form is complete until it discusses methods for contacting the investigator within the health care setting and after working hours. The name, address, phone number should appear on the consent form. Procedures to be followed should the patient require emergency treatment should be discussed.

Occasionally, investigators recruit patients by offering financial renumeration to the participant. Regardless of what the situation may be, the consent form should certainly contain a clause stating clearly that the patient will or will not be paid for his participation. The consent form must also include a statement of policy concerning financial compensation should the patient become physically harmed by the study medication. In the event of an adverse clinical experience, the patient should feel confident that he will receive excellent medical care at little or no cost to him.

The participant's anonymity must be secure at all times and a statement of this is an essential element of all consent forms. This assures the patient that no unauthorized person(s) will obtain access to his file.

The patient is supplied with an unsigned copy of the consent form, thus providing him a ready reference to protocol events at all times. An additional copy of the consent form displays the signatures of the patient and two witnesses, one of whom should not be a member of the research team. If the patient is not of legal age, a parent or guardian must also sign the consent form.

In summary, the issue of informed consent is of major significance for achieving the overall objectives in any research effort. Indeed, comprising a consent form which incorporates all of the above infomation is no miniscule task, but requires careful attention to protocol details and general research policy on human subjects. The patient who gives informed consent based on his working knowledge of the details of research procedure will be the more pleasant, cooperative participant.

D. PATIENT RECRUITMENT

Carefull study of the protocol affords the investigator information crucial to the patient recruitment effort. The inclusion-exclusion criteria set forth by the protocol succinctly defines the patient population for evaluation.

Research tactics employed by investigators in this country are many and varied, and a few of the more popular methods are appropriate to mention here

1. Begin by compiling a brief, descriptive summary of the protocol objectives.
2. Include a list of patient exclusions and circulate copies to appropriate health care facilities within the geographic area. (Examples of such facilities are general medical clinics in university health science centers, medical doctors in private practice, and centers of emergency care.)
3. When appropriate, it is often helpful to draft a recruitment letter for distribution to potential study candidates.
4. Exercise caution and discretion when recruiting patients who reside great distances from the research center, because time and travel money become obstacles for these patients and often the result is poor compliance in keeping appointments.
5. Recruitment often benefits when a computer bank of patients is available or if free screening for a specific disease such as hypertension is performed.

E. LABORATORY FACILITIES

All phases of clinical investigation entail some form of laboratory testing. Therefore, it is important that our discussion of study administration focuses momentarily on the subject of laboratory facilities. Clinical trials which are based in large hospitals or large clinics may utilize the facilities within the institution or patient samples may be sent to another "outside" laboratory. Many factors must be considered when weighing the pros and cons of using an "inside" vs. "outside" laboratory. For example, sample collection requires the purchase of materials such as urine containers, needles, vacuum tubes, Band-Aids®, alcohol swabs, and the like. As with everything else, these items may cost money which must be fed into the study budget. Private laboratories often supply these materials to the customer, but this is seldom the case with "in-house" laboratories, unless the samples are collected by laboratory personnel. Thus, the question arises as the most efficient means of collecting samples. Most investigators prefer that samples be collected by a member of their own research team, thereby circumventing problems which arise when nonteam members perform this task. Without strict adherence to the clinical protocol the entire project becomes of questionable validity.

A given laboratory's reputation for accuracy is another factor worthy of note. Both the investigator and the pharmaceutical sponsor should feel confident that the test results are accurate; the turnaround time for obtaining such results should certainly be no longer than a few days. Just how long samples are retained for purposes of rechecking questionable test results is another important point to ponder. Turnaround time lag for receiving results should not exceed the length of time samples are held. An illustration follows: the investigator draws the patient's blood sample on a Monday and receives the test results on Thursday afternoon: the laboratory receives the sample Tuesday morning, runs the test, and discards the sample 48 h later on Thursday morning. It is evident from this illustration that no opportunity exists for repeating the test, thereby causing a delay in the schedule of both patient and investigator when the patient must return to the clinic for a repeat of the test.

Clinical trials which are not conducted within the confines of a large health care delivery system present other problems when addressing the issue of laboratory facilities. The investigator must consider whether or not a given laboratory is comprehensive in its ability to perform all tests as required by a specific protocol. Patients become poor compliers when asked to report to several different locations for purposes of laboratory testing, especially when this may not be scheduled for a date other than the clinic visit appointment. Every effort should be made to coordinate clinic visits with laboratory testing.

III. THE STUDY PROPER

Thus far, our discussion of the administrative aspects of Phase III and Phase IV clinical drug trials has dealt with those aspects inherent to initiating the trial. Let us proceed now to areas of study administration which focus on the study proper.

Many investigators find that keeping an up-to-date patient listing functions as an accurate study progress report. Each patient is recorded in sequence of entry. The patient's initials, date of entry into the screening or pretreatment phase, the date on which the study drug is administered, study drug lot number or allocation number, and the patient's date of completion or date patient is aborted are facts essential to a comprehensive patient roster. Helpful also is a section for each participant which allows for miscellaneous comments should problems be encountered during the course of the clinical trial, e.g., adverse side effects and noncompliance.

Appointment scheduling is an aspect of study administration often treated with little respect. It is important that the study recorder schedule patients' visits in accordance with patients' work schedules. Discussing patient preferences at the outset and keeping time slots open for those patients expressing a desire to be seen at specific times is often helpful. For absent-minded patients, appointment reminders are frequently instrumental in improving patient attendance. One should stress the importance of keeping appointments and if necessary, telephone the tardy patient in an effort to maintain consistency in the daily clinic schedule.

A. COLLECTION OF BIOLOGICAL SPECIMENS

When a protocol requires fasting blood samples, this should be accomplished on a date other than the patient's regular clinical evaluation. A truly fasting sample demands that the patient consume nothing by mouth for a period of at least 8 to 12 h and, by definition, excludes study drug ingestion. Indeed, there exists the possibility that the test drug may interfere with the results. Again, the protocol provides the necessary guidelines for sample collection; strict adherence is mandatory.

Providing the patient with a printed instruction sheet explaining the laboratory testing schedule functions to eliminate guesswork and improve compliance. Should home specimen collections be involved, the necessary specimen containers should be supplied in advance.

Many protocols require blood sample collections at various stages throughout the study. The venipuncture experience wins no popularity contest with the participants, but most individuals accept blood drawing as a fact of life. Nevertheless, the research team member responsible for performing venipuncture must be an expert. A potentially stressful situation is easily alleviated when the participant has confidence in the individual performing venipuncture. This also applies to other laboratory tests which may cause discomfort for the patient.

B. RECORDING DATA

Data generated at each patient visit are recorded in the clinic chart and on the case report forms to facilitate recording data at the time of the patient's visit. This copy may then be filed in the clinic chart after the data are transcribed on the case report forms. Pharmaceutical companies occasionally require that the case report forms be typed, but, for those allowing the data to be handwritten, legibility is essential. The forms are proofread, signed, and dated by the investigator at his earliest convenience. It also follows that laboratory data should be accurately recorded as soon as such results become available.

Questionable lab results require verification by repeat testing, always taking care to be candid and honest with patients. If repeat testing reaffirms preexisting abnormalities, the investigator must then question and examine the patient to ascertain the etiology. For those abnormalities deemed to be of minor significance, the investigator should exercise discretion and may elect to keep the patient in the study while closely monitoring the lab values in question. When relationship to the test drug is not firmly established or when symptoms are present, further testing is indicated and the pharmaceutical sponsor is consulted to discuss all avenues of problem solving. Again, patient awareness of the situation is essential.

The accurate recording of all adverse clinical and laboratory events is paramount in all phases of drug development. The patient's assessment of the adverse experience is all important in determining the actual sequence of events and their relationship to the test agent. Therefore, it is helpful if the participant keep a log which affords information concerning signs, symptoms, date of onset, and duration of untoward side effects. He should be encouraged to discuss the problem with the investigator or other member(s) of the research team. Case report forms, of necessity, should reflect all events.

Determining a side effect relationship to the study drug is a most arduous task. Laboratory evaluation additional to those previously performed is of great assistance. Investigators must never hesitate to consult with other specialists whenever the complaint does not parallel their area of expertise. Whenever the investigator deems a positive correlation between side effects and study drug to exist, the patient may assist the investigator in determining the degree of discomfort of severity. The presence of a moderate to severe degree of discomfort necessitates removing the patient from the study. Another more conventional therapeutic is then prescribed. When the adverse experience does not greatly interfere with the patient's daily lifestyle, he is offered the option of continuing in the study, and the symptoms are treated to ensure maximum patient comfort and security. Clinical protocols outline the above procedure in greater detail and, to reiterate, strict adherence is mandatory to ensure patient safety and to achieve the general protocol objectives.

In the presence of a laboratory adverse experience unaccompanied by clinical signs and symptoms, the investigator must not overlook the possibility that the patient is taking other medications. Over-the-counter preparations are frequently the culprits and the patient must be questioned about this. Again, a patient diary may benefit such detective work. Determining whether or not the laboratory abnormality actually constitutes a study drug side effect and documenting such an event requires essentially the same procedure as mentioned in the previous discussion of adverse clinical events. Furthermore, severe adverse drug side effects mandate that open line of communication with the sponsor be maintained.

C. ADMINISTERING THE TEST MEDICATION

Pharmaceutical companies insist that all test medications be housed in locked cabinets or rooms which are locked to deny access by all except members of the research team. Additionally, maintenance of an accurate, up-to-date inventory is of great importance. Many pharmaceutical companies furnish tear-off labels which may be affixed to the case report forms; this system supplants the inventory sheet.

It is imperative that patients return all pill bottles at each visit. Many Phase III and Phase IV protocols, by design, require dispensation of new medication at each visit. Occassionally a patient may return only the pill bottle, leaving the test medication at home. Situations such as this are easily avoided by remembering to ask the individual to return all pills with the bottles.

Another salient point concerns study subjects who become lost to follow-up care. Every effort must be made to contact this person's family or a relative in an attempt to obtain the unused study medication. Case report forms should elucidate all details of the incident.

D. PILL COMPLIANCE

As previously discussed in this chapter, the evaluation of study drug efficacy is one of the principal objectives at the Phase III and Phase IV levels of clinical investigation. To achieve this end, many pharmaceutical companies require that pill counts be performed at each visit and duly recorded on the case report forms. Pill compliance may then be computed on the basis of the number of pills returned compared with the number dispensed. No accurate assessment of test drug efficacy can be accomplished if the patient fails to comply in taking his medication. Whenever pill counts are not mandatory, the conscientious investigator will accept this responsibility himself in the interest of generating reliable data. Furthermore, it is a fact that publications based on research data are of questionable validity if patient compliance determinations are ignored.

E. PATIENT DEATH

Protocols at all levels of clinical investigation set forth strict guidelines for reporting the death of a study participant. All circumstances surrounding the patient's demise must be conveyed to the drug sponsor within 24 h. Interviewing the patient's family frequently affords information concering the individual's general state of health prior to death; it is also important to determine if the deceased was medicated with drugs other than the test drug. If possible, an autopsy provides the most trustworthy information in the quest for the cause of death.

A full disclosure of all facts is appropriately recorded on the case report forms. The FDA also requires the completion of federal form number 1639 entitled "Drug Experience Report — In Confidence".

IV. STUDY CONCLUSION

Formulating plans for study termination becomes a painstaking task, especially if the clinical trial encompasses several years of investigation. Such arrangements are preferably mapped out in the early stages of the study in an attempt to, first and foremost, meet the needs of the patient and second, to authenticate the collection of all data.

Many investigators are cognizant of the sense of dependence a study patient experiences during the course of long-term study. Consider, for example, the indigent patients who, for 2 or perhaps even 3 years, are taken out of the hectic clinic atmosphere to participate in a clinical trial. For them, overcrowded waiting rooms and long hours of waiting become things of the past and the change is indeed refreshing. Therefore, it becomes the investigator's duty to prepare patients well in advance of the final visit. Discussing the various forms of medical therapy and allowing patients to participate in the selection of a conventional therapeutic agent are stratagems which often facilitate a smooth transition. Proper etiquette demands that the investigator express his gratitude to patients and reassure them that their follow-up care has been arranged. The investigator often is in a position that enables him to continue acting as the patient's primary physician. When this is not the situation, however, the investigator incurs the responsibility for assigning the patient to the care of another qualified physician, but the patient's choice of the physician should be honored whenever feasible.

The "separation anxiety" born of short-term clinical trials proves less traumatic for patients. Nevertheless, keeping the patient informed throughout the study with respect to the length of time remaining is of assistance in preparing the patient for the study's end. Again, the same courtesies afforded long-term study participants hold true for individuals completing short-term trials.

Following the collection of study data, the investigator and pharmaceutical representative meet to clarify details of study closure, as protocols are poor sources of information in this area.

Completing and submitting case report forms to the pharmaceutical sponsor constitutes one of the many steps to study closure. Original copies of these forms are accompanied by the completed patient assignment form. The FDA mandates that the investigator retain copies of these forms for a period of 2 years following study termination.[4] In addition, unused supplies and case report forms are returned to the sponsor.

All experimental medications, such as used and unused bottles, should be readied for shipment after an inventory has been effected. Occasionally, the pharmaceutical company prefers this task to be completed by their own personnel.

No clinical trial is concluded until a terminal financial statement is accomplished. The responsibility for initiating this action lies chiefly with the sponsor.

Statistical analysis of the study data customarily is performed by the pharmaceutical sponsor. There are occasions, however, when it is the investigator's desire to publish findings, particularly when a special project has been incorporated into the protocol. As stated in the previous section concerning the objectives of Phase IV protocols, such special undertakings often serve to expand and enhance the original protocol, thereby giving impetus to the evolution of new drug qualities.

REFERENCES

1. **Waife, S. O. and Shapiro, A. P.,** *The Clinical Evaluation of New Drugs,* Paul B. Hoeber, New York, 1959, 123.
2. **Ziegler, J. C.,** Clinical trial methodology, *Cancer Clin. Trials,* 89, 1978.
3. **Oberst, M. T.,** Research ethics. I. Randomized clinical trials, *Cancer Nursing,* 385, 1979.
4. Clinical Testing for Safe and Effective Drugs, Food and Drug Administration form 72-3014, Public Health Service, Food and Drug Administration, U.S. Department of Health, Education, and Welfare, Atlanta, September, 1971.
5. Drug Experience Report—In Confidence, Food and Drug Administration form 1639, Public Health Service, Food and Drug Administration, U.S. Department of Health, Education, and Welfare, Atlanta, October, 1979.

Chapter 16

MONITORING CLINICAL STUDIES

Winston Liao

TABLE OF CONTENTS

I. INTRODUCTION

As part of its emphasis on good quality assurance for clinical investigations, the FDA has published in the March 19, 1987 issue of *The Federal Register* its final rule on regulations governing the submission and review of investigational new drug applications (INDs). Contained in this document is an elaboration of the responsibilities of sponsors and investigators with respect to ensuring proper monitoring of the investigation(s). Based on this IND Rewrite, the following sections will address the primary issues involved in the monitoring of clinical studies, in particular, clinical trials.

II. RESPONSIBILITIES OF SPONSORS AND INVESTIGATORS

Prior to a discussion of the actual monitoring process, it is helpful at this point to emphasize the general responsibilities for sponsors of clinical studies as stated in the 1987 document:

Sponsors are responsible for selecting qualified investigators, providing them with the information they need to conduct an investigation properly, ensuring proper monitoring of the investigation(s), ensuring that the investigation(s) is conducted in accordance with the general investigational plan and protocols contained in the IND, maintaining an effective IND with respect to the investigations, and ensuring that FDA and all participating investigators are promptly informed of significant new adverse effects or risks with respect to the drug.

Because very often, the sponsor may contract out the conduct of a clinical trial to a third party such as a contract research organization, it is necessary for this latter group to be aware of its obligations, as designated by the sponsor of the study. Whether or not all or part of the sponsor's obligations are transferred to the third-party contractor, it is required that the transferred obligations be described in writing.

Other specific responsibilities of the sponsor are as follows:

1. Selecting investigators and monitors
2. Informing investigators
3. Review of ongoing investigations
4. Recordkeeping and record retention
5. Inspection of sponsor's records and reports
6. Disposition of unused supply of investigational drug

As the individual who will actually conduct the clinical study, the investigator is immediately responsible for administering the investigational drug to the study subject as well as for the welfare of the study subject. The general responsibilities are stated below.

An investigator is responsible for ensuring that an investigation is conducted according to the signed investigator statement, the investigational plan, and applicable regulations; for protecting the rights, safety, and welfare of subjects under the investigator's care; and for the control of drugs under investigation.

Other specific responsibilities of clinical investigators are as follows:

1. Control of the investigational drug
2. Investigator recordkeeping and record retention
3. Investigator reports
4. Assurance of IRB review
5. Inspection of investigator's records and reports
6. Handling of controlled substances

Given the above context for the responsibilities of the sponsors and investigators, the remainder of this chapter will address those areas relating to study monitoring.

III. STUDY MONITORING

As the party ultimately responsible for the conduct of the trial, the sponsor needs to be aware of all phases of the investigation beginning with prestudy preparation. This is an important aspect of study monitoring in that it outlines the overall project plan, including the specific monitoring procedures required. Among the activities of prestudy preparation are the selection of qualified (by training and experience) investigators to actually conduct the study and individuals to monitor the progress of the study; the outlining of the investigational plan, including a draft of the research protocol; the coordination of review and approval by appropriate institutional review boards (IRBs); and the drafting and compilation of study materials for the investigator(s). Central to these activities is the identification of key personnel who will be involved in the actual conduct of the trial in the clinical setting. This will help facilitate the monitoring process once the trial is initiated since it allows the study monitor to be familiar with clinic resources should problem resolution occur.

Prior to the investigator's participation in the trial, the monitor should conduct a preinvestigational visit with that investigator. While it is not necessary for the monitor to actually visit the clinic, it may be most convenient to do so in order to gain a comprehensive perspective of the physical and research environment. The primary purpose of such a visit is to assure that the investigator understands the investigational status of the drug, understands the nature of the protocol or investigational plan, and understands and accepts his obligations in conducting the clinical investigation in accordance with good clinical and research practices. At this time, the monitor should also ensure that the investigator and his staff have sufficient time and access to an adequate number of subjects to conduct the clinical investigation and to fulfill his obligations as an investigator.

In general, there are five major tasks that can be performed at this preinvestigational visit. The first involves verification of appropriate regulatory and IRB documents, including IRB approval, an IRB-approved informed consent form, and a signed investigator statement (form FDA-1572). Second, the monitor should confirm that the clinic has all the study materials, including the most current versions of the study protocol and case report forms (CRFs). Third, it is helpful to convene a protocol review meeting involving appropriate clinic personnel, including co-investigators, study management staff (for example, study coordinator, study nurse), data manager, and study pharmacist. This meeting would consist of a presentation by the monitor covering the following:

1. Brief explanation of the role of the contract research organization in the clinical trial
2. Explanation of how the clinical site will be monitored
3. Discussion of the methodological aspects of the trial, particularly the importance of patient follow up through study completion or as per protocol and the intention to treat rule
4. Review of the general study procedures: randomization (note if the study is placebo controlled), drug handling and accountability, data collection and transmission
5. Review of FDA regulations: informed consent, source documentation requirements
6. Review of adverse events reporting: what, how, when, and where to report
7. In-depth review of the study protocol, page by page, beginning with the background and objectives of the study, with emphasis on particular sections (such as inclusion and exclusion criteria, toxicity management, study discontinuation)
8. In-depth review of the CRFs, page by page, with reference to the CRF manual, when necessary, to clarify forms completion instructions and procedures

Fourth, the monitor should arrange for a tour of the clinic facilities and evaluate them accordingly. These areas include: the clinical area (note adequacy for patient management and privacy, ease of access, and patient record security); data collection area (note limited access for nonstudy personnel); pharmacy (note personnel with access to study drug(s) and drug codes/lists, drug handling and accountability procedures, and secured areas for drug storage); laboratories (note personnel for performing study-required lab tests, obtain lab normal values, and express need for updates as they occur); and other secured areas (such as CRF storage, consent form and patient files, and drug storage). Lastly, the monitor should clarify and discuss any general or specific study-related questions as well as note those that could be referred to the sponsor or to other resources at the contract research organization.

The monitor should maintain personal contact with the investigator by conducting periodic visits to the investigator at the clinical site. Meetings could be arranged with the investigator and his staff to assure continued acceptability of the facilities; adherence to the protocol; maintenance of adequate records; and submission of timely, adequate, and accurate reports by the investigator in support of the safety and/or effectiveness of the investigational drug. At these periodic visits, it is also prudent to conduct an audit of the following items:

1. IRB approval and correspondence
2. Availability of study records (such as form FDA-1572, protocol, protocol modifications, and CRFs)
3. Modifications to the protocol made by the investigator or the sponsor
4. Appropriately signed informed consent forms
5. Drug storage and accountability
6. Adequacy of facilities (note any changes since preinvestigational visit)
7. Adverse events reporting
8. Disposition of unused study materials (including study drug)
9. Source documents.

As part of the quality assurance plan for the trial, it is also necessary to conduct a review of selected patient records (including a 100% sample review depending on the phase and progression of the clinical trial). Comparisons are made between key items on the CRFs and source documents (usually the investigator's patient records or the hospital/clinic charts). Examples of such items are

1. Date the informed consent form was signed (should be prior to study start date)
2. Date the patient was entered (or randomized) into the study
3. Screening criteria or criteria for enrollment
4. Diagnoses
5. Concurrent illnesses
6. Administration of the investigational drug (including dose and frequency)
7. Concomitant medications
8. Laboratory results
9. Adverse events recorded
10. Any unreported adverse events
11. Raw data agreement with the CRF

It is during this activity that the monitor may be able to identify problems and concerns relating to the proper completion of the CRFs. Underlying this is the assurance that there is a clearly defined data-audit trail which will lead to complete and accurate resolution of all data problems which may occur during the course of the clinical investigation.

While there is no minimum standard for the frequency of such periodic visits, the monitor should be aware that the frequency should be sufficient to ensure that the obligations of the investigator are being fulfilled. However, the monitor should always prepare and maintain complete records of these visits. These records should include: the date(s) of the visit; name of the monitor; name and address of the investigator visited; a summary of the factual findings; and a statement concerning any actions taken to correct deficiencies noted during the visit. It is most important that the monitor be available for consultation at the request of the investigator and to serve as liaison and communication link between the sponsor and the investigator.

Although the site visit is a crucial component of the overall study monitoring process, internal monitoring at the contract research organization is also important. This involves proper training of all study-related personnel, including both the medical and data management staff. Familiarity with the protocol and CRFs on the part of the medical staff is critical to the interpretation of these documents by both the monitor and the clinic personnel. Additionally, the "in-house" data management staff will benefit from the clear and uniform interpretation of the protocol by the medical and monitoring staff in the processing of all incoming data from the clinic.

Internal monitoring may also be an activity conducted by either the monitor and/or data management staff with respect to regular review of selected key parameters of the study. These may include definition and verification of entry and exclusion criteria, stratification variables, dosing calculations, diagnoses and symptoms, deaths, and study terminations. A study management system may be established in order to track delinquent forms, problems forms, and/or duplicate forms. Resolution of study issues and problems through frequent communications with all parties involved in the clinical investigation is also of paramount importance and coordinated by the monitor.

IV. SUMMARY

Monitoring clinical studies is an activity that is associated with quality assurance, whether it deals with good clinical practices or good investigational methods. In part it is an assessment of the overall conduct of the clinical investigation with respect to patient management within a clinical research setting, adherence to the study protocol, and compliance with study procedures. Study monitoring is also the establishment of quality control for the complete and accurate documentation of study data, thus ensuring the integrity of the entire study. When both the sponsor and the investigator are fully cognizant of their responsibilities and obligations, then the role of the monitor in monitoring the progress of the study is clearly defined, allowing for the careful and responsible conduct of the clinical investigation.

Chapter 17

PREPARING THE NEW DRUG APPLICATION

Robert A. Paarlberg

TABLE OF CONTENTS

I. INTRODUCTION

The New Drug Application (NDA) is a document which is submitted by the sponsor (applicant) requesting FDA approval to market, via interstate commerce, a new drug for human use. The NDA contains data to show that the drug is safe and efficacious for the intended population. Basically, the NDA is prepared to support the statements in the proposed package insert. The NDA is comparable to a Product License Application for biologics or a Premarket Approval Application for devices.

Major milestones have occurred since the Food and Drugs Act of 1906 was passed:

- Federal Food, Drug, and Cosmetic Act of 1938
- Kefauver-Harris Drug Amendments in 1962
- Revision of NDA regulations in 1985

This chapter will focus on preparation of the NDA as it pertains to the revised NDA regulations of 1985. These revised regulations are also referred to as the "NDA Rewrite".

A. NDA REWRITE

The revised NDA regulations were first issued for comment in the *Federal Register* on October 19, 1982. In the preamble of the final rule which issued on February 22, 1985, the FDA responded to over 140 comments from industry, trade associations, health professionals, consumers, professional societies, and Congress.[1]

The objectives of the NDA Rewrite were to:

1. Reduce administrative delays in NDA review by permitting concurrent reviews
2. Ensure that the safety information in an NDA is fully updated before approval
3. Reduce some of the documentation contained in an NDA

B. FDA GUIDELINES

In concert with the NDA Rewrite, the FDA issued a series of content and format guidelines to assist applicants in preparing an NDA. A list of these guidelines is given in Table 1.

TABLE 1
FDA Guidelines

Guideline for the Format and Content of the Summary for New Drug and Antibiotic Applications, February 1987.

Guideline on Formatting, Assembling, and Submitting New Drug and Antibiotic Applications, February 1987.

Guideline for the Submission in Microfiche of the Archival Copy of an Application, February 1987.

Guideline for the Format and Content of the Human Pharmacokinetics and Bioavailability Section of an Application, February 1987.

Guideline for the Format and Content of the Nonclinical Pharmacology/Toxicology Section of an Application, February 1987.

Guideline for the Format and Content of the Chemistry, Manufacturing and Controls Section of an Application, February 1987.

- Guideline for Submitting Documentation for Packaging for Human Drugs and Biologics, February 1987.
- Guideline for Submitting Documentation for the Manufacture of and Controls for Drug Products, February 1987.
- Guideline for Submitting Supporting Documentation in Drug Applications for the Manufacture of Drug Substances, February 1987.
- Guideline for Submitting Documentation for the Stability of Human Drugs and Biologics, February 1987.
- Guideline for Submitting Samples and Analytical Data for Methods Validation, February 1987.

Guideline for the Format and Content of the Microbiology Section of an Application, February 1987.

Guideline for the Format and Content of the Clinical and Statistical Sections of New Drug Applications, July 1988.

The applicant should become very familiar with these guidelines early in the drug development process. Many of the guidelines provide examples of the formats to be used in the NDA. The introduction in the guidelines states "An applicant may, but is not required to, rely upon the guideline ... When a different approach is chosen, the applicant is encouraged to discuss the matter in advance with FDA to prevent the expenditure of money and effort on preparing a submission that may be determined to be unacceptable."

C. NDA TEAM
Since the NDA is the final product of the drug development process, preparation of the NDA should be the focus of all advance planning. The NDA Rewrite makes planning and coordination among various divisions within a company a necessity. The regulations now require that the various technical data be integrated into the NDA. Early proactive planning can prevent the submission of an inadequate NDA which the FDA may reject.

Because of the high degree of coordination needed within a company in preparing the NDA, the formation of an NDA team can facilitate this preparation. Members of the team would normally include representatives from regulatory, project management, clinical, control, manufacturing, drug experience, pathology/toxicology, pharmacology, biopharmaceutics, biostatistics, and medical writers (Figure 1). Representation is dependent upon the corporate structure and philosophy. Such a team would provide a forum to discuss format and content issues, data presentation, target dates, etc. The team should be aware that the NDA is a document which is written to support the statements contained in the proposed package insert (Section III. E).

It is imperative that one person or group be responsible for the coordination and assembly of the NDA. Usually this function is coordinated by the regulatory affairs department. It is helpful if the coordinator issues a "working outline" to the NDA team, which delineates the information which will be required in the NDA. The outline should also note which unit/person is responsible

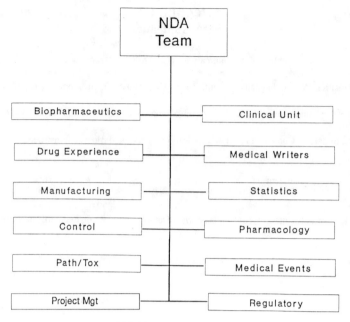

FIGURE 1. The NDA team.

for supplying the information. The outline can also be utilized in developing the comprehensive index for the NDA.

D. FDA INPUT

Input from the FDA is very crucial in the preparation of the NDA. This input can come from an end-of-Phase II conference, meetings with individual reviewers, an Advisory Committee meeting, or from the pre-NDA meeting (Section V). Any agreements or recommendations reached at any of these meetings should be documented in the appropriate section(s) of the NDA.

II. RESOURCES

In addition to the technical considerations, assembly of the NDA also requires logistical considerations. These considerations include room size, pagination equipment, and photocopying facilities.

A. ROOM SIZE

Usually, the information for the NDA arrives in "pieces". Consequently, one should have a room that can be secured and dedicated to the assembly of the NDA. Access to this room should also be limited so that the individual responsible for assembly is aware of incoming information and if any information is removed. Given the fact that NDA for new molecular entities can be 400 to 600 volumes, which equates to 160,000 to 240,000 pages, the room should provide adequate space.

B. PAGINATION EQUIPMENT

Any method for pagination can be used as long as it permits rapid access to the entire application.[2] The important phrase is "permits rapid access to the *entire* application". Hand-operated or electric "stampers" can be used. Pagination is not a trivial task; pagination on large NDAs can take as long as 2 weeks utilizing three to four people every day. It is important to consider this function in the planning matrix for the NDA.

Although the location of the "numbering scheme" is not specified in the guideline, the numbering should be placed either at the top or bottom of the page, free from any other numbering on the page. I have found it useful to number pages by item number, volume number (within the technical section), and page number (e.g., 7 1/001 = item 7, volume 1 of item 7, page 1). The page number of each volume within the technical section would start at one. The numbering scheme, however, should not be so complicated as to make it difficult for the reviewer. The other contributing areas in the company should be informed where the numbering will be located so that they do not place anything in that area. It is also important that the ink for the numbers be black or some other color which can be easily photocopied.

For large applications, one will probably have to paginate sections of the NDA as they become available. Consequently, it is imperative that one have the index (table of contents) fairly complete before proceeding to paginate.

This system of numbering minimizes pagination from being on the critical path. Upon completion of all the items of the NDA, all the volumes are numbered sequentially and the comprehensive index finalized.

C. MICROFICHE

The guidelines provide for submission of the application on microfiche; however, the reviewing division at the FDA should be consulted prior to pursuing this effort. Due to the advent of the computer-assisted submissions (Section VIII), I do not foresee microfiche being pursued by many companies.

D. PHOTOCOPYING

The applicant must have access to either a dedicated photocopier or use of a central copy center. The individuals in the photocopying center should be alerted to the amount of material needed to be copied and the expected due dates. It is also advisable that the photocopying be done in the same building in order to eliminate copies "lost in the mail".

E. VOLUME SIZE

The guidelines require that the thickness of a volume not exceed 2 in. (approximately 400 pages).[3] Applicants submitting more than 50 volumes may obtain a preassigned NDA number by contacting the Central Document Room of the FDA, Rockville, MD (301-443-0035). The Central Document Room should also be notified in advance of any large submissions.

F. NDA JACKETS

In order to facilitate review by the FDA, the guidelines require that the archival and review copies of the NDA be bound in color-coded jackets as follows:

	Color	Form number
Archival copy	Blue	FDA 2626
Review copy		
Chemistry, manufacturing, and controls	Red	FDA 2626a
Nonclinical pharmacology and toxicology	Yellow	FDA 2626b
Human pharmacokinetics and bioavailability	Orange	FDA 2626c

	Color	**Form number**
Microbiology	White	FDA 2626d
Clinical	Light brown	FDA 2626e
Statistical	Green	FDA 2626f

The NDA jackets are sent free of charge from the FDA (Forms and Publications Distribution [HFA-268], 12100 Parklawn Drive, Rockville, MD 20852). Requests should be in writing and specify the color, FDA form number, and quantity requested. Ordering of the jackets should be done well in advance of any submissions.

G. SHIPPING

The exterior of the packing carton should identify the drug name, the applicant's name, and the volume numbers. The packing carton should also identify which boxes contain the archival and review copies. The FDA recommends using boxes measuring $14 \times 12 \times 9\frac{1}{2}$ in. The applicant may wish to personally deliver the NDA to the FDA.

Full application submissions should be sent to:

Food and Drug Administration
Central Document Room
Park Building, Room 214
12420 Parklawn Drive
Rockville, MD 20852

III. THE NDA

The NDA is an official document described in the U.S. Code of Federal Regulations (CFR), Title 21, Part 314. The regulations concerning the content and format of the NDA are found in §314.50.

For a new molecular entity (NME), the regulations state that the NDA should contain the following items:

- Signed form FDA 356h
- Index
- Summary
- Technical sections
    Chemistry, manufacturing, and control
    Nonclinical pharmacology and toxicology
    Human pharmacokinetics
    Microbiology (for antibiotic drugs only)
    Clinical
    Statistical
- Samples and labeling
- Case report tabulations
- Case report forms
- Patent information

The relationship of the technical sections to the remainder of the NDA is depicted in Figure 2. The regulations require that two copies of the NDA be submitted: an archival copy and a

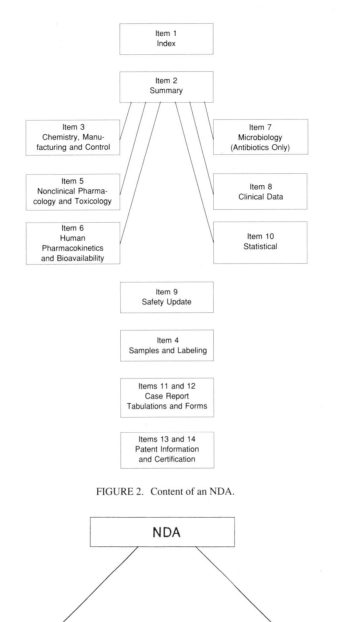

FIGURE 2. Content of an NDA.

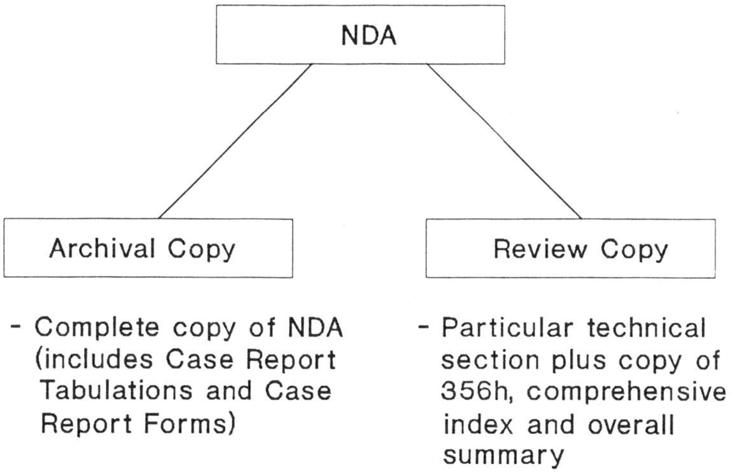

FIGURE 3. Contents of archival and review copies.

review copy. Each of these copies should be bound separately. The archival copy includes case report forms and tabulations, whereas the review copy does not include these items (Figure 3).

The review copy contains copies of the application form FDA 356h, cover letter, comprehensive index, overall summary, and particular technical section. The review copies are distributed to the individual reviewers within the agency, thus permitting concurrent reviews to occur.

The archival copy is the FDA's official file copy. During the review of the NDA, it serves as a reference source for agency reviewers. After the NDA is approved, the archival copy is retained by the agency as the official copy.[4]

A. APPLICATION FORM FDA 356h [21CFR§314.50(a)]

Every NDA must contain a signed application form. The FDA 356h form provides the basic information on the applicant and drug product. The signed form also obligates the applicant to comply with applicable laws and regulations.

The applicant is required to list on the form all Investigational New Drug Applications (INDs), NDAs or Drug Master Files (DMFs) which are referenced in the application. One should include the type of document; document number; title; document holder; and volume, pages, dates, etc.

The patent information and patent certification on the drug should be submitted on separate pages and attached to the application form (Sections III.N and III.O). The patent information and patent certification in an NDA need to be updated as appropriate for new patent numbers and exclusivity claims.

B. COMPREHENSIVE INDEX [21CFR§314.50(b)]

Every application is required to contain a comprehensive index (by volume and page number) of the overall summary, review sections, and to any supporting documentation. The comprehensive index provides a "road map" to the entire NDA for the reviewers.

As previously noted, the review copy for a specific technical section (e.g., chemistry, manufacturing and control, CMC) contains the particular technical section, comprehensive index, and overall summary. With the aid of the comprehensive index, a reviewer can request additional information from the archival copy.

C. ITEM 2— SUMMARY [21CFR§314.50(c)]

As noted in the preamble to the NDA Rewrite regulations, the summary is intended to facilitate review of the application. If a more complete summary is needed for review purposes, it should be included in the appropriate technical section.[5] The summary (also referred to as the overall summary) should be contained in one volume and is ordinarily 50 to 200 pages in length.

Each of the technical sections contains a copy of the summary volume. The summary volume is the most widely read document in the NDA and provides a crucial link to the remainder of the NDA. The summary can be used to brief advisory committee members or used to prepare the Summary Basis of Approval.

The summary "... integrates all the information in the NDA and provides reviewers in each review area, and other agency officials, with a good general understanding of the drug product and of the application. The summary should discuss all aspects of the application and should be written in approximately the same level of detail required for publication in, and meet the editorial standards generally applied by, refereed scientific and medical journals. In addition to the agency personnel who will use the summary in the context of their review of the application, advisory committee members may be furnished the summary. To the extent possible, data in the summary should be presented in tabular and graphic forms ...."[6]

The summary volume should contain a statement on the pharmacologic class, discussion of the scientific rationale, intended use and clinical benefits, foreign marketing history of the drug, summary of the technical sections, and a final discussion of benefit-to-risk considerations. Any proposed postmarketing studies should also be discussed.

The summary volume is also required to contain an annotated copy of the proposed package insert, with the annotations citing the data (volume and page number) contained in the summary volume and technical sections. It is important to remember that the purpose of the NDA is to support the statements contained in the package insert.

D. ITEM 3 — CHEMISTRY, MANUFACTURING, AND CONTROL [21CFR§314.50(d)(1)]

The method of synthesis, the testing of raw materials and finished dosage forms, the proposed packaging components, and the stability reports are specific for the new drug substance, drug product, and packaging configurations proposed in the NDA. It is essential that corporate management make a definite commitment to a manufacturing formula and dosage form early in the development of the product. The Phase III clinical studies should be conducted with the final dosage form.

In order to expedite the review of the application, the NDA Rewrite provides that the CMC section can be submitted 90 to 120 days before the anticipated submission of the remainder of the NDA. The applicant should check with the particular reviewing division before pursuing this option.

The CMC section is divided into three subsections:

- Drug substance
- Drug product
- Environmental impact

Drug substance — This section should provide a full description of the drug substance including:

- Physical and chemical characteristics and stability
- Names, structural formula, physical/chemical characteristics, elucidation of structure, and stability information
- Name and address of the manufacturer
- Materials and methods used in the synthesis (or isolation) and purification
- Process controls used during manufacture and packaging
- Characteristics and test methods for the container/closure system (only if shipped)
- Specifications and analytical methods necessary to assure the identity, strength, quality, and purity of the drug substance and the bioavailability of the drug product made from the drug substance
- A copy of the specifications and analytical methods should also be included in each of the four copies of the methods validation package (Section III.E)
- Relationship of solid-state drug substance forms to bioavailability

The applicant may also provide for the use of alternative sources, process controls, methods, and specifications. Reference to the current edition of the *U.S. Pharmacopeia* and the *National Formulary* may satisfy the requirements in this section.

Drug product— Information should be provided on:

- Components used in the manufacture of the drug product
- Composition of drug product
- Specifications and analytical methods for inactive components
- Name and address of each manufacturer of the drug product
- Manufacturing procedures and in-process controls for the drug product
- Characteristics and test methods for the container/closure system

- Specifications and analytical methods necessary to assure the identity, strength, quality, purity, and bioavailability of the drug product
- Stability data and proposed expiration dating

In addition to the information on the investigational formulations required by the guideline,[7] some reviewers have found it helpful if the applicant also includes the protocol numbers and lot numbers used in the investigational studies.

As with the drug substance, the applicant may provide for alternate components, manufacturing and packaging procedures, in-process controls, methods, and specifications. Reference to the current edition of the *U.S. Pharmacopeia* and the *National Formulary* may satisfy the requirements in this section.

Environmental impact — The applicant is required either to claim a categorical exclusion under 21CFR§25.24 or an environmental impact assessment under 21CFR§25.31 concerning the production, distribution, or disposal of any of the ingredients or the drug product itself.

The CMC section should also contain copies of the methods validation package and labeling (Section III.E).

E. ITEM 4 — SAMPLES AND LABELING [21CFR§314.50(e)]
1. Samples

The applicant submits samples at the request of the FDA. These samples are usually submitted directly to the FDA laboratories for analytical methods validation and testing.

Four representative samples are submitted; each sample has sufficient quantity to permit the laboratory to conduct the test three times. The following samples are submitted:

- Drug product
- Drug substance
- Reference standards and special reagents (except those reference standards recognized in an official compendium)

Samples of the finished market package are also requested by the reviewing division at the FDA.

The regulations specify that three copies of the analytical methods and related descriptive information (methods validation package) contained in the CMC section (Section III.D) be included in the archival copy. The guideline, however, notes that in the interest of expediting the methods validation process, the applicant is requested instead to include one copy of the methods validation package in the archival copy and three additional copies with the CMC section.[13] A statement that this option has been followed should be included in the archival copy.

The methods validation package should consist of photocopies from various pertinent sections of the NDA and retain the original pagination of the sections from which the photocopies were taken.[14] The related descriptive information includes a description of each sample; the proposed regulatory specifications for the drug; a detailed description of the methods of analysis; supporting data for accuracy, specificity, precision, and ruggedness; and complete results of the applicant's tests on the sample.

2. Labeling

The package insert is a compilation of the pertinent scientific and medical information about the drug. This document, which serves as a regulatory basis for all labeling and advertising, is a summary of the essential information that a medical professional needs in order to use the drug safely and effectively for the intended purpose.

The term "labeling" includes all information on or accompanying a drug product. The more restrictive term "label" refers to the information on the immediate container, carton, or on the shelf carton.

The package insert must meet the general requirements of 21CFR§201.56 and must contain the information in the format as specified in 21CFR§201.57:

- Description
- Clinical Pharmacology
- Indications and Usage
- Contraindications
- Warnings
- Precautions
- Adverse Reactions
- Drug Abuse and Dependence
- Overdosage
- Dosage and Administration
- How Supplied

Other sections which may be included are

- Animal Pharmacology and/or Animal Toxicology
- Clinical Studies
- References

Because the NDA is a document written to support the package insert, it is imperative that the appropriate groups within a company (e.g., marketing, medical, and regulatory) agree to the wording of the proposed insert before technical summaries are prepared. Early agreement will provide for a more consistently written document.

Labeling requirements for prescription and nonprescription drug products include the label requirements of the Fair Packaging and Labeling Act (21CFR§201.60, 61, 62, and 63); the requirements of the Drug Listing Act as they relate to the display of the National Drug Code (21CFR§207.35); the requirements for expiry dating and storage conditions as promulgated in the Good Manufacturing Practices regulations (21CFR, Part 211); and the statement of ingredients, lot number, proprietary/established names, and identification of the manufacturer, packer, or distributor as specified in 21CFR§201.10.

The applicant is required to include copies of the label and all labeling for the product (4 copies of the draft labeling; 12 copies of the final printed labeling). A copy of the labeling should also be included in the CMC section (Section III.D). Of the 12 final printed copies, usually 7 are individually mounted on $8^{1}/_{2} \times 11$-in. heavy-weight paper with the remainder of the copies enclosed in an envelope.

F. ITEM 5 — NONCLINICAL PHARMACOLOGY AND TOXICOLOGY [21CFR§314.50(d)(2)]

The NDA Rewrite requires that this section include a discussion on:

1. Studies on the pharmacological actions of the drug in relation to its proposed therapeutic indication and studies that otherwise define the pharmacologic properties of the drug or are pertinent to possible adverse effects
2. Studies of the toxicological effects of the drug as they relate to its intended clinical uses, including, as appropriate, studies assessing the acute, subacute, and chronic toxicity; carcinogenicity and mutagenicity; and studies of toxicities related to its particular mode of administration or condition of use

3. Studies, as appropriate, of the effects of the drug on reproduction and on the developing fetus
4. Any studies of the absorption, distribution, metabolism, and excretion of the drug in animals
5. For each nonclinical laboratory study, a statement that it was conducted in compliance with the Good Laboratory Practice regulations, or if not in compliance, a statement of the reason for the noncompliance

Most of the nonclinical data will have been previously submitted to the IND. For submission to the NDA and in order to facilitate NDA review, the FDA recommends reorganization, to the extent feasible, of the studies in accordance to the February 1987 "Guideline for the Format and Content of the Nonclinical Pharmacology/Toxicology Section". Formats of individual studies which were completed years before the issuance of the guideline cannot always easily be brought into conformance with the guideline. For this reason, consideration should be given to incorporating the recommendations in the guideline in future IND submissions of nonclinical studies.

Several general principles apply to submission of all pharmacology and toxicology studies:[8]

1. The entire submission should receive careful editorial and scientific review.
2. Standard abbreviations acceptable to a refereed pharmacology/toxicology journal should be used.
3. Data should be kept available by the applicant.
4. Tables and graphs should be used in reporting and evaluating the data. Tables should be appropriately identified; graphs should supplement data tables.
5. Drug code numbers should be highlighted; metabolites or reference compounds referred to by code numbers should be identified by chemical name or structure in a nearby location. Batch or lot numbers should be included where appropriate.
6. Where more than one animal species is used, the data should be presented in a specified order.
7. Studies for each species should first represent the intended route of human use followed by data for other routes.
8. In multidose studies, data should be presented in a specified order based on dose level, using specified dosage units.
9. All biological tests, laboratory determinations, and statistical methods should be described in the study report or properly referenced.
10. Drug safety study reports should contain Good Laboratory Practice statements.
11. New studies or studies not previously submitted to an IND or previous marketing application should be identified.
12. Pertinent published literature should be appended to the appropriate report or section of the application.
13. A contact person should be identified should the FDA have any questions about the data in this section.

Rather than submit studies on a chronological basis, studies should be submitted in the following order:

*   Pharmacology
*   Acute toxicity
*   Multidose toxicity (subchronic, chronic, carcinogenicity)
*   Special toxicity
*   Reproduction

- Mutagenicity
- Absorption, distribution, metabolism, excretion

G. ITEM 6 — HUMAN PHARMACOKINETICS AND BIOAVAILABILITY [21CFR§314.50(d)(3)]

This section of the NDA describes the human pharmacokinetic data and human bioavailability data. In lieu of the data, the applicant may supply information supporting a waiver of the submission of *in vivo* bioavailability data under 21CFR§320.22.

Five general types of studies are included in this section:[9]

- Pilot or background studies
- Bioavailability/bioequivalence studies
- Pharmacokinetic studies
- Other *in vivo* studies
- *In vitro* studies

The format for this section includes several tabular presentations:

- Overall comprehensive summary by study type
- Summary of all bioavailability/pharmacokinetic data and overall conclusions
- List of all formulations used in the clinical trials and *in vivo* bioavailability/pharmacokinetic studies (any significant or formulation changes for the drug product during the development period should be identified)
- Summary of the analytical method employed in each *in vivo* biopharmaceutic study
- Summary of the dissolution performance of the product
- Summary of the dissolution method and specification proposed
- Data presentations for each study report

In addition, each study report should provide documentation of the sensitivity, linearity, specificity, and reproducibility of the analytical method, including sample chromatograms, recovery studies, etc. Data analyses should include appropriate statistical analyses. Details of pharmacokinetic parameter calculations, including pharmacokinetic models and equations, should also be described and referenced.

Each study report should also contain a brief paragraph summarizing the pertinent conclusions; a statement that the study was conducted in compliance with the institutional review board regulations (21CFR, Part 56), or was not subject to the regulations; and a statement that the study was conducted in compliance with the informed consent regulations (21CFR, Part 50).

If the CMC section (Section III.D) contains specifications or analytical methods needed to assure the bioavailability of the drug product or drug substance, or both, a statement is needed in this section noting the rationale for establishing the specification or analytical methods, including data supporting the rationale.

The applicant should also provide a summary discussion and analysis of the pharmacokinetics and metabolism of the active ingredients and the bioavailability or bioequivalence, or both, of the drug product.

H. ITEM 7 — MICROBIOLOGY [21CFR§314.50(d)(4)]

The applicant must complete this section if the product is an anti-infective agent. The regulations require that microbiological data be submitted describing:

- Biological basis of the action of the drug on microbial physiology
- Antimicrobial spectra of the drug, including results of *in vivo* preclinical studies to demonstrate drug concentrations required for efficacy

- Any known mechanisms of resistance to the drug, including results of known epidemiologic studies to demonstrate prevalence of resistance factors
- Clinical microbiology laboratory methods needed to evaluate effective use of the drug

In preparing this section, the applicant should provide the following information:[10]

- Mechanism of action
- Pharmacokinetics
- Antimicrobial activity
- Enzyme hydrolysis rates
- Miscellaneous studies
- Assessment of resistance
- Clinical laboratory susceptibility test methods
- *In vivo* animal protection studies
- *In vitro* studies conducted during clinical trials
- Conclusions
- Published literature

I. ITEM 8 — CLINICAL [21CFR§314.50(d)(5)]

In July 1988, the FDA issued a final guideline for both the Clinical and Statistical sections. Several principles form the basis of this guideline:[11]

- It is important to distinguish presentation of data from the subsequent evaluation, interpretation, and analysis of those data.
- Interrelationships among data from different studies should be examined; i.e., studies cannot be considered only in isolation.
- Studies reported in the literature should be incorporated into appropriate sections of the submission.
- For most analyses, tabular listings, not case report forms, are the "raw data".
- The data base behind a table or figure must be readily ascertained.

For the Clinical section, the applicant should include the following information:

1. A description and analysis of each clinical pharmacology study, including a brief comparison of the results of the human studies with the animal pharmacology and toxicology data should be included.
2. A description and analysis of each controlled clinical study pertinent to the proposed use of the drug, including the protocol and a description of the statistical analyses used to evaluate the study; if the study report is an interim analysis, this must be noted and a projected completion date given. Controlled clinical studies that have not been analyzed in detail for any reason should be included in this section, including a copy of the protocol and a brief description of the results and the status of the study.
3. Include a description of each uncontrolled clinical study, a summary of the results, and a brief statement explaining why the study is classified as uncontrolled.
4. Include a description and analysis of any other data or information relevant to an evaluation of the safety and effectiveness of the drug product obtained or otherwise received by the applicant from any domestic or foreign source. This would include information from clinical investigations (controlled and uncontrolled) of studies of uses of the drug other than those proposed in the NDA, commercial marketing experience, reports in the scientific literature, and unpublished scientific papers.
5. Include an Integrated Summary of Effectiveness describing the data demonstrating

substantial effectiveness for the claimed indication(s). Evidence is also required to support the dosage and administration section of the proposed package insert, including support for the dosage and dose interval recommended, and modifications for specific subgroups.

6. Include an Integrated Summary of Safety describing all available information on the safety of the drug product, including pertinent animal data, demonstrated or potential adverse effects of the drug, clinically significant drug/drug interactions, and other safety considerations, such as data from epidemiological studies of related drugs.

7. Safety update reports (Section III.J) are to be submitted 4 months after the initial submission, following receipt of the approvable letter, and at other times requested by the FDA.

8. If the drug has the potential for abuse, a description and analysis of studies or information related to abuse of the drug, including a proposal for scheduling under the Controlled Substances Act. A description of any studies related to overdosage is also required, including information on dialysis, antidotes, or other treatments, if known.

9. Include an Integrated Summary of the Benefits and Risks of the drug, including a discussion of why the benefits exceed the risks under the conditions stated in the proposed labeling.

10. Include a statement that each clinical study was or was not in conformance with the institutional review board regulations (21CFR, Part 56) and the informed consent regulations (21CFR, Part 50).

11. If the applicant has transferred any obligations for the conduct of the clinical study to a contract research organization, include a statement containing identifying information for the research organization.

12. If the original subject records were audited or reviewed by the applicant in the course of monitoring any clinical study to verify the accuracy of the case reports, a list should be submitted identifying each clinical study audited or reviewed.

The clinical and statistical descriptions, presentations, and analyses are integrated into a single report. This report incorporates tables and figures into the main text, or at the end of the text; the appendices should contain the protocol, investigator information, related publications, patient data listings, and technical statistical details (e.g., computations, analyses). The integrated full report should not be derived by simply attaching a separate statistical report to the clinical report.[12]

J. ITEM 9 — SAFETY UPDATES [21CFR§314.50(d)(5)(vi)(b)]

Safety updates provide the vehicle by which the FDA is updated on the safety of the drug product following submission of the NDA. New safety information learned about the drug that may reasonably affect the statement of contraindications, warnings, precautions, and adverse reactions in the proposed insert should be included in the update.

The new safety information can arise from clinical studies, animal studies, or from other sources. Case reports are to be included for each patient who died during a clinical study or who did not complete the study because of a medical event. Planning matrices should allow for adequate resources for this activity as it can involve a considerable amount of time and personnel.

Safety update reports are required 4 months after the initial submission of the NDA; following receipt of an approvable letter; and at other times as requested by the FDA.

Prior to submitting the first safety update, the applicant should consult with the appropriate reviewing division at the FDA for details on the timing, content, and format of the report. In some cases, FDA reviewers have not wanted the 4-month update.

TABLE 2
Clinical and Statistical Sections

	Clinical	Statistical
List of investigators, list of INDs and NDAs	Yes	Yes
Background/overview of clinical investigations	Yes	Yes
Clinical pharmacology studies	Yes	No
Controlled clinical studies	Yes	Yes
Uncontrolled clinical studies	Yes	No
Other studies	Yes	No
Integrated summary of effectiveness	Yes	Yes
Integrated summary of safety data	Yes	Yes
Drug abuse and overdosage	Yes	No
Integrated summary of benefits and risks	Yes	Yes

K. ITEM 10 — STATISTICAL [21CFR§314.50(d)(6)]
The Statistical section should include:

1. A copy of the information regarding the description and analyses of each controlled study from the Clinical section along with the documentation and supporting statistical analyses used in the evaluation
2. A copy of the Integrated Summary of Safety as included in the Clinical section along with the documentation and supporting statistical analyses used in the evaluation
3. A copy of the Integrated Summary of Effectiveness as included in the Clinical section
4. A copy of the Integrated Summary of Benefits and Risks as included in the Clinical section

In addition, the Statistical section should contain a list of investigators and background/ overview of the clinical investigations.

Table 2 summarizes the information required in the Clinical and Statistical sections.

L. ITEM 11 — CASE REPORT TABULATIONS [21CFR§314.50(f)(1)]
The archival copy of the NDA is required to contain tabulations of the data from the clinical studies. The tabulations are required to include the data on each patient in each study unless the FDA has previously agreed that certain tabulations are not pertinent to the review of the safety or efficacy of the drug.

Case report tabulations are distinct from and more extensive than the tabulations of individual patient data called for as parts of the full reports of controlled clinical studies and the safety portions of reports of all studies. These case report tabulations contain, in an organized fashion, essentially all data collected in the case report. These data include:[15]

1. Effectiveness data from adequate and well-controlled trials, including all measurements made (Phase II and Phase III)
2. Data from clinical pharmacology studies (Phase I)
3. Safety data (observations, adverse events, and laboratory data from all studies)

The FDA has substituted tabulations for case report forms as the primary focus of data review. The FDA estimates that the tabulations will result in a reduction of about 75% in the number of case reports that are routinely requested, when compared to the previous requirement of full submission of case report forms.[16]

Case report tabulations may be submitted on microfiche only if the reviewing division at the FDA and the applicant agree.

M. ITEM 12 — CASE REPORT FORMS [21CFR§314.50(f)(2)]

Prior to the NDA Rewrite, the applicant needed to submit all of the case report forms. In most cases, this amounted to several thousand pages.

Since case report tabulations are submitted, the applicant is now required to submit only copies of case report forms for each patient who died during a clinical study or who did not complete the study because of an adverse event, whether or not the death or adverse event was drug related. This requirement also applies to patients receiving reference drugs or placebo.

During the course of the review, the FDA reviewing division may request additional case reports and tabulations. Failure to submit the information requested by the FDA within 30 days may result in the Agency viewing any eventual submission as a major amendment and extending the review period of the NDA.

As with case report tabulations, case report forms may be submitted on microfiche if this is agreeable to both the reviewing division and the applicant. Optical disk technology in conjunction with a computer-assisted submission is another possibility which should be explored with the reviewing division (Section VIII).

N. ITEM 13 — PATENT INFORMATION

Applicable patent numbers and expiration dates of the patents should be included by the applicant. This information is attached to the 356h form.

As a result of the Drug Price Competition and Patent Term Restoration Act of 1984, the FDA needs more information from the applicant concerning the marketing exclusivity determinations the Agency is required to make. The Act prohibits the Agency from approving or accepting submissions of certain NDA if specified criteria are met by other NDA holders. If the applicant or applicant holder believes he is entitled to some period of exclusivity, it is to their benefit to assist the Agency in making the exclusivity determinations by supplying the necessary information. This information can be included as a "Request for Exclusivity".

A 5-year period of exclusivity is available only to NMEs. A 3-year period of exclusivity is available to drug products in which the NDA contains new clinical investigations (other than bioavailability studies) that were conducted or sponsored by the applicant and were essential to the approval.

The FDA issued a policy letter on April 28, 1988 to all NDA holders and applicants:[17]

- For a 5-year exclusivity, information is needed on:

    1. Whether or not any active moiety in the drug product has ever been approved in another drug product in the U.S. either as a single entity or a combination product
    2. If not, whether or not any active moiety of the drug product has been previously marketed in the U.S., and under what name

- For a 3-year exclusivity, information is needed on:

    1. Whether or not a drug product containing all the same active ingredients with the same conditions of approval has been previously approved
    2. Whether or not, other than a bioavailability or bioequivalence study, one or more clinical investigations were submitted to support the application, and, if studies have been conducted, a certification statement that these studies were not part of a previously approved application
    3. Where these studies can be located if new clinical investigations have been previously submitted
    4. List of all published studies and publicly available reports of clinical investigations relevant to supporting the conditions of approval in the NDA

5. Certification that the applicant has thoroughly searched the scientific literature and that the list of published studies and reports is complete and accurate
6. Certification that, in the applicant's opinion, there are not sufficient published studies or publicly available reports (other than those conducted or sponsored by the applicant) to support approval of the NDA
7. Whether or not the applicant was the sponsor named in the IND(s) for each study that was submitted by the applicant and which the applicant believes is essential to approval of the NDA, identifying the IND number of each study
8. If the applicant was not the named sponsor of the IND(s), whether or not it provided substantial support for any of the essential studies

O. ITEM 14 — PATENT CERTIFICATION

Once the NDA is approved or if the drug is the subject of a formulation previously approved, the applicant needs to include a patent certification statement. This information should also be attached to the 356h form.

P. ITEM 15 — OTHER [21CFR§314.50(g)]

If the applicant references previously submitted information, complete identification should be provided for that information in this section. Accurate and complete English translations of each part of the NDA not in English are required in this section. The applicant is also required to submit a copy of each original literature publication for which an English translation is submitted.

Q. INTERNAL REVIEW

The applicant should allow appropriate time in the network for internal company review of the NDA by upper management. This time also provides an opportunity for a "naive" reader to review the application for clarity and continuity. One FDA reviewer remarked that "he felt he was the first person to see the entire submission". Considerable review time at the FDA can be saved by submitting a "quality" document.

IV. THE DRUG MASTER FILE

In order to facilitate the information supplied by an applicant, the FDA provides for some of the information to be submitted as a Drug Master File (DMF). A DMF may be used to provide detailed information about a specific facility, process, or component used in the manufacturing, processing, packaging, or storage of a product which is the subject of an NDA, IND, Abbreviated New Drug Application (ANDA), another DMF, or an Export Application.[18]

There are five types of DMF:

- Manufacturing Site, Facilities, Operating Procedures, and Personnel
- Drug Substance, Drug Substance Intermediate, and Material Used in Their Preparation, or Drug Product
- Packaging Material
- Excipient, Colorant, Flavor, Essence, or Material Used in Their Preparation
- FDA-Accepted Reference Information

The DMF can be useful in situations where the information contained in the DMF is applicable to several other applications. In this case, information can be updated in one source rather than submitting the updated information to several applications. The DMF is also useful where the applicant of the NDA is different from the holder of the DMF. In this situation, the DMF holder may have proprietary information in the DMF which he wants to protect. The confidentiality of the DMF allows this to occur. A reference to the DMF allows the FDA to review the information on behalf of the applicant.

It is important to note that the information contained in the DMF is not approved or disapproved by the FDA. This information is reviewed only in conjunction with the review of an IND, NDA, ANDA, or an Export Application.

If the applicant is going to reference a DMF from another party/company, he should ensure that the party/company is fully aware of the FDA requirements for a DMF as noted in the September 1989 Guideline for Drug Master Files. If an applicant references a DMF, the NDA is required to contain a copy of the DMF holder's letter of authorization. The letter of authorization should give the submission date(s) and page numbers for the information. An inadequate DMF can delay approval of the NDA.

The FDA does not encourage referencing DMFs in an application. Since DMFs are stored at a different site from the reviewer, the reviewer may have to wait several days before he receives the requested information from the DMF.

V. SUBMITTING AND PURSUING THE NDA

The FDA has found two meetings to be particularly helpful and productive both to agency reviewers and the sponsors. These are the "end-of-Phase II" and "pre-NDA" meetings. The FDA subsequently codified these meetings in the IND Rewrite regulations which issued on March 19, 1987.[19] The end-of-Phase II meeting has been previously addressed in this book.

A. PRE-NDA MEETING

The FDA has found from past experience that delays associated with the initial review of an NDA may be reduced by discussing with them the proposed application prior to submission of the NDA. The primary purpose of a pre-NDA meeting is to uncover any major unresolved problems, to identify those studies that the sponsor is relying on as adequate and well controlled to establish the effectiveness of the drug, to identify the presentation of the safety data, to give the FDA reviewers an overview of the application (format and content), and to discuss the statistical methodology used for the data analyses.

This meeting is arranged with the FDA reviewing division responsible for the IND. Meeting arrangements are coordinated by the Consumer Safety Officer (CSO).

In order to achieve the most comprehensive feedback from the FDA, the following information should be submitted at least 1 month prior to the meeting:[20]

- Brief summary of the clinical studies to be included
- Proposed tables for the efficacy and safety data
- Brief summary of the chemistry, manufacturing, and control data
- Brief summary of the animal data (if applicable)
- Brief summary of the biopharmaceutic data (if applicable)
- Brief summary of the microbiological data (if applicable)
- Proposed format for the application
- Proposed package insert

The FDA participants at the pre-NDA meeting would normally include reviewers from chemistry, pharmacology, biopharmaceutics, clinical, and biostatistics as well as the CSO and division director. The applicant should have the appropriate individuals present. If agreeable to both the reviewing chemist and applicant, the CMC section may be discussed at a separate meeting.

Agreements reached at the pre-NDA meeting should be recorded in the meeting minutes. As with the end-of-Phase II meeting, any agreements should also be described in the appropriate technical section of the application. It is to the applicant's benefit not to "surprise" the reviewer with data when the actual application is submitted. If the NDA classification has not been done at the IND stage, the applicant should inquire at the pre-NDA meeting how the NDA will be classified (i.e., chemical classification and therapeutic potential rating). The rating will have an impact on the review priority given by the FDA.

B. ADVISORY COMMITTEE MEETING

The FDA reviewing division may request that an advisory committee review drugs (NMEs or new indications) which have special concerns such as safety issues, adequacy of efficacy endpoints, adequacy of efficacy and safety data, or approval criteria. In addition to reviewing specific drugs, the advisory committees also discuss clinical guideline development.

For drugs, there are currently 16 advisory committees:

- Cardiovascular and Renal Drug Advisory Committee
- Gastrointestinal Drug Advisory Committee
- Drug Abuse Advisory Committee
- Peripheral and Central Nervous System Drug Advisory Committee
- Psychopharmacologic Drug Advisory Committee
- Arthritis Advisory Committee
- Oncologic Drug Advisory Committee
- Radiopharmaceutical Drug Advisory Committee
- Anesthetic and Life Support Drugs Advisory Committee
- Pulmonary-Allergy Drug Advisory Committee
- Anti-Infective Drug Advisory Committee
- Dermatologic Drug Advisory Committee
- Endocrinologic and Metabolic Drug Advisory Committee
- Fertility and Maternal Health Advisory Committee
- Antiviral Drugs Advisory Committee
- Generic Drugs Advisory Committee

In rare instances, two advisory committees may be requested to review an application.

The Advisors and Consultants Staff of the Center for Drug Evaluation and Research coordinates the 16 drug advisory committees and the 4 biologic advisory committees.

The advisory committees meet at the request of the reviewing division. As stated in 21CFR§14.1(b)(6), "...In general, a committee is utilized when FDA requests advice or recommendations from the committee on a specific matter in order to obtain an independent review and consideration of the matter ..." Normally, the committees meet twice a year.

The committees are composed primarily of physicians, pharmacologists, and biostatisticians who are recognized as experts in their field. Although the committee membership does not consist of any FDA staffers, the reviewing Division Director is present on the committee at the meeting. The Office Director may also attend the committee meeting.

If the division has requested that the application be reviewed by an advisory committee, the applicant should obtain the membership roster for the committee. The applicant may also want to determine whether or not any of the members have conducted any studies for the applicant or have any affiliations with the applicant. Any conflicts of interest should then be noted to the FDA.

Prior to the meeting, the applicant should obtain from the executive secretary the list of questions the reviewing division will be addressing to the advisory committee. The applicant should clarify any questions or issues with the reviewing division.

Whenever possible, all written information to be discussed by the applicant at the meeting should be provided to the executive secretary or other designated agency employee.[21] Applicants prepare a brochure (e.g., NDA summary volume) for the advisory committee members. This document normally consists of a summary of the efficacy and safety data as well as a copy of the labeling. The summary document must be submitted to the reviewing division well in advance of the meeting. Adequate time should be allowed for FDA review and comment.

The FDA mails copies of the brochure to the committee members if time permits; otherwise, the copies are given to the committee members when they arrive for the meeting. The mailing or distribution of the material is undertaken only by the FDA, unless the FDA grants permission to the applicant. The committee members also receive copies of the FDA efficacy and safety reviews.

The presentation by the company should be structured to answer or address the FDA's questions to the advisory committee. The presentation should be as specific as possible and follow an orderly approach through the drug development process. When appropriate, the applicant should utilize consultants and investigators to address new technologies, difficult studies, or to provide expert opinions.

Each advisory committee has its own personality. It is helpful if the applicant can attend a meeting of that advisory committee in order to learn how they conduct meetings and to determine the committee's past performance.

The applicant should ascertain the workload of the committee for the day of the presentation. The applicant will have a limited amount of time to make the presentation. It is imperative that the presentation be crisp and to the point. Speakers should be chosen who know the data. The applicant should make a scientific presentation of the data; the committee members do not want to hear a "marketing pitch" for the drug.

The importance of a good presentation cannot be overemphasized. Color slides summarizing the data in an easily read format should also be utilized. The committee members should be provided copies of the slides. New data or new analyses should not be presented at the meeting unless the committee and the FDA have given prior consent. Since the meeting is open to the public, the applicant should make arrangements to discuss confidential information in a closed session.

Although not required to do so, the reviewing division usually follows the recommendation of the advisory committee. In many instances, a committee's recommendation of nonapproval is usually because of insufficient data.

C. SUMMARY BASIS OF APPROVAL

Once an NDA is approved, safety and efficacy data are available to the public (21CFR§314.430). Since July 1, 1975, the FDA has prepared a Summary Basis of Approval (SBA) document that contains a summary of the safety and efficacy data and information evaluated by the FDA during the approval process. Preparation of an SBA would also apply to major clinical supplements to the NDA.

A draft SBA is needed for the Office of Drug Evaluation review of an NDA approval recommendation. The applicant may prepare a draft of the SBA or the reviewing division may prepare the SBA. It is usually more expeditious if the applicant prepares the draft SBA. The applicant should prepare the document from the FDA's perspective based upon the FDA reviews. The reviewing division should be consulted before preparing the SBA, since the SBA must be formatted in a particular manner.

The SBA should be submitted in hard copy as well as on a floppy diskette compatible with the FDA's word processing equipment. Following review by the division, the applicant makes the changes and resubmits the document in hard copy and floppy diskette. The Scientific Information Systems Branch (HFD-76) can be contacted regarding compatible word processing equipment.

The Pharmaceutical Manufacturer's Association has developed a guideline for an SBA.[22] The basic elements of the SBA include:

- Title page heading
- Name of applicant
- Indications for use
- Dosage form(s) and route(s) of administration
- Recommended dosage
- Manufacturing and controls information
- Stability information
- Methods validation statement
- Labeling
- Establishment inspection statement
- Environmental impact analysis report
- Pharmacology information
- Toxicology information
- Clinical study information
- Advisory committee recommendations
- Postmarketing surveillance studies

In preparing the SBA, it is also helpful to obtain copies of previous SBAs which have been prepared by the reviewing division. Since the SBA becomes available to the public, it should not contain any confidential information.

D. FDA REVIEW TEAM
In the Center for Drug Evaluation and Research, there are nine reviewing divisions:

1. Office of Drug Evaluation I
   - Division of Cardio-Renal Drug Products, HFD-110
   - Division of Neuropharmacological Drug Products, HFD-120
   - Division of Oncology and Pulmonary Drug Products, HFD-150
   - Division of Medical Imaging, Surgical, and Dental Drug Products, HFD-160
   - Division of Gastrointestinal and Coagulation Drug Products, HFD-180

2. Office of Drug Evaluation II
   - Division of Metabolism and Endocrine Drug Products, HFD-510
   - Division of Anti-Infective Drug Products, HFD-520
   - Division of Anti-Viral Drug Products, HFD-530

3. Office of the Center Director
   - Pilot Drug Evaluation Staff, HFD-007

The division directors report to the office director, who in turn reports to the center director. The director of the Pilot Drug Evaluation Staff reports to the center director.

An NDA review team is assigned once the NDA is received by the reviewing division. Normally, the FDA reviewing team will consist of:

- Medical officer
- Pharmacologist
- Biopharmaceuticist
- Chemist
- Biostatistician
- Consumer Safety Officer

The reviewing division may utilize a non-agency physician to assist in the medical review.

In some instances, the principal reviewing division may request a consult from another division (e.g., dermatologist from Anti-Infective Division).

VI. FOREIGN DATA

The NDA Rewrite provides that an application based solely on foreign clinical data (21CFR§314.106) may be approved by the FDA providing:

- Foreign data are applicable to U.S. population and U.S. medical practice.
- Studies have been performed by clinical investigators of recognized competence.
- Data may be considered valid without the need for an on-site inspection by the FDA or, if the FDA considers an inspection necessary, the FDA is able to validate the data through an on-site inspection or other appropriate means.

The FDA encourages applicants to discuss with them at the pre-NDA meeting if they intend to submit an application comprised entirely of foreign data.

In addition, the criteria for acceptance of foreign clinical studies not conducted in an IND are described in 21CFR§312.120. Deviation from the "Declaration of Helsinki" must be described. When the research has been approved by an independent committee, the applicant should also submit documentation of such review and approval, including names and qualifications of the members of the committee.

If the foreign study(s) is a pivotal trial, consideration should be given to integrating the data into the applicant's data base. This becomes very important when safety updates are being prepared.

If the information (including case report forms) is not in English, a complete translation will also be necessary.

VII. THE ABBREVIATED NEW DRUG APPLICATION

A. BACKGROUND

The Federal Food, Drug and Cosmetic Act of 1938 was passed in response to the sulfanil-amide tragedy which killed 107 persons. The major provision of the Act required drug manufacturers to demonstrate proof of safety in any new drug product prior to marketing. The mechanism to provide the safety data was via the NDA. Prescription drug products marketed before 1938 were "grandfathered".

The thalidomide tragedy in the early 1960s led to the passage of the Kefauver-Harris Drug Amendments, which strengthened the provisions of the 1938 Act. This amendment required that proof of efficacy be demonstrated in addition to the proof of safety. A provision of the 1962 Amendments enabled the FDA to require tests of efficacy for every product which was the subject of an NDA from 1938 to 1962. This resulted in the Drug Efficacy Study Implementation (DESI) project. The National Academy of Sciences/National Research Council (NAS/NRC) was asked to assist the FDA in the DESI project by evaluating for efficacy over 3500 prescription drug formulations. Review panels were then established and rated the drug products into one of the following categories:

- Effective
- Probably effective
- Possibly effective
- Ineffective

The Abbreviated New Drug Application (ANDA) procedure was subsequently established by the FDA in the *Federal Register* notice of April 24, 1970.[23] This procedure allowed additional manufacturers to meet the NDA requirements for marketing a new drug without the need for duplicating the preclinical and clinical studies previously performed by the innovator of the drug compound.

Provisions did not exist for the use of the ANDA process for drugs approved after 1962. This regulatory barrier resulted in the FDA implementing a "Paper NDA" policy via a memorandum issued by Dr. Marion Finkel, Associate Director for New Drug Evaluation, on July 31, 1978. The memorandum was subsequently published in the *Federal Register* dated May 19, 1981.[24]

In July 1983, Congressman Henry Waxman introduced a bill (H.R. 3605 — the Drug Price Competition Act) authorizing the Agency to accept generic copies of post-1962 new drugs as well as for copies of pre-1962 drugs reviewed through the DESI system.[25] The Drug Price Competition and Patent Term Restoration Act (Waxman — Hatch Act) was subsequently enacted on September 24, 1984, replacing the "Paper NDA" policy for generic versions of post-1962 drug products.

B. ANDA REQUIREMENTS [21CFR§314.55]

The FDA will accept an ANDA only if the FDA has made a finding that an ANDA is suitable for the drug product. ANDA suitability applies only to drug products that are the "same" in active ingredient, dosage form and strength, route of administration, and conditions of use as the original NDA product.[26]

If the drug product is similar, but different in one or more of the "suitability characteristics", the FDA will accept an ANDA only if the FDA has made a separate finding of suitability. In this case, the applicant submits a suitability petition requesting permission to file an ANDA. Usually, extensions of the suitability are limited to other dosage forms for the same route of administration, or to closely related ingredients. All approved products appear in the FDA publication, *Approved Drug Products with Therapeutic Equivalence Evaluations,* which is available from the Superintendent of Documents, U.S. Government Printing Office.

Each ANDA must contain information to show that the product provided for in the ANDA is the same as a listed product, patent certification information, labeling, CMC information and bioequivalence data.[27] The ANDA is also required to contain both archival and review copies.

The archival copy should contain:[28]

- Signed Form FDA 356h
- Table of contents
- CMC technical section
    Drug substance
    Drug product
    Environmental impact
- Human pharmacokinetics and bioavailability technical section
- Samples and labeling

The review copy should contain the technical sections for chemistry and pharmacokinetics. Each of these sections should be separately bound in their respective folders.[29]

ANDAs should be addressed to:

Division of Generic Drugs, HFD-230
Center for Drug Evaluation and Research
Document Control Room 17B20
Food and Drug Administration
5600 Fishers Lane
Rockville, MD 20857

ANDAs for antibiotic submissions should be addressed to:

Division of Generic Drugs, HFD-235
Center for Drug Evaluation and Research
Document Control Room 17-48
Food and Drug Administration
5600 Fishers Lane
Rockville, MD 20857

The Director and Deputy Director, Division of Generic Drugs, Office of Drug Standards, have authorization to approve ANDAs.

VIII. COMPUTER-ASSISTED SUBMISSIONS

The review process for NDAs is very complex. The culmination of the NDA is a synthesis of laboratory tests, animal studies, and clinical trials. When the NDA is submitted, the FDA is consequently left with a mass of data to review and evaluate. As a means to make the review process more efficient, the FDA and industry have been experimenting with submission of parts of the NDA in some electronic format. Thus far, four approaches have been used:

- Use of a third-party vendor
- Use of sponsor's mainframe
- Microcomputer based
- Use of FDA mainframe

In the September 15, 1988 *Federal Register*, the FDA provided guidance to sponsors who are interested in submitting a computer-assisted submission. A computer-assisted new drug application (CANDA) is defined as "any method using computer technology to improve the transmission, storage, retrieval, and analysis of data submitted to FDA as part of the drug development and marketing approval process".[30] As noted in The Electronic NDA Experiment, "The ability to analyze or inspect data by individual patients as well as data across patients and/ or studies, is an especially important and necessary feature of any proposed electronic NDA format ...".[31] Optical disk technology can allow the reviewer to simultaneously display an image of an NDA summary page and a tabular listing of data or case report form.

The Center for Drug Evaluation and Research encourages sponsors to explore the use of CANDAs. Prior to submitting a CANDA, the sponsor should discuss its plans with the Office of Management and with the reviewing division in order to obtain their "approval" to proceed with a CANDA.

Since reviewers' needs differ, the CANDA should be customized for each reviewer. Input from the individual reviewers is critical in designing the CANDA system. A side benefit of the CANDA is increased communication between the sponsor and the reviewer. In considering the type of system to be developed, the sponsor should also factor in reviewer training time and allow for intensive reviewer support during the review of the NDA.

The time saving to the primary reviewer will be the elimination of the "dead time" during a review.[32] The dead time is the time from when a reviewer asks a question to when the sponsor responds. The CANDA will allow the reviewer to formulate his own queries and get the results immediately back from the computer. This type of immediate response should allow the reviewer to gain a quicker "comfort factor" of the NDA data base as opposed to relying on a hand search of the data. Another benefit of the CANDA to the reviewer is immediate access to all of the NDA (including case report forms via optical disk) without having all of the NDA volumes in his office.

Although it is too early to quantitate the time saving with a CANDA, one trial showed that the secondary review was reduced by several months.[33] Most of the time saving will probably occur during the secondary (division director) and tertiary (office director) reviews. In addition, the FDA attempts to corroborate the clinical data in an application by conducting their own statistical analyses, which may differ from the sponsor's analyses. Having the data in an electronic format has the potential to facilitate this activity.

IX. OBTAINING FDA APPROVAL

An original NDA is delivered to the FDA Central Document Room. At this time they will stamp the transmittal letter with a receipt date. The application will then be sent to the appropriate reviewing division.

Within 60 days after receipt of the application, the Agency determines whether or not the application may be "filed". The filing of the application means that the FDA has made a threshold determination that the application is sufficiently complete to permit a substantive review (21CFR§314.101). Failure to comply with the NDA format or insufficient data can result in an application being returned.

By law, the FDA has 180 days in which to complete review of the application. Factors which slow the review process include shortage of FDA reviewers, change of FDA reviewers mid-review, amendments by the sponsor, additional data requested by the FDA, and change in FDA review priority. Tables 3 and 4 provide information on NDA approvals and submissions during the time period of 1975 to 1987. The average approval times for all NDA approvals ranged from 20.9 to 33.6 months; for all NMEs the approval times ranged from 20.3 to 39.1 months. The 5-year average (1983 to 1987) for all NMEs was 33.5 months, 27.5 months for 1A and 1B drugs, and 39.4 months for 1C drugs (Figure 4). For this same time period, review times for NMEs also varied among reviewing divisions — from 22.8 months for Anti-Infective Division to 48.5 months for Metabolism and Endocrine Division (Figure 5).

Once the application arrives at the reviewing division, the CSO distributes the copies to the reviewers according to the colored jackets (i.e., chemistry, pharmacology, biopharmaceutics, microbiology, clinical, and statistical). Copies for each of the technical sections permit parallel reviews; however, each reviewer can have a somewhat different set of priorities.

Considerable dialog occurs between the sponsor and the FDA during the review of the application. During this time, the sponsor usually amends the application to provide for additional information requested by the FDA reviewers. Two copies should be submitted — an archival copy and a review copy. For reference purposes, it is helpful if the transmittal letters have the amendments numbered sequentially. Submission of new information or a large amendment can cause the "review clock" to be reset by the FDA. Usually, the "clock" is reset at least once during the review.

FDA reviewers frequently request additional information or analyses over the telephone, which saves the time required to send a formal letter. Prompt sponsor response to FDA inquiries is critical in order to maintain the momentum of the review. Considerations should be given to submitting desk copies of the amendments to the reviewer via overnight mail, facsimile (for small amendments), or personally delivering the amendments.

The Office Directors and Deputy Directors of Drug Evaluation I and II are authorized to approve an NDA for a NME, new combination product, new indication, or sustained release product. The Division Directors and Deputy Directors are authorized to approve supplemental NDAs and NDAs for products that contain the same or different dosage form or strength, one or more active ingredient(s) identical to, or differing only in a salt or ester of the ingredient(s) of a previously approved drug product.[34] In some cases, the Office Directors may reserve their right to approve a new salt/ester, new formulation, or new indication. Approximately 75% of the NDA eventually receive approval for marketing.[35] The FDA communicates their response to the sponsor via an action letter (i.e., approvable, not approvable, or approval).

A. NDA DAY

Since the final review of the application (tertiary review) is conducted by the Director, Office

217

TABLE 3
All New Drug Applications
NDA Approvals and Submissions: 1975 to 1987

Year	No. approved	No. received	No. pending	Approval time (months)
1975	68	137	265	22.5
1976	101	127	260	24.9
1977	63	124	242	26.6
1978	86	121	244	32.2
1979	94	182	228	33.6
1980	114	162	187	21.3
1981	96	129	172	24.5
1982	116	202	257	22.4
1983	94	269	343	20.9
1984	142	217	272	24.2
1985	100	148	269	24.9
1986	98	120	204	27.9
1987	69	142	217	29.1

TABLE 4
New Molecular Entities

Year	No. approved	No. received	No. pending	Approval time (months) (all NMEs)	Approval time (months) (1A & 1B)
1975	15	25	55	22.2	
1976	24	31	56	23.2	
1977	21	27	60	30.9	
1978	22	18	51	20.3	
1979	14	18	45	37.5	
1980	12	32	50	34.5	21.7
1981	27	24	48	31.2	23.7
1982	28	35	65	28.8	14.4
1983	14	37	74	28.5	19.2
1984	22	32	83	39.1	25.8
1985	30	20	64	31.9	29.6
1986	20	29	66	34.1	32.1
1987	21	22	64	32.4	22.8

Note: It is important to note that, in 1985, the FDA revised its definition of an NME which significantly lowered the number of NMEs considered pending at the Agency. The FDA had previously defined NMEs as all "ls", but is now considering NME to refer to only the first application received for an active moiety that has neither been marketed nor approved in the U.S. Because several dosage forms of a "1" moiety may be pending at the same time, the number of pending NMEs decreased as a result of this redefinition.

Sources: New Drug Evaluation: Statistical Report April 1987, prepared by FDA, Office of Management; Personal Communication, Carol Grundfest, Director, Scientific and Regulatory Analysis, PMA.

of Drug Evaluation, the FDA is exploring ways to minimize the review time in this office. One of these possibilities has been an "NDA day". The "NDA day" consists of an intensive 1-day meeting between the tertiary reviewer, secondary reviewer, primary reviewer, and sponsor. At such a meeting the sponsor has the appropriate representatives on site to respond to any questions raised by the reviewers.

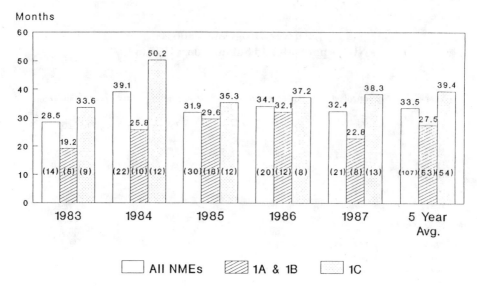

FIGURE 4. NME approvals 1983 to 1987. (From Powell, R. and Grundfest, C., PMA Study, June 1988.)

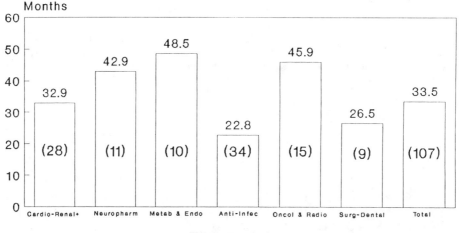

FIGURE 5. NME approvals by division 1983 to 1987. (From Powell, R. and Grundfest, C., PMA Study, June 1988.)

B. APPROVABLE LETTER

If the response from the FDA is an approvable letter, the letter usually requests changes to the physician insert, acknowledgment of an agreed upon postmarketing surveillance study(s), and a request for the final printed labeling (insert, bottle, carton). Upon receipt of the approvable letter, the sponsor should assemble the appropriate representatives within the organization (medical, manufacturing, marketing) in order to address the issues raised in the approvable letter.

The extent of the insert changes and other information requested by the FDA can lead to an intense period of negotiations between the sponsor and the Agency. Many times this is best resolved in a meeting environment between the sponsor and the Agency. Further negotiations between the sponsor and the FDA will extend the amount of time for receipt of a letter of approval.

If the sponsor is interested in maintaining the momentum of the review, it is important to respond to FDA requests in the shortest time possible. The approvable letter will state that within 10 d after the date of the approvable letter, the sponsor is required to amend the application, notify the FDA of the intent to file an amendment, or follow one of the other options under 21CFR§314.110. The FDA may also want to see copies of the introductory promotional material the sponsor plans to use at the time of product launch.

C. NOT-APPROVABLE LETTER

If the application is too deficient to approve, the FDA will issue a not-approvable letter to the sponsor. This letter will describe the deficiencies in the application. Within 10 days after the date of the not-approvable letter, the sponsor shall either amend the application, withdraw the application, or follow one of the other options under 21CFR§314.120.

D. LETTER OF APPROVAL

Following receipt of the final printed labeling and other requested information, FDA approval can take from 1 week to a couple of months, providing there are no further deficiencies. Usually, the sponsor can begin to market the product following receipt of the letter of approval. In some cases, however, the FDA may make final approval conditional upon the sponsor submitting some minor changes to the final printed labeling. Generally, the letter of approval follows an approvable letter.

ACKNOWLEDGMENTS

The author thanks the following people for providing invaluable input in their areas of expertise: D. J. Mason, G. H. Ishler, M. C. Walker, P. D. McCabe, G. N. Griffiths, F. A. Kimball, A. N. Young, Z. M. McDonald, D. L. Rosen, T. E. Nightingale, and C. C. Grundfest.

REFERENCES

1. *Federal Register*, 50(36), 7452, 1985.
2. Guideline on Formatting, Assembling and Submitting New Drug and Antibiotic Applications, Center for Drugs and Biologics, U.S. Food and Drug Administration, Washington, D.C., February 1987, 12.
3. Guideline on Formatting, Assembling and Submitting New Drug and Antibiotic Applications, Center for Drugs and Biologics, U.S. Food and Drug Administration, Washington, D.C., February 1987, 10.
4. Guideline on Formatting, Assembling and Submitting New Drug and Antibiotic Applications, Center for Drugs and Biologics, U.S. Food and Drug Administration, Washington, D.C., February 1987, 5.
5. *Federal Register*, 50(36), 7458, 1985.
6. Guideline for the Format and Content of the Summary for New Drug and Antibiotic Applications, Center for Drugs and Biologics, U.S. Food and Drug Administration, Washington, D.C., February 1987, 2.
7. Guideline for Submitting Documentation for the Manufacture of and Controls for Drug Products, Center for Drugs and Biologics, U.S. Food and Drug Administration, Washington, D.C., February 1987, 12.
8. Guideline for the Format and Content of the Nonclinical Pharmacology/Toxicology Section of an Application, Center for Drugs and Biologics, U.S. Food and Drug Administration, Washington, D.C., February 1987, 2-9.
9. Guideline for the Format and Content of the Human Pharmacokinetics and Bioavailability Section of an Application, Center for Drugs and Biologics, U.S. Food and Drug Administration, Washington, D.C., February 1987, 2-9.
10. Guideline for the Format and Content of the Microbiology Section of an Application, Center for Drugs and Biologics, U.S. Food and Drug Administration, Washington, D.C., February 1987, 4-7.

11. Guideline for the Format and Content of the Clinical and Statistical Sections of New Drug Applications, Center for Drugs and Biologics, U.S. Food and Drug Administration, Washington, D.C., July 1988, 7-9.
12. Guideline for the Format and Content of the Clinical and Statistical Sections of New Drug Applications, Center for Drugs and Biologics, U.S. Food and Drug Administration, Washington, D.C., July 1988, 49.
13. Guideline for the Format and Content of the Chemistry, Manufacturing, and Controls Section of an Application, Center for Drugs and Biologics, U.S. Food and Drug Administration, Washington, D.C., February 1987, 10.
14. Guideline for the Format and Content of the Chemistry, Manufacturing, and Controls Section of an Application, Center for Drugs and Biologics, U.S. Food and Drug Administration, Washington, D.C., February 1987, 10.
15. Guideline for the Format and Content of the Clinical and Statistical Sections of New Drug Applications, Center for Drugs and Biologics, U.S. Food and Drug Administration, Washington, D.C., July 1988, 81.
16. *Federal Register*, 50(36), 7464, 1985.
17. FDA Letter to all NDA or ANDA Holders and Applicants, July 29, 1988.
18. Guideline for Drug Master Files, Center for Drug Evaluation and Research, U.S. Food and Drug Administration, Washington, D.C., September 1989, 1.
19. *Title 21 Code of Federal Regulations* §312.47(b).
20. *Title 21 Code of Federal Regulations* §312.47(b)(2).
21. *Title 21 Code of Federal Regulations* §14.29(b)(1).
22. Guideline — Industry Prepared Draft SBA, Pharmaceutical Manufacturer's Association, 1986.
23. *Federal Register*, 35(80), 6574, 1970.
24. *Federal Register*, 46(96), 27396, 1981.
25. **Dickinson, J.,** Washington Report, *Pharmaceutical Technology*, October 1983, 26.
26. *Title 21 Code of Federal Regulations* §314.55(c)(1).
27. **Rosen, D. L.,** Understanding and Preparing ANDAs. Presented at the Educational Workshop of the Regulatory Affairs Professionals Society, July 29, 1987.
28. *Title 21 Code of Federal Regulations* §314.55(e)(1).
29. *Title 21 Code of Federal Regulations* §314.55(e)(2).
30. *Federal Register*, 53(179), 35912, 1988.
31. The Electronic NDA Experiment (1987). This report is available through the FDA. Participants: Office of Drug Research and Review, FDA; Division of Cardio-Renal Drug Products, FDA; Biometrics Division, FDA; Abbott Laboratories; Research Data Corporation.
32. Bell, R. A., FDA Perspective on CANDA's. Presented at the Twelfth Annual Meeting of the Regulatory Affairs Professionals Society, Alexandria, VA, September 28, 1988.
33. The Electronic NDA Experiment (1987). This report is available through the FDA. Participants: Office of Drug Research and Review, FDA; Division of Cardio-Renal Drug Products, FDA; Biometrics Division, FDA; Abbott Laboratories; Research Data Corporation.
34. *Title 21 Code of Federal Regulations* §5.80.
35. *Pharmaceuticals For The Future*, videotape, Institute for Alternative Futures, 1988.

Chapter 18

PRODUCT LIABILITY ISSUES IN DRUG DEVELOPMENT

William G. Pappas and Kenneth D. Sibley

TABLE OF CONTENTS

I. INTRODUCTION

In recent years, the legal shield protecting pharmaceutical manufacturers from consumers has significantly eroded. With the demise of the requirement of privity of contract between manufacturers and consumers, and the advent of strict liability in tort, pharmaceutical manufacturers have been held accountable for personal injuries to a degree that was not previously contemplated. Pharmaceutical manufacturers should therefore be aware of the legal issues involved and protective measures that can be taken to avoid liability.

II. MANUFACTURING AND DESIGN DEFECTS

A. MANUFACTURING DEFECTS

With the increasing sophistication and computerization of the pharmaceutical manufacturing industry, most drugs entering the market fall within the specific design intended by the manufacturer. Nonetheless, manufacturing defects can occur, and these defective drugs are not always detected by quality control personnel in time to prevent their entry into the marketplace. The consumer who discovers that the prescribed drug contains an improper mix of chemicals or a foreign substance may sue the manufacturer for allowing the defective product to be marketed. An actionable manufacturing defect may also consist of mislabeling product containers or misprinting warnings or instructions for drugs.

Most states have adopted a "strict liability" tort standard regarding injuries caused by improperly manufacturered or labeled drugs. In a strict liability scheme, a manufacturer of a flawed product is automatically liable if that product causes injury. The degree of care used in the manufacture and labeling of a product is irrelevant under this standard. However, other states require a showing of negligence in order to recover. To prove negligence, a claimant must show that a manufacturer failed to exercise reasonable care during the assembly process, and that such care would have prevented a defectively manufactured drug from reaching consumers. Negligence might occur at the research stage if research technicians fail to note instances in which such defects might occur, or at the preparation stage when component chemicals are mixed at improper levels, foreign substances enter the mixture, bottles are mislabeled, or instructions or warnings are misprinted. Finally, negligence can occur at the testing or quality control stage if the tests fail to reveal a product defect. A manufacturer can avoid liability for negligence (even if a defective product enters the market) when it establishes that reasonable care was taken at the research, preparation, and testing stages to ensure that the marketed products are safe.

B. DESIGN DEFECTS

While pharmaceutical manufacturers may or may not be liable for manufacturing defects, they are generally liable for every product produced with a "design defect". Design defects occur when the product, as designed, is not safe for its intended use. A product which is defectively designed is "unreasonably dangerous", and thus not fit to be placed into the marketplace. In most states, a consumer injured by such a product has a cause of action against the manufacturer.

1. Strict Liability

States relying on strict liability in tort are divided on the types of circumstances in which manufacturers should be held strictly liable for design defects. About half of these states use the "consumer expectation test", i.e., a product is unreasonably dangerous in its design if it is dangerous to an extent beyond that which would be contemplated by the ordinary consumer who purchases it.[1] Thus, under the consumer expectation test, open and obvious dangers as well as commonly known dangers will not give rise to manufacturer liability, since the ordinary consumer who purchases a product with such dangers can appreciate them.[2] The consumer expectation test could, however, hold a manufacturer strictly liable for marketing beneficial drugs if accompanied by adverse side effects caused by the design.[3]

The other states use the "danger-utility" test, i.e., a product is unreasonably dangerous only if one of the following is true:

1. The harm flowing from the product as used outweighs its benefits in terms of wants, desires, and human needs served by the product.
2. Although the harmful consequences do not in fact exceed the benefits, alternative products are available to serve the same needs or desires with less risk of harm.
3. Although the harmful consequences do not in fact outweigh the benefits, a feasible alternative design existed which contained less harmful consequences.[4]

An alternative design is feasible only if all of the following are true: the technology at the time of manufacture would have allowed for such design; it would not be unreasonably expensive; it would not impair the benefits desired by consumers; and no new danger would be created by the design.[5] If such a safer design alternative existed and the manufacturer failed to take advantage of it, the manufacturer would be held strictly liable in states which apply a strict liability standard. However, if there was no feasible alternative design under the existing state of the art at the time of manufacture, the manufacturer has a defense against a claimant who alleges a design defect. This "state of the art" defense is primarily used when technology, developed subsequent to the manufacture of a product, could have been used to employ a safer design alternative had that technology existed at the time of manufacture. This defense is not of benefit to a manufacturer if it produces a drug that is intrinsically unsafe because its benefits do not outweigh its risks, notwithstanding that the state of the art does not allow for a safer design.[6]

2. Negligence

Claimants in states that do not apply a strict liability standard are required to prove "negligence" in order to hold a manufacturer liable for injuries resulting from use of a defective product. A claimant must prove that the product was produced with a "negligent design". A negligent design occurs when the manufacturer did not exercise due care in selecting the safest design possible for its product. Design negligence at the research level may occur if the scope of the research is too limited, or if the research fails to identify safer alternative designs which exist under the state of the art. Design negligence at the product formulation stage may occur if components known to be dangerous are nonetheless added to the mixture, or if a design alternative which is not the safest possible is consciously selected. Design negligence at the testing stage may also occur if the manufacturer (1) fails to detect the dangers of the product through proper testing, (2) erroneously concludes through testing that safer design alternatives are not as safe as the one ultimately chosen, or (3) neglects the safer design alternatives that have been discovered. Manufacturers are entitled to the same "state of the art" defense in a negligence claim as in claims based on a strict liability standard.

III. WARNINGS

A. STANDARD OF LIABILITY

Some products which would otherwise be unreasonably dangerous will not be deemed so if adequate warnings are attached to the product. In a sense, an adequate warning "shields" the drug from a defective-design claim. If a warning is not adequate, this shield dissolves.

Most courts do not distinguish between strict liability and negligence standards when determining whether or not the manufacturer failed to warn consumers of possible side effects and dangers of a drug.[7] Under either theory, the courts will analyze whether or not the manufacturer exercised due care in warning users of potential dangers associated with a drug product.[8] Liability for failure to warn also may be based solely upon failure to comply with a state or federal statute.[9] However, compliance with a statute does not necessarily immunize a manufacturer from liability.[10] A manufacturer has a duty to warn of any potential dangers which could have been discovered at the time of manufacture under the existing state of the art.[11] Conversely, if the existing state of the art would not have permitted a manufacturer to discover a potential danger or side effect, liability will not attach for a mere failure to warn.[12]

B. SCOPE OF DUTY

The scope of a manufacturer's duty to warn extends to those dangers that are known or are reasonably foreseeable based upon the state of the art at the time of the marketing.[13] A manufacturer must also anticipate misuses and unintended uses of the product in a warning.[14] A manufacturer must provide directions or instructions that describe ways to avoid dangers, how to use the product safely,[15] and the precise nature of the harm likely to result if directions or instructions are not followed.[16]

C. LIMITATIONS ON DUTY

It would be counterproductive to require a manufacturer to call the user's attention to every conceivable danger, since, as the number of warnings increase, the likelihood that a consumer will notice any one in particular necessarily decreases. When a danger is open and obvious to an individual consumer, a manufacturer is not required to warn about it.[17] A danger is considered open and obvious when both the cause of harm and its severity are known to the consumer. If only the cause of a potential risk is known to the use,[18] or if only the likely cause of harm is known,[19] but the likely severity of harm is not, the danger is not considered open and obvious and the duty to warn remains.

Moreover, a manufacturer has no duty to warn about dangers that are commonly known by members of the general public.[20] Not every danger, however, can be "commonly known" as a matter of law,[21] and in most jurisdictions, fact finders decide if dangers are so common that a person of ordinary knowledge should foresee them despite the lack of warning.

D. TO WHOM THE DUTY IS OWED

The question to whom the duty to warn is owed depends on the targeted audience. The intended audience for prescription drugs and vaccines is licensed physicians and pharmacists, not consumers. Therefore, the manufacturer's duty to warn of potential dangers from prescription items usually extends only to those groups.[22] However, if the manufacturer knows or should know that the drug will be sold or administered without the intervention of an individualized medical judgment to assess the risks, the manufacturer must warn the ultimate product user as well.[23] Aside from normal dangers, a manufacturer must also warn medical or pharmacological intermediaries of exceedingly rare, idiosyncratic adverse reactions to its product if the potential harm from such reactions is likely to be severe.[24]

In contrast to prescription drugs, the intended audience for over-the-counter drugs consists of the general public. Therefore, manufacturers owe a duty to the world-at-large to warn of potential risks. This duty, however, only exists to the extent there are risks of adverse effects which might affect a large number of people, not rare reactions.[25]

E. THE ADEQUACY OF A WARNING

Several factors are considered as to whether or not a warning is adequate in a particular situation: (1) the dangerous nature of the product, (2) the use of the product, (3) the form and intensity of the warnings, (4) the burden of providing a warning, and (5) the probability that the warning will be communicated to those who may foreseeably use the product.[26] If the language of the warning does not reflect the gravity of the potential harm, the warning may be deemed inadequate.[27] Moreover, the warning must include instructions for safe use of the product as well as its potential risks.[28]

F. POSTMANUFACTURE WARNINGS

If a drug is found to have previously unknown risks or defects after its introduction into the marketplace, the manufacturer has a duty to take reasonable steps to inform product users of the newly discovered dangers.[29] Moreover, the manufacturer has a duty to use appropriate means to convey postscale warnings calculated to actually reach the user.[30] Depending on the intensity of the newly discovered danger and the size of the affected number of users, the manufacturer might have a duty to recall the product.[31]

G. REASONABLY FORESEEABLE MISUSES

An important limitation on the manufacturer's duty to warn is whether or not a misuse was "reasonably foreseeable". A manufacturer must warn potential users of any foreseeable misuse of its product.[32] Specific and singularly hazardous misuses are usually foreseeable.[33] Conversely, a manufacturer will not be held liable for failure to warn of misuses which are not reasonably foreseeable.[34]

H. PRODUCTS THAT ARE UNREASONABLY DANGEROUS DESPITE WARNINGS

Some products are so dangerous that any type of warning would be inadequate to ward off manufacturer's liability. If a product is unreasonably dangerous because its risks will inevitably outweigh its benefits, a warning describing all potential dangers, in clear and concise terms, may nonetheless be inadequate to avoid liability.[35]

I. FALSE ASSURANCES

Even if a warning is adequate to alert potential users to every danger inherent in the product, the warning may be insufficient if false assurances are given about the safety of the product. For example, an extensive advertising campaign alluding to the safety of the product may nullify any warning on the package, the product, or contained in an instruction booklet or manual.

IV. UNAVOIDABLY UNSAFE PRODUCTS

A. COMMENT K

Some products are so beneficial to society that their potential for harm is tolerated by the courts. Specifically, Comment k of Section 402A of the Restatement of Torts proposes a safe harbor for the production of "unavoidably unsafe products", thus excluding such products from the rule of strict liability. However, Comment k does not insulate manufacturers from liability for negligent design (or manufacture) of unavoidably unsafe products.

Comment k was intended to address two situations. First, a drug or vaccine may be produced which causes harmful side effects in a small but clearly identifiable class of users. It is assumed that such drugs or vaccines are properly prepared and incorporate the highest degree of skill and knowledge commensurate with the prevailing state of the art. If so, such drugs or vaccines are so beneficial to society that the product will not be deemed unreasonably dangerous. The risk of harm caused is outweighed by the risk of harm prevented.[37]

Second, new or experimental drugs are sometimes produced which cannot be properly tested except by introduction into the marketplace.[38] Such drugs would not be deemed unreasonably dangerous if they are produced in response to a genuine health crisis, and "such experience as there is justifies the marketing and use of the drug, notwithstanding a medically recognizable risk".[39] An example could be some drugs currently being produced in response to the AIDS crisis.

B. WARNINGS REQUIRED

In order to rely on Comment k, a manufacturer must attach a proper warning that adequately states the risks involved.[40] The warning must be complete, comprehensive, and comprehensible based on the manufacturer's available knowledge and the current state of the art.[41] As to drugs which fall into the first category noted above, the known side effects should be clearly identified. As to drugs in the second category (such as AIDS treatments), the fact that risks may be associated with the drug, while currently unknown, must be identified to the attending physician or the ultimate user as soon as they are known. An inadequate warning prevents reliance on Comment k notwithstanding the ultimately beneficial effects of a product.

V. SUMMARY

The potential product liability problems for drug manufactures cannot be understated. With modern "mass" tort product liability claims involving hundreds of litigants in multiple judicial forums, the financial and administrative resources of a growing drug company can quickly be drained.[42] However, as noted in this discussion, affirmative steps can and should be taken to lessen or obviate a pharmaceutical company's liability exposure.

ACKNOWLEDGMENT

The authors gratefully acknowledge the technical and editorial assistance of their colleagues: Robert W. Spearman, Robert W. Saunders, and Steven B. Epstein with Parker, Poe, Adams & Bernstein.

REFERENCES

1. Second Restatement of Torts Section 402A, Comment i.
2. **Keeton, W. Page,** *Prosser & Keeton on Torts,* 5 ed., 1984, 698—701.
3. *Ibid.*
4. *Id.*
5. *Id.*
6. *Id.*
7. **Ross, Kenneth, et al.,** *Product Liability of Manufacturers,* 1984, 43.
8. *Ibid.*
9. *Ezagui v. Dow Chemical Corp,* 598 F.2d 727 (2d Cir. 1979).
10. *Ibid.*
11. *Id.*
12. *Id.*
13. *Id.*
14. *Id.*
15. *Id.*
16. *Id.*
17. *Colson v. Allied Products Corp.,* 640 F.2d 5 (5th Cir. 1981).
18. Ross, 55—57.
19. *Ibid.*
20. *Id.*
21. *Id.*
22. *Brochu v. Ortho Pharmaceutical Corp.,* 642 F.2d 652 (1st Cir.) 1981.
23. *Reyes v. Wyeth Laboratories,* 498 F.2d 1264 (5th Cir.) *cert. denied,* 419 U.S. 1096, 95 S.Ct. 687, 42 L.Ed.2d 688 (1974).
24. Ross, 65.
25. Keeton, 687.
26. *Dougherty v. Hooker Chemical Corp.,* 540 F.2d 174 (3rd Cir. 1976).
27. *Borel v. Fibreboard Paper Products Corp.,* 493 F.2d 1076 (5th Cir. 1973) *cert. denied,* 419 U.S. 869, 95 S.Ct. 127, 42 L.Ed.2d 107 (1974).
28. Ross, 73.
29. *Schenebeck v. Sterling Drug, Inc.,* 423 F.2d 919 (8th Cir. 1970).
30. *Jones v. Bender Welding & Machine Works, Inc.,* 581 F.2d 1331, 1335 (9th Cir. 1978).

31. *Gillham v. Admiral Corp.*, 523 F.2d 102 (6th Cir. 1975) *cert. denied*, 424 U.S. 913 (1976).

32. Ross, 75.

33. *Brownlee v. Louisville Varnish Co.*, 641 F.2d 397 (5th Cir. 1981).

34. Ross, 75.

35. *Brochu v. Ortho Pharmaceutical Corp., supra.*.

36. Annotation, *Failure to Warn in Use of Vaccine*, 94 A.L.R.3d, 748, 780 (1979).

37. Restatement of Torts Section 402A, Comment k.

38. *Ibid.*

39. *Id.*

40. *See Collins v. Ortho Pharmaceutical Corp.*, 231 Cal. Rptr. 396, 195 Cal. App. 3d 1539 (1986).

41. Willigue, Sidney H., *The Comment k Character: A Conceptual Barrier to Strict Liability*, 29 Mercer L.Rev. 545, 568 (1978).

42. *See* Rubin, *Mass Torts and Litigation Disasters*, 20 Ga. L. Rev. 429 (1986); Rowe and Sibley, *Beyond Diversity: Federal Multiparty, Multiforum Jurisdiction*, 135 U. Penn. L. Rev. 7, 14-22 (1986).

Chapter 19

LEGAL ASPECTS OF PRODUCT PROTECTION

William G. Pappas and Kenneth D. Sibley

TABLE OF CONTENTS

I. INTRODUCTION

The four primary categories of intellectual property protection are trade secret, patent, trademark, and copyright protection. Each category provides a different type of legal right, with these rights varying in importance over the course of drug development.

Trade secret protection is a concern from the inception of drug development throughout the marketing of a product. Trade secret protection early in the course of development focuses on technical information, while later trade secret issues are more of a commercial nature. Patent protection issues arise early in the course of research, and continue to be present throughout product development and testing. Patent infringement issues likewise arise throughout the product development period, with final resolution ideally occurring prior to the first commercial use. Trademark issues arise at the time of first commercial sales, with maintenance and policing of the trademark required throughout the life of the product. Copyright issues can arise on various occasions during product development, but usually arise in connection with product marketing.

II. TRADE SECRETS

A. INTRODUCTION

A trade secret may consist of any formula, pattern, device, or compilation of information which is used in one's business, and which gives the business an opportunity to obtain an advantage over competitors who do not know the trade secret or how to use it.[1] Unlike patent rights, trade secret rights have an indefinite life span so long as they are not terminated by public disclosure. By their nature, property rights in a trade secret are asserted defensively rather than offensively, i.e., against someone who misappropriates or steals the information protected by the trade secret. The importance of trade secret law has grown as a result of the highly competitive market facing those industries influenced by the rapid pace of technological change. In addition, the greater propensity for employee mobility and for industrial espionage has lead to increased demand by businesses to protect vulnerable trade secrets.[2]

B. HOW TO ESTABLISH A TRADE SECRET

In order to establish a trade secret, one must usually show that (1) the information claimed to be a trade secret is subject matter that will be protected as a trade secret, (2) the information is not a matter of common knowledge in the industry, (3) reasonable precautions have been taken to maintain secrecy, (4) it is of some value, and (5) it has some definiteness or concreteness.[3]

The type of information that can be protected is broadly defined to include specific matters such as the formula of a manufactured product or the machinery for making the product, as well as general matters such as customer lists and marketing and pricing information. For example, formulas for medicines such as hair conditioner and liniment have been treated as trade secrets. Moreover, processes such as for the manufacture of gas-permeable polymers for use in soft contact lenses have also been protected as trade secrets.[4]

With respect to the requirement that the information be private, absolute secrecy is not required. For example, the information does not become public if the owner reveals its contents to another in confidence or under an express or implied duty not to disclose it. Moreover, the secrecy requirement is not breached when the information protected by the trade secret is used to develop a product that is later made available to the public — so long as the trade secret cannot be identified by merely inspecting the product. An owner will not be able to claim that knowledge is secret when (1) a competitor has previously used or is already using the information, (2) the information was known to the public prior to the misappropriation, (3) the information can be obtained from other readily available resources, (4) the "secret" can be discerned by simple inspection of the marketed article, or (5) the information has been published.

A failure to take reasonable precautions to maintain confidentiality may indicate a lack of trade secret status.

With respect to the reasonable precautions requirement, the owner does not have to establish that every conceivable precaution was undertaken. Instead, the owner may establish that information is a trade secret by showing that outside visitors were restricted from the plant where the trade secret was used, access to the information was limited on a need-to-know basis, the information was maintained in a secure location, and those who had access to the information were advised that it was confidential.

Information is considered "valuable" if it gives its owner an opportunity to obtain an advantage over competitors who do not know the trade secret or how to use it. However, some courts require that the information actually be used by the owner in order to show value. Thus, owners who were unsuccessful or unable to exploit information may not be able to show value. Nevertheless, most courts apply a broad definition of value.

The degree of the "definitiveness" of the information will vary under the circumstances. Simply stated, the matter sought to be protected must be more than a mere abstract idea even if not reduced to concrete form.

C. TERMINATION OF TRADE SECRET RIGHTS

Generally, trade secrets terminate upon public disclosure of the subject matter of the trade secret. Public disclosure includes free and unrestricted disclosure of the trade secret to employees, suppliers, manufacturers, and prospective licensees.

Significantly, the grant of a U.S. patent in which a trade secret is claimed or disclosed, or the publication of a corresponding foreign patent application, will usually terminate the trade secret. Trade secrets that are disclosed will lose their protection even if they are not claimed. However, if the patent does not disclose the details of the trade secret, trade secret protection will not be lost. Moreover, trade secrets that are only disclosed in a U.S. patent application are retained in confidence throughout the patenting process, including appeals. It is important to note that this protection is not provided in many foreign countries, where patent applications are open to public inspection.

Exceptions to the general rule that public disclosure terminates a trade secret exist where (1) the trade secret is disclosed to a person under a contract that provides for royalty payments as long as the trade secret is used, and (2) the disclosure of the trade secret was made in the course of a confidential relationship. In the case of the former, the person under contract must still make the royalty payments despite the fact that the trade secret is now public. In case of the latter, the subsequent public disclosure of the trade secret will not terminate the trade secret right. However, this rule is not followed in all states. Some courts have held that all public disclosures, except in limited circumstance, terminate trade secret rights. Others have combined the two approaches by employing a rule that permits an action for damages after a trade secret becomes public. Also, a trade secret does not necessarily become public when it is provided to a federal agency, such as the FDA, as part of the licensing process.[5]

III. PATENTS

A. INTRODUCTION

A patent grants legal rights in return for a disclosure which meets the statutory requirements of invention. The scope of these rights is defined by one or more paragraphs, called claims, set forth at the end of the patent.[6] The claims, which give the formal definition of the invention, are the focus of the attention of the Patent Office when it decides whether or not a patent application meets the statutory requirements for patentability and should be allowed, and are the focus of the attention of a court when it decides whether or not an issued patent has been infringed.

B. PATENTABILITY

The primary requirements which must be met to obtain a patent are given in five key sections of the federal patent statute, Title 35 of the United States Code. Section 101 requires that patentable inventions fall within specific categories of eligible subject matter, section 102 requires that the invention be novel (and that acts which lead to the forfeiture of patent rights have been avoided), section 103 requires the invention to be nonobvious, section 112 requires certain information on the invention to be revealed in the patent application, and section 116 concerns joint inventors. The sections which follow focus on only those portions of each of these statutory provisions which are particularly important in the drug development field.

1. Section 101

a. Subject Matter

Section 101 authorizes that grant of a patent to anyone who "invents or discovers any new and useful process, machine, manufacture, or composition of matter, or any new and useful improvement thereof ...". Common categories of eligible subject matter in the drug development field are pharmaceutically active compounds, intermediates useful for making active compounds, nucleic acid sequences, processes for making compounds, compositions comprising an active compound and a pharmaceutical carrier, methods of treating human or animal subjects, microorganisms isolated from nature, new microorganisms, and gene transfer vectors. In many foreign countries, method of treatment claims are not available, though similar coverage through claims to a "second medicinal use" may be available.[7]

b. Practical Utility

If a chemical compound is not "useful", it is not eligible subject matter and neither are methods and intermediates for preparing the compound. This requirement is known as the practical utility requirement. A new compound need not, however, be proven out through ultimate therapeutic efficacy to establish that it is useful. Instead, pharmaceutical activity in an *in vivo* or *in vitro* screening assay is sufficient if activity in that assay is reasonably correlated with therapeutic activity.[8] These same principles apply to methods and intermediates for preparing new compounds, but not necessarily to methods of treatment or pharmaceutical compositions containing the compounds. For the latter group, the Patent Office may require evidence of therapeutic activity.

c. Operability

When the utility stated in an application for a chemical compound is for the treatment of an intractable disease such a cancer, the Patent Office may take the position that the utility is an incredible utility, hold it to a higher standard of proof, and require more experimental data on the operability of the compounds. When the claims are directed to compounds, animal test data supporting activity against a specific disease can be sufficient.[9] When the compounds are not new and only method claims (or, perhaps, pharmaceutical composition claims) are presented, a different standard may apply and evidence of activity in the subject to be treated may be necessary.[10]

2. Section 102: The Novelty Requirement and Forfeiture of Patent Rights

Section 102 begins with a phrase "A person shall be entitled to a patent unless ...". It then goes on to list various events which result in the loss of patent rights. Section 102 is complex. However, in the pharmaceutical industry, obtaining foreign patent protection is important, and the rule for foreign purposes is simple: the application must be filed in the U.S. before any divulgation (e.g., even an oral presentation) of the invention to the public is made. The U.S. filing date is then the effective filing date in most foreign countries if those foreign applications are filed within 1 year.[11]

a. Section 102(a): Events Prior to the Date of Invention

Section 102(a) bars a patent when "the invention was known or used by others in this country, or patented or described in a printed publication in this or a foreign country, before the invention thereof by the applicant ...". In general, any event (be it public knowledge, a journal publication, etc.) cited against an inventor under this section can be avoided by showing that the date the invention was made was before the date of the event.

i. "Printed Publication" Defined

A paper or other record is a printed publication when people skilled in the art, through the exercise of reasonable diligence, can locate it and comprehend the invention from it.[12] Mere difficulty in locating a publication does not, however, take it out of section 102. For example, a catalogued dissertation is a printed publication, and a paper discusssed in front of 50 to 500 persons at a conference and there given to at least six people is a printed publication.[13]

ii. Disclosure Requirements for an Anticipatory Reference

A reference must *identically* describe an invention for it to anticipate that invention.[14] For example, a unique chlorosubstituted compound would not be anticipated by a reference showing a compound otherwise the same but described as "halogen substituted, such as by bromo-".[15]

An anticipatory reference must teach how to make a compound if a method of making the compound is not otherwise obvious.[16] However, it need not teach how to use the compound, even if no use is known.[17] This contrasts with the situation when one files for a patent, in which case a use for the compound must be previously known or stated.[18]

b. Section 102(b): Events Prior to the Filing Date of a Patent Application

Under section 102(b), patent rights are lost "if the invention was patented or described in a printed publication in this or a foreign country or in public use or on sale in this country, more than one year prior to the date of the aplication for patent in the United States ...". When applied to the inventors' own acts, this section acts as a statute of limitations: once one of the specified events occurs, an application must be filed within 1 year or rights to a U.S. patent are forfeited.

Issues such as the definition of a printed publication and the disclosure requirement of a reference are treated essentially the same under section 102(b) as they are under section 102(a). Section 102(b), however, presents unique issues on the definitions of "public uses" and "on sale". A use of an invention is a public use "when it is used in its natural and intended way — even though the invention may in fact be hidden from public view with such use". Thus, patent rights to a secret process for making a commercial compound are lost if an appliction for that process is not filed within 1 year of the first use.[19] An invention is considered to be "on sale" when it is first offered for sale, and not on the day it was first sold.[20]

In a few cases, activities which might appear to be "public use" events are excused under the experimental use doctrine. Under this doctrine, public use made to test the operability and effectiveness of an invention does not start the 1-year statutory filing period. A key consideration is that no commercial gain has been derived from the use.[21]

c. Sections 102(e), 102(f), and 102(g): Prior Acts of Another

Section 102(f) denies a patent when "the applicant did not himself invent the subject matter sought to be patented". This section ensures that U.S. patents can only be filed in the name of the inventor(s).

Section 102(g) deals with the situation of two separate parties *independently* making the same invention. It denies a patent when "before the applicant's invention thereof the invention was made in this country by another who had not abandoned, suppressed, or concealed it." Because this section is tied to the date of invention, it can be overcome by records which show the thought and work done in making the invention. The content of such records must meet the substantive requirements of the patent laws, and the records themselves must be properly corroborated in accordance with the laws of evidence.[22]

Section 102(e) makes an issued U.S. patent, filed by a *different* inventive entity, prior art as of its filing date. Note that, under section 122 of the patent statute, all patent applications are kept secret until they are issued. Again, prior art under this section can be avoided by showing a date of invention earlier than the filing date of the cited patent.

3. Section 103: The Nonobviousness Requirement

If the absolute bars of section 102 do not block the patenting of a prospective invention, the inquiry shifts to the test of nonobviousness posed by section 103. This section states that no patent is available if "the differences between the subject matter sought to be patented and the prior art are such that the subject matter as a whole would have been obvious at the time the invention was made to a person having ordinary skill in the art to which said subject matter pertains".

a. Defining the Prior Art

In general, any document or event which might serve as an anticipatory reference under section 102 can be used by the Patent Office to argue that an invention is obvious under section 103.[23] However, a special exception has been added to benefit groups of workers who are all obliged to assign their inventions to the same party (e.g., a corporate employer) at the time the invention is made. In this special case, the prior work of others in that group, which would ordinarily qualify as prior art under sections 102(f) or 102(g), is *not* available as prior art. This exception, in turn, raises a trap: a previously filed patent application which does not name the *identical* inventor or inventors can *still* be used as a prior art reference under section 102(e) when a patent on that application issues.

b. Prima Facie Obviousness

To show an invention *obvious* in view of the prior art and hence *unpatentable*, there must be shown (1) a motivation for making the change over the prior art, (2) an obvious method of making the new structure, and (3) a reasonable expectation that the changed subject matter will work.[24] That a line of research seems promising does not make the fruit of that research *prima facie* obvious: the courts have repeatedly said that "obviousness to try" is not the standard of invention.[25] For example, the change of an ether to a thioether link in an otherwise known molecule may be *non*obvious on its face.[26]

c. Rebutting Prima Facie Obviousness

An invention obvious on its face is nonobvious is an unexpected advantage results from the change. Showing unexpected advantages typically requires comparative tests between the invention and the closest prior art. Deciding when comparative data are sufficient is a difficult evidentiary decision.[27] For example, it has been said that showing a mere difference in degree of activity is not sufficient, yet unexpected superiorty in but one of a spectrum of common activities has been held sufficient.[28] The evidentiary problems with rebutting a *prima facie* showing of obviousness weight in favor of avoiding showing unexpected advantages and arguing that a *prima facie* case has not been established whenever appropriate.

4. Section 112: Disclosure Requirements

The disclosure requirements of section 112 specify the infomation which must be divulged in a patent application to obtain a valid patent. There are three different disclosure requirements. First, the application must give a *written description* of the invention. Second, the application must teach how to make and how to use the invention (collectively called the *enablement* requirement). Finally, the application must reveal the *best mode* of the invention.

a. The Written Description Requirement

Frequently, patent applications are filed, research continues, and a specific compound which was thought of as unimportant at the time the application was filed (or not thought of at all), turns out to be of great importance. If the original application does not give a complete written description of the currently preferred compound, a new application must be filed or new matter must be added to the original application. In either case, the new matter is *not* treated as having been filed on the original filing date. Thus, the written description requirement under section 102 is closely related to the written description requirement under section 112, it ensures that an inventor is not barred from obtaining a patent by a prior reference which does not *precisely* describe the invention — and it ensures that, if the prior reference is a patent application, that application does not provide a basis for claiming the invention.[29]

b. The Enablement Requirement

The breadth of protection to which an inventor is entitled is frequently dependent on compliance with the enablement requirement. In general, as an invention is claimed more broadly, more data or other guidance on how to make and use the invention will be required to satisfy the enablement requirement. For example, an inventor who has partially purified a physiologically active peptide, but who does not know how to purify that compound to homogeneity, may have difficulty obtaining claims encompassing the compound purified to homogeneity.[30] Deciding the question of enablement requires inquiry into a variety of different facts, including the unpredictability of the technology with which the invention is concerned and the amount of data or other guidance given in the application.[31] This issue should be analyzed before an application is filed. As explained in the patent infringement section below, if the invention is initially claimed too broadly and the claims in the application must later be narrowed to obtain an issued patent, an estoppel may be created which will prevent the patentee from arguing a broader interpretation of the claims against an infringer through the doctrine of equivalents.

c. The Best Mode Requirement

A patent application must set forth the best mode contemplated by the inventor for carrying out the invention at the time the application was filed. To show that the best mode requirement has not been met, one attacking a patent must show that the applicant knew of a better mode and *concealed* it.[32] The primary danger raised by this requirement is that the best mode might change between the time an invention is first disclosed and the time when the patent application is filed. To avoid this problem, the best mode question should be reviewed just before an application is filed.

5. Section 116: Inventors

If two or more people contributed to the making of an invention, then they are joint inventors and all must be named in an application for that invention. To be named as a joint inventor a person must collaborate in the "conception" of the invention.[33] A "conception" is "the formation, in the mind of the [inventive entity], of a definite and permanent idea of the complete and operative invention, as it is thereafter to be applied in practice ...".[34] When an invention is a chemical compound, the inventors must have in mind a use for the compound, in addition to a method of making the compound, for the conception to be complete.[35]

The patent statute provides that "inventors may apply for a patent jointly even though (1) they did not physically work together or at the same time, (2) each did not make the same type or amount of contribution, or (3) each did not make a contribution to the subject matter of every claim of the patent".[36] This permissive approach allows prior art problems which might arise from two commonly owned patent applications naming different inventive entities under section 102(e) to be solved by joining these inventions in a single application.

C. PATENT INFRINGEMENT

One who makes, uses, or sells a patented product, or carries out the steps of a patented process, in the territory of the U.S. is liable for patent infringement. Liability can also attach if one party induces another to infringe a patent, contributes to the infringement of a patent by another, or imports into the U.S. a product made by a process patented in the U.S.[37]

A patent lasts for an unextendable term of 17 years, though patents for new pharmaceutical compounds may be extended to make up for time invested in obtaining FDA approval.[38] In this same vein, it is not an act of patent infringement to make, use, or sell an invention solely for the purpose of obtaining FDA approval to sell the patented drug.[39]

Infringement is established when a court finds that an accused product or process possesses every element recited in a claim, or its equivalent.[40] Conversely, if an accused product or process lacks an element recited in a claim, then there is no infringement. If, however, an accused product does not possess all the elements of a claim, yet an equivalent element is present, then infringement may be found under the doctrine of equivalents.[41] The extent to which the literal language of claims can be broadened by the doctrine of equivalents is limited by the doctrine of prosecution history estoppel (also called "file wrapper estoppel").[42] A prosecution history estoppel arises when arguments or amendments made to obtain issuance of a patent application weigh against a broader interpretation of the claims under the doctrine of equivalents.

The sanctions available for patent infringement include injunctions, monetary damages, treble damages, and attorney's fees.[43] Monetary damages can be limited by the patentee's failure to bring suit before expiration of the statute of limitations,[44] the patentee's unexcused delay in bringing suit combined with prejudicial harm thereby caused the accused,[45] or the patentee's failure to mark patented products with a patent notice in the manner specified by the patent statute.[46] Treble damages and attorney's fees arise when infringement is "willful", or in "exceptional" cases, and can be avoided by showing good faith.[47] An affirmative duty of due care to avoid patent infringement can be a prerequisite of good faith, with a demonstration of reliance on a thorough infringement opinion given by patent counsel often crucial to a finding of good faith.[48] Finally, personal liability can arise when a corporate officer is the "moving force" behind that corporation's infringement.[49]

IV. TRADEMARKS AND COPYRIGHTS

A trademark is any word, logo, symbol, or other device affixed to a product which enables consumers to identify the souce of origin of that product or assures consumers of the quality of that product. To carry out its purpose, a trademark cannot be the generic name of a product or descriptive of that product. Instead, it should be arbitrary or fanciful, or at most only suggestive of what that product might be.[50]

Trademark infringement occurs when there is a substantial likelihood that the consuming public will be confused by a mark used on a product sold by someone else.[51] Similarly, the trademark statute is violated when the appearance of one product so closely resembles the appearance of another that it is "passed off" as that product. For example, a generic drug maker who designs capsules to duplicate the appearance of an established product can be held vicariously liable for the violation which occurs when pharmacists dispense the generic drug as the established product.[52]

To be federally registered, a trademark must first be used on a product sold in interstate commerce. In the drug industry, however, prior to this first sale, considerable effort is devoted to selecting a mark. Legal counsel must clear the mark as noninfringing and be satisfied of the registrability of the mark; marketing personnel must be satisfied that the mark fits the company's promotional plan for the product on which it is to be used. Trademark rights exist for as long as the mark is used, but constant monitoring of the requirements of the trademark laws and the potentially infringing conduct of others is required to avoid forfeiture of the mark.

A serious issue, once the marketing of a product begins, is the counterfeiting of that product. The trademark act provides powerful remedies for counterfeiting, including the ability to seize counterfeit goods from another without prior notice.[53]

Copyright protection is available for works of authorship fixed in a tangible medium of expression,[54] and is infringed when someone makes a substantially similar copy of the protected work.[55] Common pitfalls in protecting copyrighted matter include the failure to properly mark works with a copyright notice[56] and the failure to obtain written agreements on who owns the protected work when those works are made for hire.[57]

The copyright laws do not play a major role in protecting the fruits of drug development. Potential areas are publications arising from drug research and, importantly, the protection of sales and advertising materials once commercialization of a new drug begins.

V. CONCLUSION: EFFECTIVE PROTECTION OF DRUG DEVELOPMENT TECHNOLOGY

An effective strategy for protecting drug development research requires advanced planning and creative use of state trade secret law, federal patent law, and international treaties concerning the protection of intellectual property. Seven considerations should be kept in mind.

First, *approach protential infringement problems with care.* An infringement opinion should be obtained before any new product or process is commercialized. An infringement analysis early in the course of technology development may help avoid future infringement problems.

Second, *aggressively search the technical literature.* High-quality technical information is expensive, but crucial to a successful patent program — or to any technical venture. Special effort should be made to search both U.S. and foreign patent literature, as this literature contains information which is different from and often more current than information found in other sources.[58]

Third, *consider trade secret protection.* Since the patent laws often require public disclosure of information that would terminate trade secret rights, the two options tend to be mutually exclusive. Among the factors that should be considered in utilizing trade secret protection are (1) whether or not the patentability requirements can be met, (2) whether or not an issued patent can be successfully defended, (3) whether or not the patented technology can be developed independently by others, and at what cost, (4) whether or not the 17-year life of a patent is preferable to the potential infinite life of a trade secret, (5) whether or not the secret subject matter might be independently developed and patented by another, (6) how much information must be disclosed in the patent application, (7) the scope of patent protection which can be obtained, and (8) whether or not the technology is of such speculative worth that the filing and other expense of obtaining a patent, as opposed to the in-house steps required to protect a trade secret, is a consideration. An alternative to both trade secret and patent protection is to simply make the technology publicly available to all.

Fourth, *consider the data the Patent Office may request.* After a patent application is filed, data may be required to meet the enablement requirement to obtain claims of the desired breadth, evidence of unexpected advantages may be required, and evidence of operability may be required. The burden of such requirements, or a strategy for avoiding them, should be addressed as early as possible.

Fifth, *file patent applications early.* For defensive purposes (i.e., establishing rights to at least the best mode), an early filing date is critical. For offensive purposes (i.e., obtaining claims of significant breadth), a carefully prepared patent application is critical. To simultaneously accommodate these two goals, one approach is to file a brief, narrow U.S. application early. A more extensive "offensive" application can be filed when a strategy is better thought out and more data are collected (though it should be filed within 1 year).

Sixth, *implement a cost-effective foreign patent program.* The costs of drug development are so great that patent protection in at least some foreign markets is very desirable. While the cost of securing foreign patent protection can be high, these costs can be deferred into the future (hopefully, to a time when the desirability of proceeding is more clear) by using the Patent Cooperation Treaty.[59]

Seventh, *build a patent portfolio.* Because patents must be sought at a time in product development when the ultimate market for the product is uncertain, patents are of speculative, but high, potential value. Investing in a patent portfolio reduces this speculation. Moreover, it is easier for a competitor to avoid a single patent (while still benefiting from your technology) than it is to avoid a portfolio of patents.[60] Finally, by building a patent portfolio, inventors gain experience in the patent law and familiarity with the "prior art" by shaping and building the prior art — an exercise which is, in the final analysis, the ultimate object of the patent laws.

ACKNOWLEDGMENTS

The comments and assistance of Richard S. Faust, Joseph H. Heard, James D. Myers, and Ellen A. Page of Bell, Seltzer, Park & Gibson, and Robert W. Saunders and Robert W. Spearman of Parker, Poe, Adams & Bernstein are acknowledged with appreciation.

REFERENCES

1. Restatement of Torts, 757, Comment (b) (1939).
2. Hutter, Legal theories and recent development, in *Protecting Trade Secrets,* Practising Law Institute No. 244, 1986.
3. *Ibid.*
4. Milgrim, 12 *Business Organization,* Trade Secrets, §2.09[1][a] (1987) and 2.09[2][a].
5. Annotation "What Constitutes 'Trade Secrets and Commercial or Financial Information Obtained from a Person and Privileged or Confidential', Exempt from Disclosure under Freedom of Information Act (5 USC §552[b][4]), 21 ALR Fed. 224 (1974).
6. 35 USC §112; 2 D. Chisum, *Patents* §§8.01-8.06, 1988.
7. *International Chemical Practice,* 13 AIPLA *Quart. J.* 1 et seq. (1985).
8. *Brenner v. Manson,* 383 U.S. 519, 86 S. Ct. 1033, 16 L. Ed. 2d 69 (1966); *Cross v. Iizuka,* 753 F.2d 1040, 224 U.S.P.Q 739 (Fed Cir. 1985).
9. *Ex parte Chwanq,* 231 U.S.P.Q. 751 (Bd. Pat. App. 1986); *Ex parte Krepelka,* 231 U.S.P.Q. 746 (Bd. Pat. App. 1986).
10. **Lassen, E.,** *Chemical Practice Pharmaceutical Utility Subcommittee: Subcommittee Report to the Chemical., Practice Committee, AIPLA Midwinter Meeting, Orlando, Florida,* January 29, 1987.
11. *Manual for the Handling of Applications for Patents, Designs, and Trademarks Throughout the World,* Manual Industrial Property B.V., Amsterdam, Holland, Suppl. March 1988.
12. In re *Wyer,* 655 F.2d 221, 226, 110 U.S.P.Q. 790 (C.C.P.A. 1981).
13. See re *Hall,* 781 F.2d 897, 228 U.S.P.Q. 453 (Fed. Cir. 1986); *Massachusetts Institute of Technology v. Ab Fortia,* 774 F. 2d 1104, 227 U.S.P.Q. 428 (Fed. Cir. 1985).
14. In re *Arkley,* 455 F.2d 586, 587, 172 U.S.P.Q. 524 (C.C.P.A. 1972).
15. *Bigham v. Godtfredsen,* 857 F.2d 1415, 8 U.S.P.Q. 2d 1266 (Fed. Cir. 1988).
16. See *Akzo N.V. v. U.S. International Trade Commission,* 808 F. 2d 1471, 1479 (Fed. Cir. 1986).
17. In re *Donohue,* 632 F.2d 123 (C.C.P.A. 1980).
18. See In re *Moore,* 444 F.2d 527, 170 U.S.P.Q. 260 (C.C.P.A. 1971).
19. 2 D. Chisum, *Patents,* §6.02[5][a] (1988).
20. *Buildex Inc. v. Kason Industries Inc.,* 849 F.2d 1461, 7 U.S.P.Q.2d 1325 (Fed. Cir. 1988).
21. U.S. Department of Commerce, *Manual of Patent Examining Procedure,* §§2128.01-2128.07, 5th ed., 1983.
22. See, e.g., *Horton v. Stevens,* 7 U.S.P.Q. 2d 1245 (Bd. Pat. App. 1988); generally B. Collins, *Current Patent Interference Practice,* 1987.
23. See, e.g., *E.I. DuPont de Nemours & Co. v. Phillips Petroleum Co.,* 849 F.2d 1430, 7 U.S.P.Q. 2d 1129, 1134 (Fed. Cir. 1988).

24. See generally R. Armitage, *Chemical Patent Practice — Drafting the Patent Application,* 60 n. 49, paper prepared for American Intellectual Property Law Association Basic Chemical Practice Seminar, held at the Crystal Gateway Marriott, Oct. 8, 1986.
25. In re *Goodwin,* 576 F.2d 375, 198 U.S.P.Q. 1, 3 (C.C.P.A. 1978), see also In re O'Farrell, 853 F.2d 894, 7 U.S.P.Q.2d 1673 (Fed. Cir. 1988) (reviewing molecular biology of recombinant DNA technology).
26. In re *Grabiak,* 769 F.2d 729, 226 U.S.P.Q. 870 (Fed. Cir. 1985); see generally H. Wegner, *Prima Facie Obviousness of Chemical Compounds,* 6 APLA Quart. J. 271 (1978).
27. Comment, *PTO Practice: Spinning the Wheels of Evidence,* 70 J. Pat. Off. Soc'y 505 (1988); Comment, *PTO Practice: Ignorance May not be Bliss,* 67 J. Pat. Off. Soc'y 93 (1985).
28. Compare In re *Merck & Co., Inc.,* 800 F.2d 1091, 231, U.S.P.Q. 375 (Fed. Cir. 1986) *with In re Chupp,* 816 F.2d 643, 2 U.S.P.Q. 2d 1437 (Fed. Cir. 1987).
29. *Bigham v. Godtfredsen,* 857 F.2d 1415, 8 U.S.P.Q.2d 1266 (Fed. Cir. 1988).
30. *Hormone Research Foundation v. Genetech Inc.,* 8 U.S.P.Q.2d 1377 (N.D. Cal. 1988).
31. In re *Wands,* 858 F.2d 731, 8 U.S.P.Q.2d 1400, 1402-04 (Fed. Cir. 1988); see generally K. Sibley, *Factual Inquiries in Deciding the Question of Enablement,* 70 J. Pat. Off. Soc'y 115 (1988).
32. *Randomex v. Scopus Corp.,* 849 F.2d 585, 7 U.S.P.Q.2d 1050, 1052 (Fed. Cir. 1988).
33. In re *Hardee,* 223 U.S.P.Q. 1122, 1123 (Comm'r. Pats. 1984).
34. *Coleman v. Dines,* 754 F.2d 353, 224 U.S.P.Q. 857, 862 (Fed. Cir. 1985).
35. *Kondo v. Martel,* 220 U.S.P.Q. 47, 50 (Bd. Pat. Int. 1983); but see *Rey-Bellet v. Engelhardt,* 493 F.2d 1380, 181 U.S.P.Q. 453, 456 (C.C.P.A. 1974) (whether or not the conception of a chemical compound requires a conception of utility is an open question).
36. 35 USC §116; see also *Monsanto Co. v. Kamp,* 269 F. Supp. 818, 154 U.S.P.Q. 259 (D.D.C. 1967).
37. See Process Patents Amendment Act of 1988, Pub. L. No. 100-418, §9003, 102 Stat. 1563-64 (1988).
38. See 35 USC §§155-156; see also *Fisons plc v. Quigg,* 8 U.S.P.Q.2d 1491 (D.D.C. 1988).
39. See 35 USC §271(e); see also *Eli Lilly & Co. v. Premo Pharmaceutical Laboratories,* 4 U.S.P.Q.2d 1080 (D.N.J. 1987) aff'd, 843 F.2d 1378 (Fed. Cir. 1988).
40. *Perkin-Elmer Corp.v. Westinghouse Electric Corp.,* 822 F.2d 1528, 3 U.S.P.Q.2d 1321, 1325 (Fed. Cir. 1987).
41. See *Pennwalt Corp. v. Durand-Wayland Inc.,* 833 F.2d 931, 4 U.S.P.Q.2d 1737, 1739 (Fed. Cir. 1987); see also *Graver Tank & Mfg. Co. v. Linde Air Products Co.,* 339 U.S. 605, 70 S. Ct. 854, 94 L. Ed. 1097 (1950).
42. See *Bayer Aktiengesellschaft v. Duphar International Research B.V.,* 738 F.2d 1237, 1243, 222 U.S.P.Q. 649, 653 (Fed. Cir. 1984).
43. 35 USC §283.
44. 35 USC §286.
45. See, e.g., *Leinoff v. Louis Milona & Sons, Inc.,* 726 F.2d 734, 741, 220 U.S.P.Q. 845 (Fed. Cir. 1984); see generally 4 D. Chisum, *Patents,* §19.05 (1988).
46. 35 USC §287; see also *Devices for Medicine, Inc. v. Boehl,* 822 F.2d 1062, 1068, 3 U.S.P.Q.2d 1288 (Fed. Cir. 1987).
47. *Radio Steel & Mfg. Co. v. MTD Products, Inc.,* 788 F.2d 1554, 229 U.S.P.Q. 431, 434-35 (Fed. Cir. 1986).
48. *Underwater Devices, Inc. v. Morrison-Knudsen Co.,* 717 F.2d 1380, 219 U.S.P.Q. 569 (Fed. Cir. 1983).
49. See *Power Lift, Inc. v. Lang Tools, Inc.,* 774 F.2d 478, 227 U.S.P.Q. 435 (Fed. Cir. 1985); *Orthokinetics, Inc. v. Safety Travel Chairs, Inc.,* 806 F.2d 1565, 1 U.S.P.Q.2d 1081 (Fed. Cir. 1986).
50. See generally 1 J. McCarthy, *Trademarks and Unfair Competition,* Chap. 2 (2d ed. 1984).
51. 2 J. McCarthy, *Trademarks and Unfair Competition,* Chap. 23 (2d ed. 1984).
52. See *Ciba-Geigy Corp. v. Bolar Pharmaceutical Co.,* 747 F.2d 844, 224 U.S.P.Q. 349 (3d Cir. 1984); see also *Inwood Laboratories, Inc. v. Ives Laboratories, Inc.,* 456 U.S. 844, 102 S. Ct. 2182, 72 L. Ed.2d 606, 214 U.S.P.Q. 1 (1982).
53. See 15 USC §1116(d); see also M. McCoy and J. Myers, *Ex parte Seizure Order Practice After the Trademark Counterfeiting Act of 1984,* 14 AIPLA Quart. J. 237 (1987).
54. 17 USC §102; see generally 1 M. Nimmer, *The Law of Copyright,* §§2.01-2.19 (1988).
55. 17 USC §106; see generally 3 M. Nimmer, *The Law of Copyright,* §13.01-13.09 (1988).
56. 17 USC §§401-406.
57. 17 USC §201(b).
58. See R. Maizell, *How to Find Chemical Information,* 245-51 (2d ed. 1987).
59. See generally World Intellectual Property Organization, *PCT Applicants Guide* (1985).
60. See P. Morgan and J. Friedman, *Probabilities of Losing as to at Least One Patent in Multi-Patent Litigation,* 68 J. Pat. Off. Society 498 (1986).

Chapter 20

THE IMPACT OF BIOTECHNOLOGY ON THE PHARMACEUTICAL INDUSTRY

Mark D. Dibner

TABLE OF CONTENTS

I. INTRODUCTION

In a recent analysis by Pharmaprojects, the thousands of therapeutics in development, from preclinical to those fully launched in 1988, were ranked in 35 categories.[1] For the second year, biotechnology-related therapeutics made up the highest ranking, representing 842 therapeutics, while the next highest category, anticancer/immunological drugs, had only 302 products. Moreover, the drugs classified as biotechnology have 620 products in the preclinical area with the next highest classification having only 182 products in preclinical development.[1] Only 32 biotechnology drugs were counted as launched, however, compared with 49 anti-inflammatory drugs launched worldwide in 1988.[1]

This predominance of biotechnology in pharmaceuticals is echoed in the U.S. The Pharmaceutical Manufacturers' Association (PMA) counted 97 biotechnology-related drugs and vaccines in various stages of clinical development in late 1988, with only nine of these reaching the U.S. market (see Table 1).[2] These 97 compounds were being developed by 54 companies with such familiar names as Upjohn, Sterling, and Merck, and newcomers to the industry, such as BioTechnology General, Amgen, and Genentech.[2] Established corporations in other industries, such as Du Pont and Eastman Kodak, have also begun diversification into pharmaceuticals, in part through support of biotechnology.[3]

Not all therapeutics will be proteins or the products of genetic engineering. In fact, whether or not the products of genetic engineering will have a tremendous impact on the pharmaceutical industry has been questioned for some time.[4] Given the number of recombinant DNA-derived compounds in development or clinical trial, it is likely that the originally predicted billions of dollars in revenues from biotechnology-based drugs will be realized. Moreover, many of these drugs address new markets, such as the treatment of arthritis, a cure for cancer or AIDS, or acceleration of bone growth and wound healing, all increasing the total worldwide market for therapeutics and giving new life to a mature industry. These revenues have attracted pharmaceutical companies to the new technology. Another benefit these companies should gain by involvement in biotechnology is a greater ability to develop classical pharmaceuticals. By being able to produce natural, physiologically active proteins, their receptors, and other structures in great quantity, new chemical compounds that mimic or interact with these molecules will be discovered.[4]

The advent of biotechnology has thus brought the industry new compounds, new markets, new collaborators, and new competitors. This chapter will explore the advent of the biotechnology industry, pharmaceutical development in the small firms, involvement of the large pharmaceutical corporations in biotechnology, and trends for the industry.

II. THE U.S. BIOTECHNOLOGY INDUSTRY

Since the discovery of new techniques in genetic engineering and hybridoma production in the early 1970s, more than 600 start-up firms have been founded to work with biotechnology.[5] Although biotechnology will have tremendous impacts on a variety of industries, from chemicals to energy to agriculture to electronics, the initial products to reach the marketplace have been diagnostics, followed by the few therapeutics and vaccines mentioned above.[3] As the first "wave" of biotechnology, health care accounts for more than half of the biotech firms founded.[3,6] Today, the average biotechnology firm is only 9 years old, has 102 employees, earns $16 million in revenues, and is not profitable.[7] These are young companies undergoing very expensive research and development activities; most have not yet brought a major product to market.

In pharmaceuticals, with typical development times of 10 years and development costs often breaking $100 million, biotech firms need to find the resources to withstand these extreme costs. In the early 1980s, there was an abundance of venture capital and public funding for biotech

TABLE 1
Biotechnology-Derived Drugs in Development

Company/companies	Trade name	Product	Indications	FDA status
I. Approved Drugs				
Armour	Monoclate®	Factor VIII:C	Hemophilia	Approved
Eli Lilly	Humulin®	rDNA human insulin	Diabetes	Approved
Genentech	Humatrope®	rDNA somatropin	HGH deficiency in children	Approved
	Protropin®	HGH	HGH deficiency in children	Approved
	Activase®	t-PA	Acute myocardial infarction	Approved
Hoffmann-La Roche	Roferon®-A	IF-α2a	Hairy cell leukemia, Kaposi's sarcoma	Approved
Merck	Recombivax® HB	Hep-B	HEP-B VX	Approved
Ortho Pharmaceutical	Orthoclone® OKT3	MAB	Kidney transplant rejection	Approved
Schering-Plough	Intron® A	IF-α2b	Hairy cell leukemia, genital warts, Kaposi's sarcoma	Approved
II. Anticoagulants/Thrombolytics				
Collaborative Research/Sandoz		Prourokinase	Heart attack	II/III
Genetics Institute/Wellcome Biotechnology		t-PA	Acute myocardial infarction, thrombosis, acute stroke, pulmonary embolism	II/III
III. Colony Stimulating Factors (CSF)				
Amgen	Nupogen	G-CSF	Chemotherapy effects, AIDS, leukemia, aplastic anemia	II/III
		GM-CSF	Adjuvant to chemotherapy	II
Genetics Institute/Sandoz		GM-CSF	Chemotherapy, AIDS, aplastic anemia, bone marrow transplant	II/III
Hoechst-Roussel/Immunex		GM-CSF	Numerous: chemotherapy, AIDS, leukemia, Hodgkin's	I
Schering-Plough		GM-CSF	Chemotherapy, adjunct to treatment of infectious diseases	I/II/III
		GM-CSF	AIDS	
IV. Dismutases				
Bio-Technology General/Bristol-Myers		SOD	Reperfusion injury in acute myocardial infarction, renal transplantation	II

TABLE 1 (continued)
Biotechnology-Derived Drugs in Development

Company/companies	Trade name	Product	Indications	FDA status
IV. Dismutases				
Bio-Technology General/Bristol-Meyers		SOD	Oxygen toxicity in premature neonates	I/II
		SOD	Inflammatory disease: arthritis, colitis	I
Chiron/Pharmacia, Inc.		SOD	Reperfusion damage	III
Sterling Drug/Enzon		PEG-SOD	Reperfusion injury, kidney transplant	II/III
V. Erythropoietins (EPO)				
Amgen	Epogen	EPO	Dialysis anemia	App. submitted
	Epogen	EPO	Chronic renal failure	Human clinicals
Chugai-Upjohn/Genetics Inst.	Marogen	EPO	Anemia	App. submitted
Ortho Pharmaceutical	Eprex	EPO	Chronic renal failure, AIDS, anemias, pre- and postsurgical	Human clinicals
VI. Human Growth Hormones (HGH)				
Bio-Technology General		HGH	Human growth deficiency in children	App. submitted
Genentech	Protropin®	HGH	Chronic renal failure	I/II
	Protropin®	HGH	Burns	I
VII. Interferons (IF)				
Exovir	Exovir HZ® Gel	IF-α (topical)	Recurrent genital herpes	App. submitted
	Exovir HZ® Gel	IF-α (topical)	Oral herpes	III
	Exovir HZ® Gel	IF-α (topical)	Genital warts	II
Hoffmann-La Roche	Roferon®-A	IF-α2a	AIDS-related Kaposi's sarcoma	App. submitted
	Roferon®-A	IF-α2a	Chronic myelogenous leukemia, renal cell carcinoma	Clinical trials
Interferon Sciences		IF-α	Genital warts, genital herpes	App. submitted
Schering-Plough	Intron® A	IF-α2b	Many cancers and other indications	App. submitted
	Intron® A	IF-α2b	Ovarian cancer, viral hepatitis, transitional cell bladder cancer	III
Viragen	Alpha Leukoferon	Human leukocyte IF-α	Leukemia, AIDS, renal/bladder cell carcinoma, herpes	App. submitted
Wellcome Biotechnology	Wellferon®	IF-α	Hairy cell leukemia, severe papillomavirus-induced infections	App. submitted

Company	Product	Type	Indication	Phase
Triton Biosciences	Betaseron®	rDNA Human IF-β	AIDS, ARC, multiple sclerosis	III
Triton Biosciences	Betaseron®	rDNA Human IF-β	Venereal warts	I/II
Amgen	Immuneron®	IF-γ	Cancer, infectious disease	II
Biogen	Immuneron®	IF-γ	Rheumatoid arthritis, renal cell carcinoma	II/III
Biogen		IF-γ	Venereal warts	I/II
Genentech		IF-γ	Cancers (small-cell lung, melanoma, colorectal)	III
Interferon Sciences		IF-γ	Scleroderma	I
Amgen		IF-consensus	Cancer, infectious disease	II/III

VIII. Interleukins (IL)

Company	Product	Type	Indication	Phase
Amgen/Johnson & Johnson		IL-2	Cancer immunotherapy	II
Biogen/Glaxo	Bioleukin®	IL-2	Cancer immunotherapy	I
Cetus		PEG IL-2	Cancer	I
Cetus	Proleukin®	IL-2	Cancer	III
		IL-2	Cancer immunotherapy	I
Collaborative Research		rDNA Human IL-2	Cancer immunotherapy	In clinical trials
Hoffmann-La Roche/Immunex		rDNA IL-2/LAK	Cancer immunotherapy (LAK cell therapy)	In clinical trials
Hoffmann-La Roche		rDNA IL-2/Roferon-A	Cancer immunotherapy	In clinical trials

IX. Monoclonal Antibodies (MAB)

Company	Product	Type	Indication	Phase
Becton-Dickinson	Anti-Leu-2	MAB	Renal-allograft rejection	I
Becton-Dickinson	Anti-Leu-2	MAB	Prevention of graft vs. host disease	II
Bristol Myers/Oncogen		MAB-L6	Lung cancer	I
Centocor	Centoxin	MAB	Septic shock	III
Centocor	Panorex	MAB	Colorectal cancer, pancreatic cancer	II
Centocor	Ovarian RT	MAB	Ovarian cancer	I
Cetus		Antiplatelet MAB	Antiplatelet prevention of blood clots	I
Cytogen Corporation	Centorex	MAB	Breast cancer	I
Cytogen Corporation		OncoRad MAB	Ovarian cancer	I
Cytogen Corporation		OncoScint CR 103 MAB	Colorectal cancer	III
Cytogen Corporation		OncoScint OV 103 MAB	Ovarian cancer	II/III
Eli Lilly		KS 1/4-DAVLB MAB	Cancer	In clinical trials
Genetics Institute/NeoRx		ADDC agent MAB	Colorectal cancer	I
Immunex/Becton-Dickinson		Anti-IL-2 receptor MAB	Prevention of graft-host disease in bone marrow transplant	II
Immunomedics/Johnson & Johnson		MAB	Colorectal cancer	II

TABLE 1 (continued)
Biotechnology-Derived Drugs in Development

Company/companies	Trade name	Product	Indications	FDA status
		IX. Monoclonal Antibodies (MAB)		
Lederle	MAB	Cancer	In clinical trials	I
NeoRx		Rhenium-186 MAB	Colorectal cancer	I
		Melanoma I-131 MAB	Malignant melanoma	I
		Ovarian I-131 MAB	Ovarian cancer	I
		Pseudomonum MAB	Ovarian cancer	I
Ortho Pharmaceutical	Orthoclone® OKT3	MAB	Heart and liver transplant rejection	App. submitted
Pfizer/Xoma	Xomen®-E5	MAB	Septic shock	III
Xoma	XomaZyme®-Mel	MAB	Melanoma	II
	XomaZyme®-791	MAB	Colorectal cancer	II
	XomaZyme®-H65	MAB	Bone marrow rejection, transplant graft vs. host disease	III
	XomaZyme®-H65	MAB	Rheumatoid arthritis	I
		X. Peptides		
California Biotech/Wyeth	Auriculin®	Atrial peptide (injectable)	Acute congestive heart failure	II
Immunetech		Pentigetide (aerosol)	Asthma	I
		Pentigetide (injectable)	Allergic rhinitis	App. submitted
		Pentigetide (nasal spray)	Allergic rhinitis	App. submitted
		Pentigetide (ophthalmic)	Allergic conjunctivitis	III
		T-Cell mod. peptide-80	Auto-immune diseases	I
Nova Pharmaceutical/SmithKline		Bradykinin antagonists	Common cold (nasal spray)	II
Wyeth-Ayerst	Anaritide	Vasomotor peptide	Congestive heart failure	II
		XI. Tumor Necrosis Factors (TNF)		
Biogen		TNF	Cancer	I
Cetus		TNF	Cancer	II
		TNF/IL-2	Cancer	I
Genentech		TNF	Cancer	II

XII. Vaccines (VX)

Company	Product	Type	Indication	Status
Amgen/Johnson & Johnson		Hepatitis-B VX	Hepatitis-B	III
Biogen		Hepatitis-B VX	Hepatitis-B	I
Connaught/Integrated Genetics		Hepatitis-B VX	Hepatitis-B	II
Genentech/SmithKline Beckman		Hepatitis-B VX	Hepatitis-B	II
SmithKline Beckman	Engerix-B	Hepatitis-B VX	Hepatitis-B	App. submitted
Bristol-Myers/Oncogen		HIVAC-le VX	AIDS	I
MicroGeneSys	VaxSyn™ HIV-1	AIDS VX	AIDS	In clinical trials
Praxis Biologics		VX for H. Influenzae	H. Influenzae type B	III
Ribi Immunochem Res.		Cancer VX	Malignant melanoma	II
SmithKline/Walter Reed Army Inst.		Malaria VX	Malaria	I (4)

XIII. Other Products

Company	Product	Type	Indication	Status
Alpha-1 Biomedicals		Thymosin alpha-1	Hepatitis VX adjuvant, chronic active hepatitis-B	II
Alpha-1 Biomedicals		Thymosin alpha-1	Influenza VX adjuvant, lung cancer	III
Baxter Healthcare/Genetics Institute		Factor VIII-C	Hemophilia	I
Baxter Healthcare/Genetics Institute		rDNA Factor VIII	Hemophilia	I/II
Chiron		EGF	Eye surgery, wound healing	III/II
Chiron/Ethicon		EGF	Wound healing	II
Chiron Ophthalmics		Fibronectin	Eye-wound healing	II
Chiron/Ciba-Geigy		Insulin-like GF I	Bone growth	I
Cooper Laboratories		rDNA α1-antitrypsin	Congenital emphysema	II
Enzon		PEG-ASP Asparaginase	Childhood acute lymphoblastic leukemia	II/III
Genentech	PEG-ADA	Adenosine deaminase	Severe combined immune deficiency syndrome	App. submitted
	RCD4	rDNA soluble human CD4	AIDS, ARC	I
Genzyme	Ceredase	Glucocerebrosidase	Gaucher's disease	II
Immunobiology Res. Inst.	Timunox	Thymopentin TP5	HIV infections, atopic dermatitis	II

Notes:
1. This table is modified from *Update: Biotechnology Products in Development*, October 1988, Pharmaceutical Manufacturer's Association.
2. Not included are drugs/indications that were not registered with the FDA by autumn 1988.
3. Common abbreviations in this table and in Table 2 are as follows: ABS - antibody(ies); AIDS - acquired immunodeficiency syndrome, HTLV-III, HIV; ANF - atrial natriuretic factor/peptide; CSF - colony stimulating factor; DX - diagnostic(s); EGF - epidermal growth factor; ELISA - enzyme-linked immunosorbent assay; EPO - erythropoietin; FGF - fibroblast growth factor; GM-CSF - granulocyte macrophage colony stimulating factor; HCG - human chorionic gonadotropin; HEP-B - hepatitis B; HGH - human growth hormone; IF - interferon (IFα = interferon-alpha, etc.); IGF - insulin-like growth factor; IL - interleukin (IL-2 = interleukin-2, etc.); MAB(S) - monoclonal antibody(ies); RX - therapeutic(s), drug(s); SOD - superoxide dismutase; TGF - T-cell growth factor; TNF - tumor necrosis factor; TPA - tissue plasminogen activator; VX - vaccine.

firms, but this source was greatly curtailed by the stock market crash of October 1987.[6] A primary source of funds for these companies has been through strategic alliances with pharmaceutical companies and other large corporations (see section below).

The support of biotechnology-related research by the U.S. government is the strongest in the world, more than ten times its nearest competitor nation. From this basic research, many U.S. biotech firms emerged, often founded by U.S. academic researchers.[8] More of these firms were founded in the U.S. than in Europe or the Far East, and companies worldwide have relied on U.S. biotech firms for access to biotechnology R & D.

III. PHARMACEUTICAL COMPANY INVOLVEMENT

The development of recombinant DNA-based therapeutics is not limited to the small biotech firms. Many of the products to reach the market have been brought out by the pharmaceutical companies, such as Lilly's Humulin® (human insulin) or Merck's Recombivax®-B (hepatitis-B vaccine) or Roche's Roferon® (interferon-α2a).[2] Only one biotechnology firm, Genentech, has products on the market. In contrast, only 26 of the 88 products in clinical trial listed in Table 1 are from the large pharmaceutical companies.

Pharmaceutical companies became involved in biotechnology later and move more slowly in that direction than the biotech firms. Whereas a new biotech firm is founded to work with biotechnology, the established corporations have to hire or train a new scientific team and build the required laboratory facilities. Through a combination of strategies, pharmaceutical companies have hastened their entry into biotechnology.[9]

IV. STRATEGIC ALLIANCES

With new markets and hundreds of new therapeutics being developed through biotechnological processes, pharmaceutical companies will undoubtedly play a major role in the development and marketing of these new drugs. During the last 5 years, almost all major pharmaceutical companies worldwide have added biotechnology to their ongoing activities.[10,11] Until the early 1980s, the vast majority of pharmaceutically related biotechnology products were developed by the small biotech firms. The large corporations had the choice of playing catch-up or joining with the small firms to gain quicker access to the products. In essence, they adopted both strategies — simultaneously developing in-house expertise and forming strategic alliances with biotech firms. Indeed, most of the first pharmaceuticals developed using genetic engineering were joint efforts, such as Lilly's human insulin (developed with Genentech) or Schering-Plough's interferon-α2b (developed with Biogen).

These alliances take a variety of forms and have ranged from simple research contracts to the acquisition of a biotechnology firm.[5,9] Examples of these alliances from 1988 appear in Table 2. Alliances provide the larger corporations with early access to the products of biotechnology and give the small biotech firms needed capital to remain solvent during their long initial period of high expenses and essentially no product sales. These strategic alliances have both benefits and liabilities, as described in following sections.

A. RESEARCH CONTRACTS

The simplest form of access to biotechnology is a contract to perform research in the development of a specific product. Costs can vary, from tens of thousands of dollars to a few million dollars. It is not uncommon for a pharmaceutical company to have multiple research contracts with biotech firms, picking research projects from a variety of firms along the lines of company interest. The terms of such contracts vary greatly, especially with terms of ownership of the products of research. With the fierce competition in the biotechnology industry, it is likely that a corporation can find a biotech firm working on any product, but the firms' competitive positions on products vary greatly and need to be examined closely by the potential partner.

TABLE 2
Strategic Alliances: Biotechnology and Pharmaceuticals

U.S. Company[a]	Second company	Product[b]	Action[c]
	Two U.S. Companies		
A H Robins	American Home Products	RX	A
Advances Polymer Systems	Ortho Pharmaceutical	Retinoid RX	J
Agouron Pharmaceutical	Eli Lilly	Novel RX	E
Alza	Merrell Dow	Anti-smoking RX	J
Amgen	Cetus	IL-2	L
Applied Biomedical Sci	Medi Matrix	Skin RX	A
Athena Neurosciences	Eli Lilly	RX	J
Biotechnology General	DuPont	HGH	J
Biotechnology General	SmithKline	HGH	M
Biotherapeutics	Baxter Healthcare	Cancer RX	J
Biotherapeutics	Xoma	Cancer RX	J
California Biotech	Genentech	Surfactant	J
California Biotech	Metabolic Biosystems	Diabetes RX	V
California Biotech	Wyeth-Ayerst	Atrial peptides	L
Cambridge Bioscience	Cetus	CSF	L
Cellular Products	Cetus	CSF	M
Centocor	Velos	MAB RX	L
Cetus	Triton Biosciences	IF-beta	J
Chemex	Upjohn	Skin RX	L
Chiron	Mimesys	Growth factors	J
Collagen	Bristol-Myers	TGF-beta2	J
Collagen	Target Tharapeutics	RX Delivery system	A
Cooper Development	Cooper Life Sciences	Alpha-1 antitrypsin	LA
Dow Chemical	Essex Chemical	Chemicals, RX	A
Epitope	Eastman Kodak	Cancer DX/RX	J
Epitope	Ingene	AIDS RX	J
Ethicon	Vestar	Anti-inflammatory RX	J
Fluoromed	Otisville Biopharm	RX	A
Genelabs	SRI International	AIDS RX	JR
Genentech	Vestar	RX proteins	J
Genetics Institute	Schering-Plough	GM-CSF	M
Genetics Institute	Syntex	Novel RX	J
ICN Pharmaceuticals	Eastman Kodak	RX	A
IDEC Pharmaceuticals	NY Life Insurance Co.	AIDS RX	R
IGI	Rorer Group	RX	J
Immune For Life	Monoclonal International	AIDS RX	J
Immunex	Eastman Kodak	IL-7, IL-4	JE
Immunogen	Dana Farber Cancer Institute	MAB	L
Immunogen	Merck	Lung cancer RX	M
Ingene	Eastman Kodak	Cancer RX	J
Invitron	Rorer	Factor VIII:C	J
Invitron	Searle	TPA	L
Invitron	SmithKline	AIDS RX	JE
Lasalle Laboratories	Schering-Plough	Gynecological RX	J
Lyphomed	Vestar	RX, RX delivery	J
Metabolic Biosystems	Pfizer	Diabetes RX	R
Mimesys	Warner-Lambert	EGF, NGF	JM
Neorx	Eastman Kodak	Cancer RX/DX	L
Neorx	Mallinckrodt	Cancer DX/RX	ME
Northfield Labs	Quest Biotechnology	Hemoglobin	L
Nova Pharmaceutical	SmithKline	RX	E
Oncogene Science	Pfizer	TGF beta-3	J
Osteotx	Rorer	Osteoporosis RX	R
Quest Blood Substitute	Baxter Healthcare	Blood substitute	L
Quidel	Baxter Healthcare	DX	M

TABLE 2 (continued)
Strategic Alliances: Biotechnology and Pharmaceuticals

U.S. Company[a]	Second company	Product[b]	Action[c]
Two U.S. Companies			
Repligen	Applied Immunesystems	rDNA protein A	J
Rhomed	Biomira	MABS for DX, RX	J
Sterling Drugs	Eastman Kodak	RX	A
Synergen	Ciba-Geigy	Elastase inhibitor	M
Techniclone	American Cyanimid	Antibodies	E
Vestar	Bristol-Myers	Liposomes	J
Xoma	Pfizer	MAB	M
Canada			
American Cyanamid	Quadra Logic	Cancer RX	JE
DDI Pharmaceuticals	Allelix	RDNA SOD	J
Elkins-Sinn	Quadra Logic	RX	J
Nova Pharmaceutical	Allelix	RX for AIDS	R
Verex Labs	Galen Pharma	RX	L
Vipont Research Labs	Plant Biotechnology Inst	Antiplaque RX	J
France			
Cytogen	Clonatec	RX, DX	L
Xoma	Sanofi	Immunotoxins	L
Italy			
Bio-Response	A. Menarini	TPA	L
Liposome Technology	Montedison	RX	J
Summa Manufacturing	Erbamont	Anticancer RX	A
Japan			
Biotech Research Labs	Ajinomoto	RX	R
California Biotech	Daiichi Seiyaku	Alzheimer's RX	J
California Biotech	Kaken Pharmaceutical	FGF	M
California Biotech	Mitsubishi Kasei	RX	M
Chemex	Takeda	Antiallergy RX	L
Epitope	Olympus Corp.	AIDS MABS	J
Gen-Probe	Chugai Pharmaceutical	RX	M
Genentech	Calpis Food Industry	Renal growth factor	L
Genentech	Mitsubishi Kasei	TPA, albumin	L
Genetics Institute	Chugai	EPO	L
Genetics Institute	Suntory	TPA	M
IGI	Otsuka Pharmaceuticals	RX	L
Immunetech	Tanabe Seiyaku	RX	JE
Ingene	Green Cross	Cancer DX/RX	J
Integrated Genetics	Kyowa Hakko Kogyo	MSF	M
Merck	Tanabe Seiyaku	RX	J
Regenetron	Sumitomo Chemical	RX	JE
Schering-Plough	Essex Nippon	GM-CSF	J
Upjohn	Chugai Pharmaceutical	EPO, G-CSF	V
Warner-Lambert	Kyowa Hakko	Anticancer RX	JM
Netherlands			
Quidel	Maatschappij Voor Ind.	RX	E
Rhomed	Syngene	Colorectal cancer RX	J

TABLE 2 (continued)
Strategic Alliances: Biotechnology and Pharmaceuticals

U.S. Company[a]	Second company	Product[b]	Action[c]
Sweden			
Bristol-Myers	Pharmacia Ophthalmics	Eye growth factor	J
Chiron	Pharmacia	SOD	JM
Genentech	Kabigen	IGF-I	L
Genesia	Kabivitrum AB	RX	J
Switzerland			
Amgen	Hoffmann-La Roche	G-CSF	M
Amgen-Kirin	Cilag	EPO	L
BioTechnica International	Hoffmann-La Roche	Vitamins	R
Cetus	Hoffmann-La Roche	IL-2	E
Creative Biomolecules	Alcon Laboratories	Growth factors	J
DuPont	Hoffmann-La Roche	Cancer RX	J
Immunex	Hoffmann-La Roche	IL-2	J
Interferon Sciences	Hoffmann-La Roche	Genital wart RX	LE
Ribi Immunochem	Hoffmann-La Roche	VX for tumors	JR
Schering-Plough	Sandoz	GM-CSF	J
SmithKline	Symphar	Cardiac RX	J
Verax	Sandoz	RX	J
United Kingdom			
American Cyanamid	Celltech	Cancer RX/DX	J
Biogen	Glaxo	IL-2, GM-CSF	J
DuPont	Xenova	RX	J
Lederle	Celltech	Cancer RX	J
McNeil	British Biotechnology	Cholesterol RX	R
Pfizer	British Biotechnology	Endothelium	JR
Pharmatec	Wellcome	Retrovir	R
SmithKline	Bio-Technology Ltd.	TPA	J
Upjohn	Beecham	Clot dissolver	JM
West Germany			
Genetics Institute	Boehringer Mannheim	EPO	M
Immunex	Hoechst	GM-CSF	J
Immunogen	E. Merck	Lung cancer RX	L
Lectec	Beiersdorf	Skin RX	J
Phillips Petroleum	Bissendorf	Peptides	JR
Repligen	E. Merck	Platelet factor 4	J
Squibb	Boehringer Ingelheim	ACE Inhibitor	M

Notes: These are representative samples of companies working together on biotechnology products for the period January 1988 through January 1989 in actions involving therapeutics. The source of these actions is the North Carolina Biotechnology Center's Actions Database.

[a] Company 1 is always a U.S. company. Company 2 is from the country indicated. If two U.S. companies are involved, the smaller of the companies is listed first.

[b] See product abbreviations list in Table 1.

[c] Codes for actions are A, acquisition; E, equity purchase; J, joint interaction, usually unspecified; L, licensing agreement; M, marketing agreement; R, research contract.

B. JOINT VENTURES AND PARTNERSHIPS

An extension of a research contract can range from a contract for jointly developing a therapeutic to forming a new business venture to work on the project. Examples of the latter are the formation of Kirin-Amgen to develop erythropoietin and the formation of Genencor by Genentech and Corning. These arrangements represent a higher level of commitment between partners and may provide more limited returns to each partner.

C. LICENSING AND MARKETING AGREEMENTS

The average biotechnology firm is still in the stage of performing mostly research and development and has not yet brought a major product to market. It has not had the need, and likely not the resources, to develop full-fledged marketing or production teams. Pharmaceutical companies are the more likely candidates to market the early products of biotechnology, and numerous licensing and marketing agreements have been formed, some of which are listed in Table 2. Once again, these contracts are highly variable in their terms, including length of time and geographic location. It is not uncommon for a biotechnology firm to have marketing agreements with a U.S. pharmaceutical company for North America, as well as a European company and a Japanese company for European and Asian marketing rights. An example of this is Genetics Institute's erythropoietin development with marketing in the U.S. through Chugai-Upjohn, in Europe through Boehringer Mannheim, and in Asia and elsewhere through Chugai.[5]

D. EQUITY PURCHASES AND ACQUISITIONS

It has been common practice for corporations to take equity positions in biotech firms, often accompanying or following other alliances with the small firm. Schering's 20% stake in Biogen is an early example and has led to those companies' joint development of interferon products. Companies such as American Cyanamid, Becton Dickinson, Du Pont, Eastman Kodak, Eli Lilly, Johnson & Johnson, and Syntex have purchased equity positions in multiple biotech firms.[3]

To date, there have been relatively few acquisitions of biotech firms by pharmaceutical companies. The purchases of Hybritech by Eli Lilly and Genetic Systems by Bristol-Myers in 1985, costing over $300 million each, are among the few examples of major acquisitions in biotechnology.

Before October 1987, biotechnology stocks were valued at a high price, perhaps grossly overpriced, making acquisition an expensive route for getting expertise in biotechnology. Acquisition also has some drawbacks: limitation to the focus of the acquired firm; problems of fitting an entrepreneurial organization into a large, established corporation; and retaining key personnel after the acquisition. Regardless, acquisition can give a pharmaceutical company ready access to a team of researchers with biotechnology expertise, some products in development, and perhaps a strong competitive position with one or more key products.

Pharmaceutical companies have used multiple forms of strategic alliances and, conversely, the more advanced biotech firms have formed strategic alliances with numerous corporations. These alliances have been the hallmark of the development of U.S. biotechnology.

This transfer of technology from the small U.S. biotech firms to larger corporations for subsequent commercialization is not limited to transfer to U.S. corporations. Numerous alliances with foreign or subsidiaries of foreign-based corporations have also occurred, as can be seen in Table 2. Many of these alliances confer marketing rights for local markets, while others are for product development or worldwide rights.

V. ISSUES AND TRENDS

The impact of biotechnology on pharmaceuticals may be significant, but it is not without major issues. The final outcome is not yet clear. With intense competition in the industry, especially for the development of therapeutics, uncertain regulatory and patent questions, intense competition from abroad, and the financial fragility of many U.S. biotech firms, many issues are yet to be resolved.

A. INTENSE COMPETITION

With the lure of substantial markets for therapeutics made with genetic engineering, it is understandable that many players have joined in the race to develop the same product. For example, tissue plasminogen activator (t-PA), once cited with a $500 million market potential, has attracted dozens of companies in many alliances.[3] What is in question is how many companies will be able to receive a substantial return on their investment in t-PA. It is unlikely that more than a handful will be able to recoup their millions of dollars in expenses in t-PA development. Similarly, intense competition can be seen in the development of many other therapeutics, including interleukins, interferons, and growth hormones.[3,5,12] Sales of biotechnology-derived therapeutics may reach the predicted billions of dollars by the turn of the century, but these sales are unlikely to sustain all of the biotech firms and all of the pharmaceutical corporations working on these products.[7,12]

Biotechnology has not only the fierce competition between companies described above, but has attracted new competitors into the arena. The growth of therapeutics markets due to the advent of biotechnology is certainly to be accompanied by new competitors in the industry. Corporations not previously tied with health care, such as Du Pont or Monsanto, have used biotechnology as a means of diversifying into pharmaceuticals. The U.S. pharmaceutical industry was considered to be a mature industry, with only one major company, Syntex, founded in the last 50 years. Now, to a large degree via biotechnology, the players are changing. Some of the biotech firms will emerge as major competitors.

B. PATENT AND REGULATORY ISSUES

The therapeutics made with genetic engineering have introduced new questions and considerations related to their manufacture, use, and regulation. The U.S. Food and Drug Administration (FDA) has made efforts to work with the companies developing these products in order to resolve the regulatory process involved.[13] This is especially important for the new firms that do not have a history of working with the FDA.

The patenting of genetically engineered therapeutics (and other products of biotechnology) is further from resolution. At least 6000 patent applications await decision at the Patent and Trademark Office, and the wait for decisions is almost double the normal time.[12] A shortage of examiners with the proper training is cited as the basis of this backlog, and only recently have measures been taken to train personnel. This backlog may be especially costly to the smaller biotech firms, with patents being considered as a form of value owned by these firms.[7,12]

Issues related to patents also remain to be resolved. The scope of patents for biotechnology-derived therapeutics has not been determined. For example, will Genentech be able to maintain a monopoly in the sale of t-PA due to its early patent position and regulatory approval? Or will other companies be able to make t-PA by other means, such as in different cells or with minor modifications, thus circumventing Genentech's patent position?

C. INTERNATIONAL COMPETITION

Competitiveness in biotechnology on a national scale has been the focus of much recent attention. Government agencies in Japan, West Germany, the U.K., and other countries have created programs for the development of biotechnology. They include targeting areas of research, fostering technology transfer to industry, and developing fermentation processes, separations, and downstream processing, among others.[10] Similar programs have yet to be developed in the U.S., but have been the subject of numerous congressional hearings and public concern. Competition from abroad is likely due more to strengths in industry than from government programs, but these programs help to assure involvement in key areas related to national need.[7,10,14]

The U.S. has enjoyed early leadership in the basic research related to biotechnology, but scientific discovery is many steps removed from its related commercialization. With only a handful of therapeutics from genetic engineering now in the marketplace, it is too early to tell which country will emerge as the leader in the commercialization of therapeutics. Japan has many corporations working with therapeutics and a strong history of fermentation-based production, and is likely to emerge as a strong competitor in biotechnology worldwide.[9,10] Moreover, the Japanese pharmaceutical industry has shown signs of strengthening — in a 1987 to 1988 study, of the 11 pharmaceutical companies worldwide showing the largest pharmaceutical sales increase, 6 were Japanese (and none were from the U.S.).[15] What was once considered the "commanding lead" of the U.S. in biotechnology may no longer be valid.

VI. CONCLUSIONS

Biotechnology has begun to make its mark on the pharmaceutical industry. Many new products are in development, opening up new markets. The breakthroughs in science related to biotechnology will lead to new methods of drug discovery. Pharmaceutical companies have included biotechnology in their drug discovery process and have entered numerous business alliances related to biotechnology. The nature of the pharmaceutical industry will change with corporations diversifying into health care and the stronger biotechnology companies growing into pharmaceutical companies. In turn, these occurrences will factor into national competitiveness in the global economy.

First, we need to resolve patent issues and clarify the regulatory process for biotechnology. Many of the financially fragile biotech firms will not survive the intense competition. Many more strategic alliances are likely to be formed, and biotechnology will be another front in high-technology where the Japanese may take over as the global leader. Perhaps most importantly, new therapies will evolve to cure diseases not previously curable, and new vaccines will help curb a wide variety of major ailments. We have an exciting decade ahead of us.

REFERENCES

1. SCRIP, Review Issue 1988, p. 13.
2. Pharmaceutical Manufacturers' Association, *Update: Biotechnology Products in Development,* October 1988.
3. **Dibner, M. D.**, *Biotechnology Guide U.S.A.: Companies, Data and Analysis,* Stockton Press/Macmillan, New York, 1988.
4. **Vane, J. and Cuatrecasas, P.**, Genetic engineering and pharmaceuticals, *Nature (London),* 312, 303, 1984.
5. The North Carolina Biotechnology Center maintains three databases on commercial biotechnology: The *Actions Database* has more than 3500 records of actions taken between companies, such as licensing agreements and research contracts; the *Companies Database* contains detailed information on more than 600 U.S. companies working with biotechnology; and the *Japan Database* contains detailed information on 250 Japanese corporations working with biotechnology.
6. **Burrill, G. S. and the Arthur Young High Technology Group**, *Biotech '89: Commercialization,* Mary Ann Liebert Publishers, New York, 1988.
7. **Dibner, M. D. and White, R. S.**, Biotechnology in the United States and Japan: who's on first?, *Biopharm,* 2(2), 22, 1989.
8. **Dibner, M. D. and Lavrich, C. C.**, Doing business with Japan: an analysis of partnerships. *Bio/Technology,* 5, 1029, 1987.
9. **Dibner, M. D.**, Corporate strategies for involvement in biotechnology, *Biofutur (Paris),* July/August 1987, 47.
10. U.S. Congressional Office of Technology Assessment, *Commercial Biotechnology: An International Analysis,* U.S. Government Printing Office, Washington, D.C., 1984.
11. U.S. Congressional Office of Technology Assessment, *New Developments in Biotechnology (4): U.S. Investment in Biotechnology,* U.S. Government Printing Office, Washington, D.C., 1988.
12. **Naj, A. K.**, Clouds gather over the biotech industry, *Wall Street Journal,* Jan. 30, 1989, B1.
13. **Baum, R. M.**, Biotech industry moving pharmaceutical products to market, *Chem. Eng. News,* 65(29), 11, 1987.
14. **Dibner, M. D.**, Biotechnology in Europe, *Science,* 232, 1367, 1986.
15. SCRIP, Review Issue 1988, 7.

Chapter 21

TO START A BIOTECHNOLOGY COMPANY

G. Steven Burrill

TABLE OF CONTENTS

I. INTRODUCTION

In this chapter, we shall review the path from a promising laboratory invention to a functioning biotechnology business. Review is timely because biotechnology continues to offer new commercial possibilities as we approach 1990, although the rules of the game have somewhat toughened since the mid-1970s, when the commercial promise of the new biotechnologies first became obvious. At that time, entrepreneurial scientists and venture capitalists were witnessing a revolution in the laboratory, and they foresaw a corresponding revolution in the marketplace. They were not wrong.

The accomplishments of the first generation of companies are impressive. They also represent a mixed blessing for new companies. On the one hand, the pioneers have demonstrated how to go about building a biotech company. On the other hand, new companies seeking investor attention and top-flight scientific staff must compete with the well-established first-generation companies for these scarce resources. Be that as it may, the experience of scientists, executives, and business advisors responsible for the successes of the first generation provides a realistic guide to what is required today to start a biotech company. Their experience will be reflected in this chapter.

Unlike many chapters in this volume, what I have to offer is not "hard science", nor can it be rigidly systematic. Building a biotechnology business, like building a business of any type, requires clearly identifiable skills and assets, passes through recognizable stages of growth, and faces well-known hurdles, but the environment in which a company has to operate is full of uncertainty. Business competitors, both American and foreign, can be counted on to do the unexpected; regulatory agencies are apt to change the rules; the general economy and Wall Street, safely ignored by lab scientists, are likely to have considerable impact on the freedom of a new biotech company to do what it thinks it should be doing.

A note of caution, then, at the outset: to start a new biotechnology company is a great endeavor, never an easy one, which locks the scientist-executive into relationships of a very different kind from the classic struggle for knowledge that attracted him or her to science in the first place. The venture can be fascinating, it can render important services to humanity, and it can be extremely profitable. But only one of these factors is virtually guaranteed the newcomer: it *will* be fascinating.

II. THE INVENTION

Biotech companies start with an invention or series of inventions. From the mid-1970s to the early 1980s, the invention could be a technique of broad scope and essentially unproved commercial value. It was enough for a group of eminent scientists to decide to found a company dedicated to monoclonal antibody technology, to recombinant DNA, and/or to protein chemistry. The broad technology came first, it was matched — sometimes a little vaguely — to commercial goals, and the race was on. At this early stage, the selling point was as much the revolutionary technology itself as the products it might generate and the markets it might capture. Venture capitalists and private investors, soon followed by public-equity investors, caught the excitement and extended substantial financial resources to those equipped with the credentials to commercialize the technology.

This was an easier climate in which to start a company than the climate today. Biotechnologies now form the basis for some 1500 existing companies engaged in human health care, veterinary health care, agricultural improvement, food processing, lab instrumentation, and smaller niches such as hazardous waste processing. The combined weight of these companies in the marketplace is not so easily displaced to make room for start-ups, although the market is not closed and opportunity still audibly knocks. Owing to their presence in the marketplace, considerable experience has accumulated, so that potential investors are more knowledgeable than they could be a decade ago. Their questions are more pointed, their doubts more pervasive. Today, the invention must be more than a thrilling technology breakthrough. The new company needs to be precise about products it intends to manufacture and market, and about the competitive marketplace in which its products will have to generate revenues. *To the new company today, market understanding has become as important as technology.*

III. EVALUATING THE COMMERCIAL PROMISE OF THE INVENTION

Not all interesting inventions justify the attempt to found a company around them. The scientist who has made a breakthrough needs to consider carefully just where that breakthrough belongs in the scheme of things. There are vast differences between an invention, a product, and a company. An invention can be brilliant, but it may not offer a broad enough platform to build a commercial enterprise. A commercial product can be outstanding, but it may not command a sufficient market to support a company. "One-product companies" are notoriously fragile because they run the risk of being unable to develop a successful second generation of products. Let us consider some of the questions that need to be asked to evaluate the commercial promise of the invention.

Should it be taken to the university licensing office and licensed out in due course to an existing company involved in biotechnology, pharmaceuticals, chemicals, agriculture, energy, or food? This is an honorable outcome for a significant invention of limited scope.

Coldly considered, is the breakthrough really part of a larger process which has already been commercialized? Should it therefore be offered to a company that has shown vigorous interest in that process?

Can the invention be converted into a market-ready commercial product or products within a reasonable time frame at reasonable cost? A $100-million, 10-year development period for a human therapeutic that will ultimately serve a $5-million market is, in commercial perspective, obviously unworkable. On the other hand, that much financing and time is tolerable for a product that is likely to earn annual revenues of $100 million or more when it reaches the marketplace.

Is the breakthrough a singularity rather than a fertile source of further developments and multiple applications? By way of illustration, I often draw the contrast between a tulip and a rosebush: the tulip is a beautiful single blossom, while the rosebush — no less beautiful — will produce clusters of blossoms, each blooming at a different point in time.

Is the breakthrough subject to "scale-up" from laboratory procedures and quantities to commercial manufacturing procedures and quantities?

Is the invention patentable? The patent disputes currently rife in the biotechnology industry dramatize that this issue needs to be thought through, although there are uncertainties in patent law, particularly with regard to recombinant products, which will only be resolved in the course of time.

Are there daunting barriers to market entry? Other technologies or alternative answers to the same problem may bar the way. Owing to a scarcity of distribution channels or other constraining factors, the target market may be less accessible in fact than it first seems.

IV. THE INVENTOR AS BUSINESSPERSON

Let us hypothesize that the invention passes all the tests: it is patentable, it can be scaled up for manufacturing, it has multiple applications, it matches an identifiable market need or needs, the market opportunity justifies projected development costs, and there are no insuperable barriers to market entry. At this point the scientist or founder group needs friends. *Stars lose, teams win* — this is virtually a law of high-tech business development. There is nothing inimical in this law to the mores of the scientific community, in which research papers are signed by numerous participants. On the other hand, scientists characteristically admire "the great man" — the groundbreaking investigator with a sustained record of achievement. There is need for "the great man" in commercial biotechnology, but such persons ignore at their peril the requirement to build a great team.

The first stop in gathering a team of professionals with varied skills is very probably an advisor well versed in commercial biotechnology and general business and finance. It has been my privilege to play this midwifing role for many scientists, and on the basis of experience I have developed a rather brutal rule of thumb concerning my first meeting with them: if they choose to spend the first half-hour talking science and science alone, I seriously doubt that they should persist in trying to start a business. On the other hand, if the scientist addresses with clarity the technology, the market opportunities, the R & D milestones, and the team that can make it all happen, a listener cannot help but respond. One has to *assume* that the science can be completed successfully — the molecule can be cloned and expressed, the procedure scaled up. The business discussion starts from there.

The inventor as businessperson is turning toward a new world — a world disciplined by such concepts as return on investment, risk/reward, and strategic planning. He or she is setting out to build an *organization* with a complex internal structure and external relations with investors, analysts, regulators, the scientific community, competitors, business partners, news media, and the general public. The organization will be a demanding focus of attention for years to come — and if the scientist sitting with me does not show much interest in creating that organization in our first meeting, it is unlikely that the personal characteristics are all there to make a go of it. A great scientist is not necessarily an entrepreneur, nor need he be. But if he wants to found a biotechnology company, business has to matter to him.*

In time, he will unquestionably team up with seasoned business executives to operate the company. Meanwhile, there is a business to plan. Even when experienced managers come on board, biotechnology businesses do better when the scientific and management forces understand each other and know how to minimize agenda differences.

V. ROLE OF THE BUSINESS ADVISOR AND OTHER PROFESSIONALS

The business advisor to whom the entrepreneurial scientist turns can help him or her begin thinking realistically about the business that needs to grow up around the invention. How much money will it take to get started? And into the marketplace? How much time? How large an organization? What are the regulatory requirements? What is the patent situation? What is the competitive situation? What existing companies are likely to benefit from the R & D effort in view — and might therefore be willing to help finance it? Among the scientist's friends and acquaintances, who might be interested in helping finance the venture in return for a share in the company? Among colleagues, who should be persuaded to join what must be a genuinely prestigious scientific advisory board? How many skilled post-docs are ready to move from the

---

* To some participants, the patterns of business life are as fascinating as the patterns explored by science. A business is, in effect, a living organism generated from the single cell of a powerful idea. Differentiating into multiple related structures with distinct functions, it is endowed with its own internal metabolism and relates to its environment in increasingly complex ways. It inevitably meets internal and external crises — Darwinian episodes that challenge its survival and force adaptive change. The analogy can be drawn out, but without further elaboration the point may be clear that the scientist as businessperson need not think of himself or herself as moving into a compromised, excessively materialistic world where sound values and critical thinking are irrelevant. On the contrary, biotechnology companies of the first generation have developed original, humane, and broadly influential patterns of business organization. These are discussed at some length in Ernst & Young's annual surveys of the biotechnology industry, available from local offices of Ernst & Young.

university laboratory to the company laboratory? At least in preliminary ways, these are all questions that need answers.

When the time comes, the business advisor will also put the entrepreneur in touch with legal counsel, needed to give the business a proper form. In addition, if the advisor is not a CPA, he will almost certainly be able to provide the name of an accountant experienced in new business development, ideally one who is thoroughly familiar with the industry. An accountant's skills are just as critical as legal counsel's from this point forward.

The question will naturally arise: Doesn't this early-stage professional service cost money? The answer cannot be better put than "yes and no". The entrepreneurial scientist needs to build an army; he or she is the person with the vision, and that vision needs to be persuasively shared. If this broadening of "ownership" takes place, the professionals who have begun to share the vision might be persuaded to share the risks, too. They may be willing to postpone, in effect, some or all of their earnings until the business has taken shape and it can afford to compensate them. On the other hand, this contingency basis is a topic for negotiation; hence the "yes and no". Entrepreneurs do well to reflect that even if they don't pay out a dollar of their own funds at this early stage, they *are* paying many dollars in terms of the personal time required to work toward founding their business.

At the proper time, the principal advisor and his colleagues will probably be in a position to make introductions to reliable investors — venture capitalists, private sources, corporations interested in ground-floor investments in significant new biotechnology. Few scientists have sufficient personal financial resources to start a biotechnology company, although a Master-Card, so to speak, and personal savings are surprisingly relevant at this early stage. Generally speaking, there is a necessary passport to locating capital: a persuasive business plan.

VI. BUSINESS PLANNING

The process of business planning is as important, even more important, than its outcome. The bound document that results from planning is a necessary financing tool; for venture capitalists and other financial sources, it will in many instances represent their sole introduction to the company. But moving through the planning process in cooperation with a business advisor/ CPA, a lawyer, and fellow scientists provides an invaluable reality check at the level of detail, where the fate of companies is actually decided.

I want to stress that there is no need to reinvent the wheel where business planning is concerned. Sound business-planning manuals exist. To read one is good homework, although not a substitute for the participation of experienced planners in the actual process.* That such manuals exist is a clear indication that the entrepreneurial scientist is moving at this point into terrain familiar to business people, although perhaps new to him personally.

The business plan may be 20 pages or 200 pages long. Whatever its length, the venture capitalist who typically sees dozens each week is almost certain, initially, to read just the opening Executive Summary and, at a stretch, another section or two for *signs* of commercial promise. Clearly, those first pages are crucial. They need to convey scientific vision and commercial promise persuasively. Beyond this, there is no telling which sections of the plan will have that bellwether quality for venture capitalists with 5 minutes to invest in exploring the scientist's dream of a lifetime. Some turn to the scientific advisory board for familiar names that implicitly guarantee the quality of the company's science. Others are primarily interested in estimates of market size and time-to-market, because science that can't be converted into products and reach

---

* *The Ernst & Young Business Plan Guide* (John Wiley & Sons, New York, 1987) is my own firm's manual. There are, of course, other useful manuals.

attractive markets within a reasonable time is of dubious commercial value, however thrilling in concept.

Whatever the venture capitalist's approach to appraising quickly the potential of a business plan, the plan needs to be conceived and written with care throughout. The goal is to induce the venture capitalist or any promising investor to take the plan home for an attentive reading — and give the scientist a call the next morning. A business plan is a door-opener, not a document that closes an agreement. For this reason among others, it need not be glossy and elegant. Some venture capitalists regard an expensive-looking publication as a sign of spendthrift ways, although this is factually a rare trait among scientists more likely to be driving into the business world in a battered station wagon than in a 12-cylinder Jaguar.

VII. ISSUES FOR PLANNERS TO CONSIDER

A full outline of the "ideal" business plan need not be incorporated in this article, in light of the existence of well-detailed manuals. However, some background comments may be useful. In structure (see the table), the business plan generally begins with a clear, brief Executive Summary and continues with topics ordered to reflect the priorities of experienced investors. Hence, the marketing section precedes the technology/R & D section — not a sequence likely to satisfy a scientist's priorities, standard nonetheless.

Sequence of Topics in a Biotechnology Business Plan

1. Executive summary
2. Table of contents
3. Company description
4. Market analysis and marketing plan
5. Technology: research and development
6. Manufacturing/operations
7. Management and ownership
8. Organization and personnel
9. Funds required and their uses
10. Financial data (historical data if relevant, 3- and 5-year projections)
11. Administrative considerations (e.g., company name)
12. Appendices or exhibits (as required, e.g., resumes of key managers)

A. RISK STEP-DOWN POINTS AND CONTROL

As noted earlier, the Executive Summary is a key component of the plan. It should include data on (1) the purpose of the business (e.g., to develop and market innovative diagnostics for human disease), (2) the market size, (3) key people, (4) significant product features, (5) product development milestones, (6) competitive advantages, such as patents, and (7) financial goals, such as "achieving $1 million in sales in 1992". Technical, operational, and financial milestones should be presented — in this section as elsewhere in the document—as risk step-down points. These are the points in time at which specific risks are neutralized either by achieving milestones or by tactical withdrawal from efforts that have proved less promising than expected.

A strong, well-communicated awareness of risk step-down points can encourage potential investors to have confidence that the founders understand what is necessary to achieve their goals and have a clear sense of how to proceed. The founders need to demonstrate that they will know how to *control* the new business from day 1. It is a common experience of biotechnology companies to go a certain distance down a research path, encounter unexpected barriers to commercial development or scientific understanding, and at that point cut their losses. They may cancel the research program, sell it to a company better positioned to pursue it, or scale back to a level of effort and expense that seems realistic in light of the obstacles encountered. This is management, and biotech companies need management willing and able to exercise control over science, finance, and every other component of the business.

B. DISTINCTIVE COMPETENCE

The section of the business plan dedicated to a company description details the intended field of business; products, services, and markets; and the firm's *distinctive competence*. The importance of assessing and persuasively stating the firm's distinctive competence cannot be overstressed. To dramatize the need for this unique capability, some have described distinctive competence as a firm's "unfair advantage". Virtually all markets addressed by biotechnology are competitive, more so now than a decade ago. At that time, newly founded biotech firms took the field with success against established pharmaceutical and agricultural enterprises for two reasons: their distinctive competences in new technologies (about which larger companies had adopted a wait-and-see attitude) and their entrepreneurial initiative in converting new science into commercial products. Today, the "majors" are skilled in biotechnology, and first-generation biotech firms have achieved a decade or more headstart. In this environment, distinctive competence is a critical success factor.

C. DELIVERING TO THE MARKETPLACE

The section on market issues is likely to be one of the longest and most thorough in a successful business plan. It will need to address the character of the industry now, in 5 years, in 10 years; industry trends; major anticipated customers; market segments targeted for penetration by the new company's products; market size and share; and many other issues. This section provides a platform for the founders to convey their practical knowledge of the commercial environment which their company will address. As such, this section is a primary test by which many potential investors will measure the attractiveness of the venture. It is also a section where, to the detriment of the overall document, naivete often disguises as commercial aggressiveness. For example, to point out that a $1 billion market exists for a given product, and that 10% market share would yield $100 million in sales, is a weak statement without convincing information about *who* will actually buy the product, *why* the product will command their attention, and what distribution channels can actually be used or developed to bring the product efficiently to customers.

The acceptance of a product in the marketplace ultimately determines the company's success — this is a law of business of which experienced early-stage investors in biotechnology are acutely aware. There are two corollaries: (1) *The key issue in the technology business is the barrier to entry,* and (2) *The product will not sell itself.* These observations are for the most part self-explanatory, although easily enough lost from sight as the founding scientist pushes forward. However, the concept of entry barriers deserves further comment.

Certain barriers are obvious and accepted by industry, while others may be hidden and potentially damaging to commercial success. In the category of obvious, accepted barriers, FDA oversight of the approval process for human therapeutics and diagnostics is often criticized in its details, but virtually no one wants to dispense with sensible execution of this responsibility on the public behalf. This is a known barrier, and the requirements it imposes are familiar to regulatory professionals, however much FDA policy evolves from year to year.

Hidden barriers can change from year to year and product to product. To recognize them in time and address them vigorously requires management and market experience — and luck. Americans are taught to think that it suffices to "build a better mousetrap" for customers to beat a path to your door. Not true. Consider a marketplace already saturated with mousetraps that work adequately. The fact that a somewhat better mousetrap reaches market may not be a compelling reason for users pleased with the current model to spend money on the new one. We needn't think in fictional terms to continue this line of thought. Technology changes very rapidly in the desktop computer industry — but businesses and individuals already heavily invested in desktops move a good deal more slowly than the rate of technology change. A major innovation may not capture major market share, although it is intrinsically deserving.

Another hidden barrier, more common in biotechnology than many think, is the risk of being blindsided. The risk is not so much that a competitor will bring to market a directly comparable product (this can be expected to occur sooner or later in profitable market niches). The risk is that a competitor's product will virtually sweep away all need for one's own. The legendary example is the buggy whip — hardly worth perfecting any further in the 1900s, when the automobile was poised to dominate personal transportation. These dynamics potentially exist today in the markets served by biotechnology; for example, a company focused on achieving a therapeutic intervention may find that its market all but vanishes if a competitor develops an effective vaccine.

Distribution can also pose a hidden barrier to market success. A product that is literally perfect for certain regions of the Third World may never reach the Third World because distribution systems are inadequate and/or customers in the region may have little foreign exchange to spend on the product.

In summary, the business planning process is an important occasion for foresight and prudence. Some biotechnology businesses will not, and should not, pass this test. The entrepreneurial scientist will best serve his or her long-term interest by making a dignified retreat because planning has revealed barriers which it would be reckless to address. The scientific agenda, however brilliant and medically astute, may not be broad enough to justify the founding of a company. Distribution channels may be scarce. The planning process is meant in part to uncover whatever serious difficulties may exist.

Some projects will pass this test with flying colors and move on to the next stage: financing.

VIII. FINANCING STRATEGY

Early-stage financing for a biotechnology business is a matter of planning, making connections, negotiating, and concluding well-structured agreements. It is also a matter of abandoning old conceptions and routines that succeeded for the entrepreneurial scientist as director of an academic laboratory. The primary financing routine for an academic lab is the grant-winning process, typically pitched to a 3- or 5-year cycle that entails worry, effort, and peer review over the span of a year or so, followed by a longer balmy period when the laboratory can go about its work without financial worries. Further, given the magnitude of challenge in basic research, the measure of success at grant renewal time is not so much victory as significant progress.

Much of this familiar, although not easy, financing routine is irrelevant to commercial biotechnology. The timing of refinancings is unlikely to be so tidy, but that is the least of the differences worth noting. The major difference is that early-stage investors in commercial biotechnology, unlike government and foundation grantors, generally do not step back into the shadows while R & D proceeds. Major early investors are likely to demand — and deserve — a major management role, usually a seat on the board of the new company; they may conceivably dominate its management in many respects; and they will be looking for significant dollar-and-cents returns on their investment within a defined time horizon. Venture capitalists typically want a minimum return of ten times their investment within 5 years. They are gamblers who recognize that among 20 investments only 2 or 3 may be winners, and these few may be quite enough to carry their portfolio, but they understandably have high expectations of all of their investments.

Owing to the powerful influence of financing sources on company strategy and operations, it is not too much to say that *financing strategy drives business strategy*. This statement may be counter-intuitive and even distasteful to entrepreneurial scientists who wish to found a business in order to reach precise product-development goals. The implication is that founders will be free to pursue product development goals only to the degree that major financing sources agree with those goals. *He who has the gold rules* — or at least imposes compromises, timetables, even the abandonment of R & D projects, however promising their results at some indefinable future date. Because financing strategy will almost inevitably drive business strategy during the early years, the founders need to connect with venture capitalists and other investors who will share the dream and the mission — without much alteration of substance.

The founders should realize that venture capital, despite its prestige and leading role in the development of commercial biotechnology, is only one among a number of potential financing sources. There are always financing alternatives, some more desirable at a given time. The price and availability of money from different sources is always changing. The agendas by which large pools of investment capital are managed can vary widely. In this perspective, the goal is to achieve a marriage between the founders' agenda and that of the finance professionals who control investment capital.

Large corporations interested in investing in a biotech start-up with an intriguing R & D program may be somewhere "out there". It is part of the founders' job, with their advisors, to investigate this possibility very carefully — and to cover the country, if need be, giving what is commonly called a "dog and pony show" which conveys the company's promise to potential investors. In some economic climates (and not others), bank loans are a reasonable financing source. Private placements may, with luck, be available at a cheaper price than professional venture capital. Government and institutional grants, while almost never adequate on their own to the founding of a business, may provide some seed money. All of these possibilities, and still others, need to be considered by the founders in cooperation with a qualified financial advisor.

IX. NEGOTIATING THE DEAL

Let us assume that a strong business plan and vigorous follow-up efforts have brought the founders to the table with a venture capitalist seriously interested in financing the start-up company. The venture capitalist may bring in others from the profession to complete the financing, as well as passive investors who participate in the venture capitalist's deals. Whatever the circumstances, this first money is the most expensive which the founders will encounter in the lifetime of their firm. They must frequently give up 40 to 60% of the company in the first round of financing, in return for a sum approaching $2 million. A second round, for comparable or greater sums, is likely to occur about a year after start-up at a valuation which, if all has gone well, reflects the increased value of the company — particularly if, at the time of the financing, demand among venture capitalists for promising biotech start-ups is strong.

There are likely to be no more than three or four rounds of financing before it becomes wise to introduce other sources of capital, for example, public equity markets, corporations, and debt. The founders do well to seek enough financing in the first two rounds to accomplish the primary goals; additional rounds should be regarded as a contingency. Refinancings should correspond to milestones — risk step-down points — which demonstrate the company's capability and continuing promise. Venture capitalists and experienced investors are always looking not just at one company, but at *everything else* they could be doing with their funds.

The best rule of thumb for negotiation is that there are no rules of thumb; everything is negotiable. However, there are some operating principles well worth following. In the first place, leadership in the negotiation process cannot be delegated even to financial advisors and lawyers with the firm's welfare very much at heart. Only the founding scientist and his or her direct co-workers can make final decisions, although qualified advisors are not only useful, but necessary.

A second principle is to conduct negotiations as an equal of those who sit across the table. Venture capitalists and other experienced investors in biotechnology are typically successful and oversee large pools of capital. They may have participated in the founding of first-generation biotechnology companies which have gone on to win worldwide fame — but they are not visionary molecular biologists or protein chemists, not Nobel Prize winners or members of the National Academy, not inventors. They are there to help the founding scientist achieve commercial success, and as such they are equals in the venture, not more, not less.

Be willing to compromise. What the founders want and what investors want are both abstract until the negotiation process generates a middle ground where their desires can be coordinated in a deal that is fair to all parties, indulgent to none. An ugly but truthful business phrase is fully applicable here; there is no free lunch. The investor takes a greater risk by investing in a biotech start-up than by buying a Treasury bond — and expects a comparably greater return on investment. The founders would like to maintain ownership of the lion's share of the company — but, to look ahead, they are likely to own no more than 10 to 15% of the company by the time it goes public. The rest will have been traded for capital resources. In light of this fact, "control of the company" should not be allowed to become a prickly issue in the founders' minds. To the truism "He who has the gold rules", we might add this corollary: Where there is no gold, there is no company. A small piece of a sizable pie is as attractive as a large piece of a small one.

Be willing to walk away with nothing. Some investors may want too large a piece of the company; others may be unwilling to meet the company's real needs. Whatever the obstacle, it needs to be recognized without regret. Obtaining capital may not be easy — biotechnology is, after all, only a bit player in the worldwide, efficient market for capital. The risks of investing in biotechnology are high; the rewards, while potentially great, are attended by this risk. Investors always consider return on investment and may calculate the risk/reward ratio in ways that may seem excessively prudent or unimaginative to those seeking capital. However, provided that the company has genuine commercial promise, it will in time find its investors.

X. BUILDING THE BUSINESS

The deal has been struck. The founders are now at the helm of their own company, supported scientifically by a strong scientific advisory board and strategically by a board of directors that may include the lead venture capitalist as chairman. There is enough money in the bank for the first year of operations, and a sound business plan is ready to be put into practice. Economical working space has been found. The time has come for serious company building.

An entrepreneur shared with me, some years later, his initial feeling of dismay as he scanned an empty office and pondered his company, which at that moment consisted of a desk, a telephone, a secretary, and himself. It is possible to work one's way up from there, as that individual did very successfully. For its first few years, the company cannot help but be what is derisorily called "a science project" by scientists and executives who have gotten past that stage. It will be an R & D house with the challenging task of mastering the difficulties of product development and building a real business while maintaining investor confidence.

The founder needs to build the team. The investment in *people* is extraordinarily important — initially senior scientists, gifted post-docs, and business managers. Varied talents will be needed as the business develops — expertise in finance, operations, manufacturing, marketing, and sales, as well as supporting staff in these areas. Quite a few professional services can be obtained on a consulting basis — for example, regulatory expertise and information technology expertise need not be brought in house for quite a few years, but access to these skills is critical. In due course, investments in manufacturing space and instrumentation will be made. All investments need to be made with an eye to preserving capital because biotechnology invariably takes longer and costs more than foreseen on its way to market. Just as there needs to be a business plan to start the company, there needs to be an operations plan to carry the business forward. The plan outlines the goals and objectives for the business and presents an organizational chart for reporting relationships, administrative activities for conducting the business, and the research and development milestones for product development.

The key to successfully building the business is balance. I like to compare this balance of skills to the legs of a stool. The presence of a Nobel laureate may be crucial for a company's progress, but so too is a manufacturing director who has come up through the ranks in the pharmaceutical industry, or a regulatory consultant who has been schooled by years of experience with the relevant agency.

A little opportunism along the way will not be amiss. *Tactics are more important to success than strategy.* The overarching business plan that helped the company get started needs to be followed flexibly, even defied when an unexpected but excellent opportunity shows up. An established corporation may be interested in a strategic alliance to market the company's products, or see a product through the regulatory process *and* market it. A foreign company may unexpectedly show interest. A research effort slated to yield a supporting tool for other research may turn out, surprisingly, to generate a market all its own. These unforeseen events, and others like them, call for tactical intelligence.

On the other hand, too much flexibility can destroy the company's focus. While it may be tempting, for example, to sell some reagents here and there, the company was presumably not founded to sell reagents. Managers do well to remember that short-term revenues, however useful, cannot substitute for achieving major product development milestones.

The venture should be fun. This may seem a childish criterion; there will, of course, be days and probably months of worry. But, on the whole, the experience of guiding a biotechnology business is enlivening and even joyful for those who welcome the calculated risk and are willing to do everything possible to keep the odds in their favor.

XI. GOING PUBLIC

The day may come when the company is ready to go public. Publicly financed companies come under different constraints than they experience at the earlier stage when venture capital and other private sources provided their primary financing. Wall Street demands quarterly growth, steady progress, and highly visible achievements against milestones; only this type of performance keeps investors and analysts happy. On the other hand, the venture capitalists and other private investors who involve themselves early in a company's efforts are virtual "insiders", perhaps even board members, who personally follow the company's progress. They are unlikely to demand such a tightly patterned performance, provided that real progress is being made. Early investors may well be prepared to see the company spend heavily on R & D to hit that homerun — to develop the product or products that will generate massive profitability.

A successful public offering is likely to give venture capitalists who helped start the company their anticipated return. Accordingly, they may happily cash out and look for another biotech start-up equally worthy of financial backing. On the other hand, founders and early participants in the firm typically do not cash out; they want to continue developing the business. But because they are now paper millionaires, they will be tempted to count their "money" and regard themselves as winners.

They are not yet winners. True, their paper has some value — but it will be wallpaper 3 years later if they do not get on with the real work of the company, which is to bring to market important, innovative products which generate noticeable profits and command respectable market share. The genuine winners see through their first wealth and continue building the company until it is a self-sufficient enterprise capable of financing its own research. Then the founding entrepreneurs can begin dreaming again. What new product to pursue? What new technology to develop? What real needs can be met by this real company?

Chapter 22

GLOBAL CONSIDERATIONS IN THE DEVELOPMENT AND PRODUCTION OF PHARMACEUTICALS

J. David Tucker and James W. Parker

TABLE OF CONTENTS

I. INTRODUCTION

The globalization of pharmaceutical markets is a trend of the eighties which will continue and increase as we approach the next century (Figure 1).

Developing and producing pharmaceuticals to meet global needs poses many problems not encountered when considering the needs of a single country. The technological challenges of drug development and production are made more complex by cultural, political, economic, and infrastructural factors which vary widely around the world.

This chapter will provide some brief observations on the international pharmaceutical scene. These will include the environmental factors which must be considered and understood in order to successfully develop and produce pharmaceutical products to meet worldwide needs.

II. THE INTERNATIONAL PHARMACEUTICAL BUSINESS

A. SCOPE AND MAGNITUDE

The scope of the international pharmaceutical business encompasses bulk drugs (pharmaceutical chemicals), pharmaceutical dosage forms for human and veterinary use, agricultural products containing drugs, and medical devices and diagnostic products and services. This review will concentrate on pharmaceutical dosage forms.

The countries of the world may be classified economically as low income, middle income, capital surplus, centrally planned economies, and industrialized countries (Table 1). The economic level of each country profoundly affects drug availability and consumption patterns, and technological capacity to develop and produce drugs.

There is a great disparity between the developed world and the developing countries in the consumption of pharmaceuticals (Table 2) and in health care expenditures generally (Table 3).

Although population growth is more rapid in developing countries than in the developed nations, pharmaceutical consumption is increasing most quickly in the developed countries (Figure 2).

Large differences also exist in the use of various therapeutic classes of drugs between individual countries and between developed and developing nations (Table 4).

Multinational pharmaceutical companies based principally in the U.S., Western Europe, and Japan play a key role in developing, manufacturing, and distributing pharmaceuticals to meet the needs of global markets. They dominate the pharmaceutical economics of all country categories (Table 5). These companies have the financial and technological resources essential to the development of new drugs.

The policies of some developing countries discourage the risk capital needed for new drug development and for developing local technology. Except in the industrialized countries, indigenous pharmaceutical companies play little or no role in developing new products. Their quality standards and manufacturing practices tend to lag behind those of the multinationals.

Although universities play a relatively minor role in the development of new drugs, their role in basic research is essential to drug research and development by pharmaceutical companies.

With some exceptions such as the National Institutes of Health in the U.S., government organizations have not made a major contribution to new drug discovery.

Drug innovation, manufacturing and distribution expertise, and financial resources are thus concentrated in the multinational pharmaceutical companies.

B. TRENDS AND DEVELOPMENTS

The economic and political climates strongly influence the willingness and ability of the multinational pharmaceutical industry to invest in and develop drugs for each country or market. In pursuing their needs and aspirations, each country in turn attempts to set policies within the context of its resources, political systems, and national priorities.

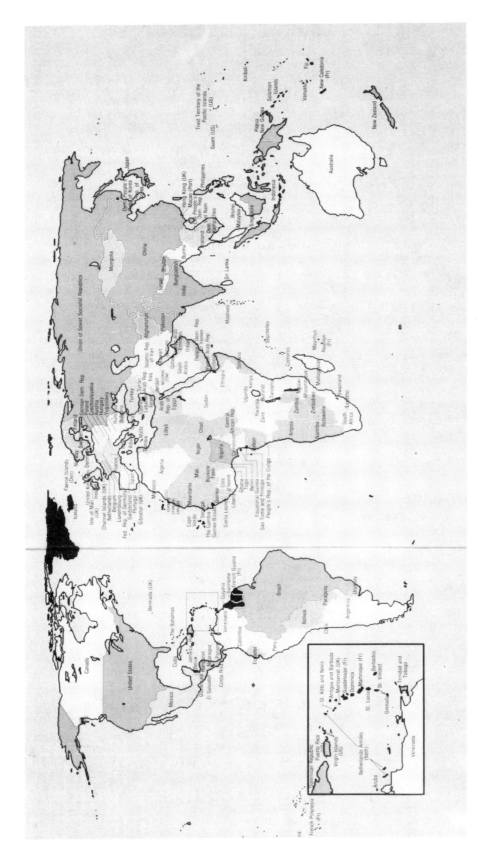

FIGURE 1. World map. (From *The World Bank Atlas*, 21st. ed., The World Bank, Washington, D.C. 1988. 4. With permission.)

269

TABLE 1
Country Classifications

Low-Income Countries

Afghanistan	India	Pakistan
Bangladesh	Indonesia	Rwanda
Benin	Kenya	Sierra Leone
Bhutan	Laos PDR	Somalia
Burundi	Lesotho	Sri Lanka
Burma	Madagascar	Tanzania
Cambodia	Malawi	Uganda
Central African Republic	Mali	Upper Volta
Chad	Mozambique	Vietnam
Ethiopia	Nepal	Yemen Arab Republic
Guinea	Niger	Zaire
Haiti		

Middle -Income Countries

Algeria	Ghana	Mauritania	Spain
Angola	Greece	Mexico	Sudan
Argentina	Guatemala	Morocco	Syrian Arab Republic
Bolivia	Honduras	Nicaragua	Thailand
Brazil	Hong Kong	Nigeria	Togo
Cameroon	Iraq	Panama	Trinidad & Tobago
Chile	Iran	Papua New Guinea	Tunisia
China, Republic of	Israel	Paraguay	Turkey
Colombia	Ivory Coast	Peru	Uruguay
Congo, People's Republic of the	Jamaica	Philippines	Venezuela
Costa Rica	Jordan	Portugal	Yemen PDR
Dominican Republic	Korea, Republic of	Romania	Yugoslavia
Ecuador	Lebanon	Senegal	Zimbabwe
Egypt	Liberia	Singapore	
El Salvador	Malaysia		

Capital Surplus Oil Exporters

Kuwait
Libya
Saudi Arabia

Centrally Planned Economies

Albania
Bulgaria
China, People's Republic of
Cuba
Czechoslovakia
German Democratic Republic
Hungary
Korea, Democratic Republic of
Mongolia
Poland
U.S.S.R.

Industrialized Countries

Australia
Austria
Belgium
Canada
Denmark
Finland
France
Germany, Federal Republic of
Ireland

TABLE 1 (continued)
Country Classifications

Industrialized Countries

Italy
Japan
Netherlands
New Zealand
Norway
South Africa
Sweden
Switzerland
U.K.
U.S.

Reprinted from *The Pharmaceutical Industry and the Third World*, Pharmaceutical Manufacturer's Association, Washington, D.C. With permission.

TABLE 2
Value of Drug Consumption Per Capita in 1976 and 1985 in Developing and Developed Countries (US$)

	1976	1985	Annual growth rate (%)
Developed countries	29.0	62.1	8.8
Western Europe	34.0	54.5	5.4
North America	36.3	106.3	12.7
Eastern Europe	17.0	24.5	4.1
Japan	35.6	116.3	14.0
Developing countries	31.4	5.4	5.0
Asia	2.4	4.2	6.3
Africa	3.0	4.9	5.7
Latin America	11.2	13.8	2.3
World	10.3	19.4	7.2

Source: *Global Study of the Pharmaceutical Industry*, unpublished UNIDO document, ID/WG, 331/6, 1980; IMS Marketletter, August 11, 1986; estimates of the WHO secretariat. Reprinted from *The World Drug Situation*, World Health Organization, Geneva, 1988, 13. With permission.

TABLE 3
National Expenditure on Health as % of GNP

Country category	Total as % GNP
Low Income	
India	1.0
Ethiopia	0.8
Kenya	1.7
Middle Income	
Philippines	0.5
Iran	0.6
Brazil	0.5

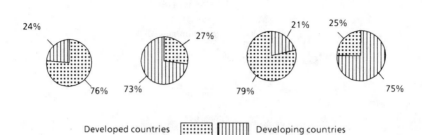

FIGURE 2. Geographical distribution of world drug consumption and population, 1976 and 1985. Percentages are based on the IMS Marketletter, August 11, 1985, p.15; UNIDO data bank; and estimates of the WHO Secretariat. (From *The World Drug Situation*, World Health Organization, Geneva, 1988, 8. With permission.)

TABLE 3 (continued)
National Expenditure on Health as % of GNP

Country category	Total as % of GNP
Centrally Planned Economies	
Hungary	3.0
U.S.S.R.	3.5
Industrialized	
Italy	8.0
West Germany	8.0
U.S.	7.9

Note: In general, developed countries spend 5 to 8% of GNP of
health care, of which 10 to 20% represents expenditure on
pharmaceuticals. Figures vary more in low-income countries,
but pharmaceutical expenditure rarely rises to US $2 and often
accounts for up to 50% of total health care. Figures relate to
1975 or latest available year.

Reprinted from *The Pharmaceutical Industry and the Third World*, p.
32, Pharmaceutical Manufacturer's Association, 1155 Fifteenth St.
N.W., Washington, D.C. 20005. With permission.

TABLE 4
Leading Therapeutic Classes by Sales Through Retail
Pharmacies in Selected Developed and Developing Markets

Country/class	Market share (%)	Country/class	Market share (%)
Brazil		**Japan**	
Systemic antibiotics	14	Systemic antibiotics	26
Cough and cold preparations	6	Vitamins	6
Vitamins	6	Antirheumatics	4
Antispasmodics	4	Antacids	4
Sex hormones	4	Hematologicals	4
Analgesics	3	Hospital solutions	4
Antirheumatics	3	Cardiac therapy	3
Psycholeptics	3	Cytostatics (anticancer)	3
Psychoanaleptics	3	Psycholeptics	3
Cholagogues/hepatic protectors	3	Cholagogues/hepatic protectors	3

TABLE 4 (continued)
Leading Therapeutic Classes by Sales Through Retail
Pharmacies in Selected Developed and Developing Markets

Country/class	Market share (%)	Country/class	Market share (%)
Pakistan		**U.S.**	
Systemic antibiotics	25	Psycholeptics	9
Vitamins	13	(tranquilizers/sedatives)	
Cough and cold preparations	5	Analgesics	8
Analgesics	5	Systemic antibiotics	7
Nutrients	3	Cough and cold preparations	6
Antianemics	3	Vitamins	5
Antidiarrheals	3	Hypotensives	4
Antacids	3	Diuretics	4
Tuberculostatics	3	Sex hormones	4
Antispasmodics	3	Antirheumatics	3
		Psychoanaleptics	3
Philippines		**West Germany**	
Systemic antibiotics	19	Cardiac therapy	11
Cough and cold preparations	12	Psycholeptics	6
Vitamins	8	Peripheral vasodilators	5
Analgesics	6	Cough and cold preparations	5
Tuberculostatics	5	Analgesics	4
Nutrients	5	Vasoprotectives	4
Antiasthmatics	3	Systemic antibiotics	4
Antidiarrheals	3	Hypotensives	4
Topical steroids	2	Sex hormones	3
Antacids	2	Antidiabetics	3

Venezuela

Country/class	Market share (%)
Systemic antibiotics	14
Vitamins	8
Cough and cold preparations	7
Analgesics	4
Sex hormones	4
Topical steroids	3
Antianemics	3
Psycholeptics	3
Systemic steroids	3

Note: Values were measured by sales through wholesalers.

Reprinted from *The Pharmaceutical Industry and the Third World*, Pharmaceutical Manufacturer's Association, Washington, D.C. With permission.

National priorities which affect the availability and cost of pharmaceuticals include:
Technological development — Most developing countries set a high priority on developing local technological skills. This, together with balance of payments and other economic concerns, has resulted in restriction or prohibition of pharmaceutical finished goods importation in, for example, most of Latin America.

TABLE 5
Share of Pharmaceutical Market Held by Indigenous Companies

Country category	Pharmaceutical market (U.S. $ millions 1976)	Indigenous companies (%)	Foreign companies (%)
Low Income			
India	625	30	70
Pakistan	95	20	80
Indonesia	250	30	70
Middle Income			
Philippines	190	30	70
Brazil	1120	27	73
Venezuela	280	30	70
Capital Surplus Oil Exporters			
Saudi Arabia	90	0	100
Centrally Planned Economies			
Hungary	250	75	25
U.S.S.R.	3750	80	20
Industrialized			
Italy	1850	45	55
West Germany	3380	65	35
U.S.	8180	85	15

Reprinted from *The Pharmaceutical Industry and the Third World*, Pharmaceutical Manufacturer's Association, Washington, D.C. With permission.

Employment — Concerns over unemployment in countries such as France lead to policies which require or encourage local production of pharmaceuticals.

Improved health care — Health services, including drug needs, are a universal priority. Concerns over costs lead to price controls in many countries, limiting the attractiveness of these markets. Price controls also limit the profits which are available for reinvestment in research.

Balance of payments — Concerns over negative balance of payments are increasing, especially among the poor, oil-importing nations. As a result, pharmaceutical and other exports are encouraged. Brazil, for example, offers tax incentives to pharmaceutical exporters. Spain requires exportation as a condition of approving a pharmaceutical foreign direct investment.

Basic manufacturing — Several countries require local production of a pharmaceutical basic chemical in addition to local pharmaceutical compounding. They wish to develop the use of indigenous raw materials, and to reduce costly basic drug imports. In Indonesia, for example, foreign pharmaceutical investors must make a commitment to basic drug manufacturing.

Research and development — Several countries require or encourage local R & D to develop technology and as a matter of national pride. This can pose difficult and costly problems to the developer of pharmaceuticals for global markets. In some countries, local clinical trials of new drugs may suffice. But, in Japan, for example, it is necessary to conduct toxicological and other more basic research for new drug registration.

Countries wishing to control foreign pharmaceutical investment find the means to do so in spite of tariffs and other international agreements. This can be and is accomplished by early (or

TABLE 6
Association Member Countries

ANCOM	ASEAN	CACM	CARICOM	COMECON
Bolivia	Indonesia	Costa Rica	Antigua	Bulgaria
Colombia	Malaysia	El Salvador	Barbados	Cuba
Ecuador	Philippines	Guatemala	Belize	Czechoslovakia
Peru	Singapore	Honduras	Dominica	German Democratic
Venezuela	Thailand	Nicaragua	Grenada	Republic (G.D.R.,
			Guyana	East Germany)
			Jamaica	Hungary
			Montserrat	Mongolia
			St. Kitts-Nevis	Poland
			Anguilla	Romania
			St. Lucia	U.S.S.R.
			St. Vincent	
			Trinidad-Tobago	

EEC	EFTA	LAIA, ALADI	OECD	
Belgium	Austria	Argentina	Australia	Japan
Denmark	Finland	Bolivia	Austria	Italy
France	Iceland	Brazil	Belgium-Luxembourg	Netherlands
Greece	Norway	Chile	Canada	New Zealand
West Germany	Portugal	Colombia	Denmark	Norway
Ireland	Sweden	Ecuador	Finland	Spain
Italy	Switzerland	Mexico	France	Sweden
Luxembourg		Paraguay	Germany	Switzerland
Netherlands		Peru	Greece	Turkey
Portugal		Uruguay	Iceland	U.K.
Spain		Venezuela	Ireland	U.S.
U.K.				

Note: ANCOM = Andean Common Market; ASEAN = Association of Southeast Asian Nations; CACM = Central American Common Market; CARICOM = Caribbean Community Secretariat; COMECOM = Council for Mutual Economic Assistance (C.M.E.A.); EEC = European Economic Community; EFTA = European Free Trade Association; LAIA = Latin American Integration Association; ALADI = Asociaciòn Latinoamericana de Integraciòn; OECD = Organization for Economic Cooperation and Development.

delayed) product registration, granting favorable (or low) pharmaceutical prices, limiting profits or restricting remittances to the parent company, or listing (or not listing) a new product in a formulary system or reimbursement program.

The political climate and political stability of a country strongly influence foreign pharmaceutical investment. Highly unstable areas such as Central America are unattractive currently, in spite of the needs of these countries. The spread of international terrorism makes several other countries unattractive.

The infrastructure of each country has a great influence on the success of a pharmaceutical development or manufacturing venture. This includes the availability of qualified professional and skilled people, communications systems, transportation, ability to import and export, currency stability and convertability, availability of services, and so on.

C. NATIONAL, REGIONAL, AND SUPRANATIONAL ORGANIZATIONS

Regional economic associations affect the development and production of pharmaceuticals in their member nations by regulating internal and external commerce (Table 6). The European Economic Community (EEC) is the most successful of these groups.

The 12 countries of the EEC have agreed to an economic integration plan referred to as "Europe 1992". This plan will permit the free movement of goods, services, capital, and labor within the EEC, with common external tariffs. The plan provides many problems and opportunities for developers and producers of pharmaceuticals. Product registration will be standardized, either by mutual recognition or by the development of a central "European F.D.A." Inspection reciprocity is planned. Pharmaceutical price erosion is anticipated, but many nontariff trade barriers are being eliminated. Production rationalization within the EEC will provide economies of scale to manufacturers.

Space does not permit a review of the other country associations. Their aims are the economic growth of the regions represented, and this can present both problems and opportunities for the astute developer and producer of pharmaceuticals.

Among supranational organizations, several agencies of the United Nations actively influence the development, production, and distribution of pharmaceuticals globally. Their main efforts are directed toward the developing countries. Agencies involved include the UN Conference on Trade and Development; the UN Industrial Development Organization (UNIDO); the UN Economic and Social Council; the UN International Children's Emergency Fund; and the UN Center on Transnational Corporations.

The Organization for Economic Cooperation and Development (OECD), among other things, provides funding for health care resources in developing countries.

The World Health Organization (WHO) directly influences the development, production, and availability of pharmaceuticals in the developing countries, and worldwide. WHO policies and programs are influenced by the politics of the third world nations. However, cooperation between the WHO and the multinational pharmaceutical industry has greatly increased in recent years. The industry is providing training for health care personnel and is increasing emphasis on drugs to treat tropical diseases. Accommodation is being reached on "essential drug lists" for developing countries.

Dr. Hiroshi Nakajima was appointed Director General of the WHO in July 1988. In an interview published in the September 1988 issue of *Health Horizons*,[1] Dr. Nakajima described his vision of the private and public sector working together for a better quality of life. A prime emphasis will be on Essential Drug Programs for the developing countries, a limited list of drugs considered most essential for the poorest countries. He stated: "The first step is to define health priorities in the context of a country's public health policy. Then the government has to be in a position to guarantee the distribution of selected drugs to the majority of the population." He went on to say: "The role of WHO is to help each country formulate its own pharmaceutical policy. It is at the stage of devising these policies that the different interested parties — governments, consumers, pharmaceutical industry, medical associations — must participate in the setting up of health care systems. In this context, WHO is ready to see that this collaboration takes place and to coordinate joint efforts".

"...What I expect from the pharmaceutical industry are efforts in the priority areas, such as tropical diseases, AIDS, and children's diseases, as well as in the improvement of local and regional infrastructures, the training of health care personnel, and their education in the use of medicines and quality control."

At the national level, health authorities and regulations have a significant and direct effect on local pharmaceutical activities.

An increasing number of countries control drug usage through formulary or reimbursement systems, such as the "limited list" in the U.K. Requirements for adverse drug reaction reporting and for postmarketing surveillance are increasing. Drug prices are controlled, directly or indirectly, by most of the governments of the world.

Food and drug regulations describe product registration, good manufacturing practices (GMPs), compliance inspections, and other requirements.[2] While in many cases requirements are similar, the application and enforcement of standards vary widely. In enforcing GMP standards, indigenous companies may be treated more leniently than foreign multinationals.

Pharmaceutical manufacturer's associations play an important role in pharmaceutical operations in many countries. While organized to further the economic interests of their members, they usually foster high standards which advance the local product quality and technology.

National pharmacopeias delineate standards for commonly used components and pharmaceutical products. Because of the considerable resources needed to produce and revise a national pharmacopeia, several countries adopt the USP/NF. The European Pharmacopeia has replaced several country standards. The existence of several pharmacopeias describing the same material can pose problems for the developer of drugs to meet global needs.

D. OTHER WORLDWIDE TRENDS

Most countries have adopted standards of GMPs. The most demanding GMP standards in terms of requirements and application are in the U.S., Canada, Western Europe, and Japan. Several countries use the much more general WHO standards with widely varying application and enforcement. There is a trend, however, to global adoption and enforcement of the most demanding of the GMP standards. This includes the concepts of process validation.

There is also a tendency toward standardization of other food and drug regulations, in the direction of the most demanding. Reciprocity between countries in plant inspection and product registration is also on the increase.

Many developing countries are forming governmental food and drug units and will be no longer willing to accept new-product data from other countries. Most already require "free sale" certification from the country of origin to ensure that only safe and effective drugs are imported.

The trend toward mandating the use of pharmaceuticals identified only by generic name is also increasing.

Drug patent protection and intellectual property rights, which motivate and fund innovation, is very limited or under threat in many countries. These trends limit profits and thus the research risk capital essential to new drug development.

These are some of the worldwide trends of which the drug developer must be aware. The forecast seems bleak: crippling third-world debt, inflation, population growth, political instability, and a widening gulf between the industrialized and poor nations. These factors provide further challenges to the developer of drugs for world markets.

III. REGIONAL REVIEW

Some brief observations on the state of pharmaceutical technology, innovative capability, and infrastructural support are provided below.

A. NORTH AMERICA

The U.S. and Canada constitute the largest pharmaceutical market in the world and lead the world in drug consumption. The North American share of world markets is increasing (Tables 7 and 8).

American research investment, and the resulting number of new drugs introduced, also leads the world.

In Canada, the pharmaceutical industry is dominated by U.S. multinationals who have absorbed many local companies. Research investment is increasing in Canada, however, in response to government patent extension and other incentives. The Canadian Health Protection Branch, which regulates the drug industry, is an effective and well-regarded agency which enjoys plant inspection reciprocity and other collaboration with the U.S. Food and Drug Administration.

The U.S./Canada Trade Agreement will eliminate existing tariff barriers to trade in pharmaceuticals. It will also result in some restructuring of the industry in Canada, with possible reductions in U.S. manufacturing investment in Canada.

TABLE 7
World Consumption of Pharmaceuticals by Region
(US$ Billion, at Manufacturer Price)

	1976	1985
North America	8.761	28.141
Western Europe	13.111	22.000
Eastern Europe	6.197	9.600
Japan	4.020	14.038
Oceania	0.480	0.700
Latin America	3.689	5.600
Africa	1.268	2.700
Asia	2.920	6.600
China	2.600	4.700
TOTAL	43.046	94.079

Sources: *Global Study of the Pharmaceutical Industry*, unpublished UNIDO document ID/WG, 331/6, 1980; IMS Marketletter, August 11, 1986; *Pharmaceutial business opportunities with China*, SCRIP, 1987. Excluding China and Japan. (Reprinted from *The World Drug Situation*, World Health Organization, Geneva, 1988, 8. With permission.)

TABLE 8
The 20 Largest Drug Markets, 1976 and 1985 (Excluding Eastern Europe)

1976			1985		
Country	Sales (US$ billion)	% of world market	Country	Sales (US$ billion)	% of world market
U.S.	7.900	18.3	U.S.	26.451	28.1
Japan	4.020	9.3	Japan	14.038	14.9
Federal Republic of Germany	3.410	7.9	Federal Republic of Germany	5.995	6.4
France	2.700	6.3	China	4.700	5.0
China	2.600	6.0	France	4.465	4.7
Italy	1.900	4.4	Italy	3.671	3.9
Spain	1.320	3.0	U.K.	2.348	2.5
Brazil	1.210	2.8	India	1.775	1.9
U.K.	1.030	2.4	Canada	1.690	1.8
Mexico	0.774	1.8	Brazil	1.408	1.5
Canada	0.672	1.6	Spain	1.397	1.5
Argentina	0.654	1.5	Mexico	1.248	1.3
Belgium	0.536	1.2	Argentina	1.211	1.3
India	0.508	1.1	Republic of Korea	1.013	1.1
Australia	0.411	1.0	Egypt	0.707	0.75
Republic of Korea	0.400	0.9	Belgium	0.694	0.70
Sweden	0.400	0.9	Switzerland	0.605	0.65
Netherlands	0.364	0.85	Australia	0.580	0.60
Switzerland	0.330	0.75	Islamic Republic of Iran	0.513	0.55
Venezuela	0.282	0.65	Netherlands	0.506	0.50
Total of top 20 drug markets	31.421	73	Total of top 20 drug markets	75.015	73
Global total	43.046	100	Global total	94.100	100

Sources: *Global Study of the Pharmaceutical Industry*, unpublished UNIDO document, ID/WG. 331/6, 1980; IMS Marketletter, August 11, 1986, 15; *Pharmaceutical business opportunities with China*, SCRIP, 187. (Reprinted from *The World Drug Situation*, World Health Organization, Geneva, 1988, 8. With permission.)

B. LATIN AMERICA

The Latin American countries are characterized by heavy foreign debt, high inflation, high population growth, and chronic infrastructural problems. As a result, per capita drug consumption is static or declining. Although pharmaceutical industry development and government policies vary between countries, the multinationals are strong or dominant throughout Latin America.

In Mexico, local companies also have a strong position. Finished goods importation is virtually prohibited, requiring local pharmaceutical investment. Local basic drug production is encouraged or required for major products. The technological level is relatively high, but GMP and other drug regulations are loosely enforced. As in much of Latin America, there are frequently differences between the standards applied to local companies and those applied to foreign companies.

The Central American pharmaceutical industry is largely foreign. Government policies permit some importation, and are less restrictive than in Mexico. Local technology is not as well developed, and there are difficulties obtaining skilled technical personnel, raw and packaging materials meeting pharmaceutical standards, equipment service and parts, etc. Little research is done. Government standards are loosely applied.

In South America the major countries — Venezuela, Colombia, Brazil, and Argentina — restrict or prohibit pharmaceutical finished goods importation to develop local industry and technology and reduce balance of payments problems. Problems with quality components, services, import permits, etc., are common. Dealings with the various government agencies involved in a pharmaceutical enterprise are slow and complex. Technological levels are good and qualified professional people are available, although scarce in rapidly industrializing countries such as Brazil, Venezuela, Chile, and Ecuador.

Political and economic instability is a constant problem throughout most of Latin America, creating an unfavorable climate for pharmaceutical investment. Argentina, for example, is still struggling with rampant inflation and a stagnant economy.

The remaining least-developed South American countries more seriously lack the infrastructure necessary to support high-technology industry. The indigenous pharmaceutical industry in, for example, Ecuador and Bolivia, is relatively primitive. Government policies tend to increasingly restrict importation to protect local companies and conserve scarce foreign exchange.

C. WESTERN EUROPE

In Western Europe, the pharmaceutical industry is highly advanced technologically and economically. In some countries, local companies rather than foreign multinationals are predominant. New product development and pharmaceutical processing innovation are very active, especially in England, Germany, and Switzerland. In these countries, some of the largest pharmaceutical multinationals in the world are based: Imperial Chemical Industries, Boots, Burroughs-Wellcome, and Glaxo in the U.K.; Ciba-Geigy, Roche, and Sandoz in Switzerland; Hoechst and Boehringer-Ingleheim in Germany. Many of these companies are also actively expanding in the U.S.

These companies have the experience and the resources to develop and market new products globally, to achieve significant processing innovation, and to develop and implement advanced standards of GMPs.

As described earlier, the pharmaceutical industry, as with all business in Europe, is being profoundly affected by the economic integration plan described as "Europe 1992".

This will create a single pharmaceutical market estimated at $34 billion, in the 12 EEC countries, with a population totaling 320 million.

The mechanism for new-product registration has not yet been agreed upon. One option is mutual recognition of the regulatory authority of each country; creation of a central European Drug Agency is also being considered.

The current wide disparities in drug prices will diminish, and prices (and profits) are likely to decrease under government pressures to control drug reimbursement and other health care costs. Pressures for generic and therapeutic substitution will increase.

The 1992 plan poses threats of "Fortress Europe" to non-European pharmaceutical companies. A strong presence in Europe will be essential to compete in this changing environment. This includes manufacturing and research within Europe, as well as marketing and distribution. The foreign investor, however, will be rewarded by more uniform regulatory requirements and the opportunity to achieve economies of scale through production rationalization.

D. EASTERN EUROPE AND THE SOVIET UNION

The Eastern bloc countries have made little contribution to the advancement of pharmaceutical technology and the development of new drugs. Western pharmaceutical sales to this area are modest, and will remain so because of the limited ability of the Council for Mutual Economic Assistance (COMECON) to accumulate hard currency for Western imports.

Under Mikhail Gorbachev, the U.S.S.R. is attempting "perestroika", a major restructuring of the Soviet system towards a consumer-oriented market economy. Health care improvement, including the pharmaceutical sector, has been declared a high priority. The Soviets hope to acquire Western pharmaceutical technology and management skills through joint ventures with Western companies. These companies will produce basic drugs and dosage forms using Soviet or Eastern European components, utilizing Western GMPs and technology. Each venture must export to "hard" or convertible currency countries in order to repatriate profits and to import raw materials and equipment.

The Eastern European countries have similar problems of low technology levels, poor quality drugs, lack of convertible currency, and foreign debt. Poland has enacted a new joint venture law. Other countries are upgrading their pharmaceutical technology under licensing agreements with Western companies.

E. MIDDLE AND NEAR EAST AND AFRICA

Most of this region suffers from the economic and infrastructural problems common to the third world. There is very little indigenous pharmaceutical industry, and almost no innovation. The oil-producing countries have the funds to import and distribute pharmaceuticals developed and registered in other countries.

In Saudi Arabia, the Saudi Pharmaceutical Industries and Medical Appliances Company is constructing a "state-of-the-art" plant to supply the Gulf States with essential drugs of high quality, using a major European company as consultant.

The nonoil producers, however, have a serious and growing problem in providing their people with even the most basic drugs. The lack of drugs and other health care products and services to combat the tropical disease, malnutrition, and other problems of the region is an unsolved problem.

Some countries in this region employ policies which discourage foreign pharmaceutical investment. This further exacerbates their already serious problems.

India has a well-developed indigenous pharmaceutical industry, but much of the population has very limited access to drugs.

The Union of South Africa has the most developed drug industry in the continent, due to heavy multinational investment. The uncertain political future of this country, however, is discouraging further investment. U.S. law prohibits new investment.

F. PEOPLE'S REPUBLIC OF CHINA

With the warming of relations between the People's Republic of China and the U.S., opportunities for increased trade in pharmaceuticals have developed. The Chinese are interested in acquiring pharmaceutical technology and are encouraging scientific and technical exchange. They are also interested in exporting basic pharmaceutical raw materials.

The Chinese are encouraging pharmaceutical manufacturing joint ventures as a means of acquiring Western technology and for increasing exports. They have created "special economic zones" with the necessary infrastructural support and duty exemption for these projects. As with the Soviet bloc countries, problems are created by low technological levels and limited convertible currency availability.

G. JAPAN

Japan is one of the largest and most rapidly developing pharmaceutical markets. Their quality standards and "zero defects" approach to pharmaceutical elegance are exceptionally stringent. Japan has many restrictions on the use of excipients, colorants, and preservatives of which the developer of drugs must be aware. Japanese research capability is strong and increasing, most notably in the field of biotechnology. Many of the large multinational Japanese pharmaceutical companies are aggressively expanding their global operations, with the strong support of the government.

H. FAR EAST

This is a very diverse region, culturally, economically, and technologically. Australia and New Zealand have an advanced pharmaceutical industry dominated by foreign multinationals. The current slow economic growth of these countries has resulted in pharmaceutical price controls and other restrictions which may not be in their best long-term interests.

Most of southeast Asia has a relatively undeveloped local pharmaceutical industry, with new products made available almost exclusively by multinationals. Some, such as Indonesia, exercise very strict controls over foreign multinational investment. Others, such as Thailand, have more liberal trade controls.

The Philippines provides a relatively receptive atmosphere to foreign pharmaceutical companies, and utilizes U.S. FDA regulations. Enforcement, however, is variable, and current economic problems are restricting business.

The Republic of Korea strictly limits foreign pharmaceutical investment and prohibits most finished goods importation. Local companies are at a relatively low technological level. Korea typifies the exceptional difficulties encountered by the developer and marketer of pharmaceuticals in much of Asia due to a poor technological base and limited infrastructure. However, industrial growth and modernization are making Korea a more attractive pharmaceutical market.

Taiwan, or, as they prefer to be called, The Republic of China, has a booming economy, a good technological base, and an excellent supply of people trained in pharmaceutical sciences. Although many restrictions exist, they are eager to continue to acquire Western pharmaceutical technology.

These brief comments on worldwide pharmaceutical activities barely scratch the surface of a complex and ever-changing global picture. Comprehensive reference material on each country is readily available. Local pharmaceutical associations can provide invaluable data to those who, forewarned, wish to pursue the development of pharmaceuticals to meet the needs of global markets.

IV. RESEARCH AND DEVELOPMENT TO MEET THE NEEDS OF GLOBAL MARKETS

A. NEEDS OF REGIONAL MARKETS

Overall growth in worldwide demand for pharmaceuticals in the next 20 years will average 8.5% yearly, rising from an estimated $75 billion in 1980 to $270 billion by the year 2000, according to a published report, "Opportunities for Pharmaceuticals in the Developing World over the Next Twenty Years", by Information Research Ltd.[3] Some highlights from the 116-page report follow.

TABLE 9
Present and Future Markets for Drugs
by Region (1980 to 2000) (Values in $ Billion)

	1980		1985		1990		1995		2000	
	Value	%	Value	%	Value	%	Value	%	Value	%
Western Europe	25.35	33.8	29.0	30.5	45.50	35.0	57.60	32.0	71.25	28.5
North America	14.70	19.6	25.20	26.5	25.35	19.5	29.34	16.3	33.75	13.5
Asia	17.10	22.8	21.18	22.3	31.20	24.0	47.70	26.5	70.00	28.0
Eastern Europe	12.15	16.2	12.83	13.5	17.55	13.5	29.34	16.3	49.50	19.8
Latin America	3.30	4.4	3.80	4.0	5.46	4.2	7.92	4.4	12.00	4.8
Africa	1.73	2.3	2.09	2.2	3.64	2.8	6.30	3.5	11.25	4.5
Oceania	0.67	0.9	0.90	1.0	1.30	1.0	1.80	1.0	2.25	0.9
Total world	75.00	100.00	95.00	100.00	130.00	100.00	180.00	100.00	250.00	100.00

From *Scrip World Pharmaceutical News*, July 28, 1980. Information Research Limited update, January 23, 1989. With permission.

TABLE 10
Relative Importance of Developed and Developing Countries
as Drug Markets (1980 to 2000) ($ Billion)

	Developed countries	Countries with central economies	Developing countries	% Developing
1980	52.50	12.15	10.35	13.8
1985	69.50	12.83	12.67	13.3
1990	92.05	17.55	20.40	15.7
1995	119.38	29.34	31.28	17.4
2000	151.20	49.50	49.30	19.7

From *Scrip World Pharmaceutical News*, July 28, 1980. Information Research. Limited update January 23, 1989. With permission.

During these two decades a number of radical changes affecting the pharmaceutical industry are forecast—ranging from the shifting pattern of demand from the developed to the developing countries, to factors such as political involvement, socio-economic forces, pricing, profits, and the structure of the industry.

The report also stresses the growing importance of the more populous and less developed regions, which were believed to account for between 12 and 15% of world usage of pharmaceuticals, rising to at least 25% by the end of this century. The estimated demand for all types of drugs in the main regions of the world, along with anticipated changes in each region in world markets, is given in Table 9. These markets are further divided into developed and developing countries, as shown in Table 10.

Most of the current top 15 countries in terms of demand for pharmaceuticals are expected to maintain their relative positions in world markets, with significant increases in the Far East. Changes in the leading ten pharmaceutical markets to the year 2000 are given in Table 11.

Taking into account the levels of self-sufficiency predicted for the various developing countries, the report points out that those with the largest markets will not necessarily be the leading markets from the point of view of exports from the developed countries. The report also assesses the specific problems and requirements of developing countries, stressing that the

TABLE 11
Changes in the Leading National
Pharmaceutical Markets to 2000

Country	$ Million		
	1979	1990	2000
U.S.	11,360	21,060	33,500
Japan	8,760	20,550	38,500
West Germany	5,000	9,270	14,670
France	4,330	8,030	12,765
Italy	2,380	4,410	7,015
U.K.	2,000	3,700	5,895
Brazil	1,890	7,830	20,775
Spain	1,570	2,910	4,630
Argentina	1,400	3,835	7,475
Mexico	907	3,780	10,025
Total world	64,570	150,000	270,000

From *Scrip World Pharmaceutical News*, July 28, 1980. With permission.

major factor which hinders greater usage of pharmaceuticals is the restriction on demand imposed by limited national health care facilities. As little as 1 to 2% of the gross national product (GNP) is allocated to health care, compared with between 5 and 10% of the greater GNP of developed countries. It is pointed out that considerable funding from the WHO will be necessary.

The most important drug requirements of developing countries will continue to be for antibiotics, cough and cold preparations, vitamins, analgesics, hormones, and tonics. This will change, however, in line with greater urbanization and industrialization. In few of these countries will adequate facilities be available to treat the whole population to a high level of protection against disease and illness.

The Conference of Experts on the Rational Use of Drugs held under the auspices of the WHO in Nairobi in 1985 acknowledged the need for more information on the drug situation at the global and national levels, and requested WHO to provide this information as part of its revised drug strategy.[4] In 1988, the World Drug Situation report was issued by WHO. The Nairobi conference may be considered the benchmark for development and revision of drug distribution policies. The report describes global supply and demand, i.e., production and consumption of drugs in the world and their geographic distribution. The report also describes situations in individual countries and steps taken to improve distribution. The pharmaceutical industry is promoting infrastructures to inventory and distribute drug supplies.

There seems to be a paradox when it comes to the therapeutic needs of less developed countries. It is true in general, in less developed parts of the world, that emphasis needs to be placed on antibiotics for infectious diseases, and steroids because they are widely used for a variety of conditions. There are many parts of the world where the therapeutic needs for antibiotics, birth control products, and drugs for parasitic diseases are greatly needed. Yet, even in these countries, despite the overwhelming needs of the mass of the population, there is still a market for sophisticated products in that small class of economic elite. That is even true in a country as poor as India, for example, and certainly true in Latin American countries.

There is one exception, of course, to all this poverty in these developing countries, and that is the oil-rich countries — the OPEC countries. They have money and they are spending it building hospitals and systems for delivering health care. This is not the case, however, for all those who have oil. Nigeria, for example, has oil, but they have so many problems that it is only helping them marginally.

TABLE 12
Estimated Demands for Drugs by Therapeutic
Group 1980 to 2000

Therapeutic group	Values in $'000 Million		
	1980	1990	2000
Antibiotics	8.25	18.00	40.50
Cardiovasculars	6.00	15.00	32.40
Antiarthritics	3.75	10.50	24.30
Psychotherapeutics	3.00	9.00	18.90
Analgesics	2.25	4.50	8.10
Cough and cold preparations	2.25	4.50	5.40
Diuretics	1.50	3.00	5.40
Steroids	1.50	4.50	10.80
Estrogens	1.50	4.50	10.80
Cancer chemotherapeutics	1.50	7.50	27.00
Others	43.50	69.00	86.40
Total	75.00	150.00	270.00

From *Scrip World Pharmaceutical News*, July 28, 1980. With permission.

There are many authorities who feel that with the exception of antibiotics, steroids, and a small number of antiparasitic drugs that do work for certain indications, the real needs of the developing countries are not primarily pharmaceutical. They still relate to classical problems of nutrition and sanitation.

B. CATEGORIES OF RESEARCH AND DEVELOPMENT

As far as the future of the world pharmaceutical industry as a whole is concerned, the previously mentioned report "Opportunities for Pharmaceuticals in the Developing World Over the Next Twenty Years" assesses the direction in which R & D is progressing, the requirements for specific product groups, and also the changes factors like these will bring about in the structure and characteristics of the industry.[5]

The major areas for intensified R & D into new drugs during these two decades are expected to be anticancer agents and antivirals, with the more immediate target being in the field of further broad-spectrum antibiotics. Six more areas which are reputed to offer the best commercial opportunities in the coming years are cardiovasculars, products for the treatment of conditions associated with the aging process (particularly antiarthritics and antirhematics), gastrointestinal agents, antiallergics, tropical medicine, and drugs for mental illness. The estimated demand for drugs by therapeutic group is given in Table 12.

Foreign-parent pharmaceutical competitors are not lagging very far behind in their own drug development activities in the U.S. (not taking into consideration compounds licensed to U.S.-based companies). Activities of Japanese companies in drug development are being carried out mainly through licensing agreements with U.S.-based companies. However, some of them are increasing their own presence in the U.S., staffing offices with small numbers of personnel to study U.S. drug regulatory procedures, to make contact with competitors, and to establish contact with possible investigators for clinical trials. There is an increasing amount of activity and interest on the part of Japanese pharmaceutical companies in gaining a foothold in the U.S. An additional indication of that trend can also be seen in the fact that increasingly, laboratories and manufacturing facilities in Japan are being designed (and sometimes inspected by U.S. FDA personnel) to conform with FDA, GMP, and good laboratory practice (GLP) standards. Other foreign countries (e.g., Sweden) are following the FDA's GMP/GLP rulings quite closely and are requiring such practices from their laboratories. This may be due to the fact that the U.S. FDA is showing a lenience toward accepting data from foreign "nonpivotal" clinical studies as supportive evidence in U.S. new drug applications (NDA). Though a "World NDA" document is many years away, there seems to be an increasing tendency toward communication and data/concept sharing among drug regulatory agencies worldwide.

Several U.S. pharmaceutical companies have publicized their commitment to the use and exploitation of recombinant DNA research and methodology, either in-house or by agreements with academic or other scientific laboratories in the U.S. and abroad. In general, the whole concept of biotechnology is being capitalized at a rapidly increasing rate.

At least one company is strengthening its commitment to viral disease research and cell biology by extending its physical facilities. It has a commitment to drug development for the less-developed countries in the area of vaccines. For the development of new indications and new formulations for marketed drugs and product license renewal, companies are increasingly using overseas clinical trials to supplement their U.S. trials.

Worldwide expansion seems to have continued as a dominant theme among U.S. pharmaceutical companies for various reasons, such as diversification into new businesses by acquisitions, or in facilities expansion for manufacture and research. Pharmaceutical companies have been directing their attention to Western Europe, but Eastern Europe has also attracted some attention, and so has Japan.

Eastern Europe is showing a growing demand for drugs to treat cardiovascular, central nervous system, and gastrointestinal disorders. Trade agreements are the avenue being cautiously used by both U.S. and other European companies.

Among foreign pharmaceutical companies, increasing emphasis is also being placed on international expansion — as well as on cost control, coordination of worldwide R & D activity, company and drug acquisition/licensing activity for complementing their existing product/research lines, etc. Western European companies appear to have overcome a fear they had of the enormous U.S. market and are rapidly increasing their participation in it. They are aggressively pursuing their personal entry into the U.S. via acquisitions of generic manufacturers, research/medical organizations, or specialty houses. Their activities are not limited to the U.S. European companies are looking to further expansion in other European countries, and Japanese companies are slowly testing the European research waters.

Pharmaceutical companies' management seems to be becoming more practical in the areas of new market entry, joint ventures, licensing, and joint marketing. Developing countries wishing to pursue their nationalism will emphasize local production of pharmaceuticals and will likely become more aggressive in seeking out partnerships with experienced manufacturers in developed countries.

In general, the third-world countries accept the verdict of the sophisticated countries when it comes to the acceptability of preclinical data. There are a small number of less sophisticated countries which require local clinical trials as a condition of registration, if not across the board, then at least in certain special fields. Argentina and Korea are examples. Even the Philippines is now leaning in this direction. This has to be a matter of national pride. The authors are not aware of any underdeveloped countries that require preclinical work-up in their country. They accept the verdict of the Western regulatory bodies in that respect.

In terms of strategies for initial clinical study of new chemical entities, U.S. pharmaceutical companies are closing the time gap between initial clinical testing in the U.S. and initial clinical testing overseas of compounds discovered in U.S. R & D labs. U.S. companies do not necessarily repatriate compounds initially discovered in their foreign R & D subsidiaries to the U.S. for first clinical trials. That the introduction of new chemical entities abroad usually precedes their U.S. introduction is a well-publicized fact, and the resultant drug lag has been the subject of numerous studies. As U.S.-based companies become worldwide in their operations, greater advantage is being taken of more expeditious drug review process in foreign countries to date, with the likelihood of earlier market introduction. Also, the greater tendency which the U.S. FDA is displaying toward consideration of foreign clinical data from nonpivotal studies in support of an NDA is another impetus for earlier clinical trials overseas.

C. DOSAGE FORM DESIGN

When an attempt is made to determine the marketability of a drug for the global market, both the active ingredient and dosage form must be considered. An example is an anticholesteremic where a country like Japan does not have a great concern. Attempts to market compounds such as this may also not be successful in poor countries. They are more concerned with infant mortality rate, approaches to population control in various forms, nutritional needs, problems with sanitation, and any advances made for a better quality of life and better standard of living for the general population. However, for cultural reasons, contraceptives and abortifacients cannot be successfully marketed in some countries.

As far as the marketability of a compound for a specific therapeutic use is concerned, it would appear that Europe and the U.S. are very similar in what they need — hypertension, for example, is a big problem for both. Japan is concerned about cardiovascular and ulcer problems. The diets of different regions of the world must also be considered. Diets are very different in Oriental countries when compared to Europe and the U.S. The need for an anticholesteremic, then, becomes apparent. Reference to Table 4 will illustrate leading therapeutic classes for selected developed and developing markets. Table 12 lists estimated demands for drugs by therapeutic group from the year 1980 through 2000. There are political and cultural problems in the third world, particularly when one considers family planning and contraception. India is a good example, where the population density is very high. Since 1947 when India achieved independence until the present, their population has almost doubled — from 350 million to 683 million. These numbers are overwhelming. There are probably about 100 million women of child-bearing age included. A system to deliver some type of contraceptive technology to these women is almost impossible to implement at this time. Nevertheless, India is very sensitive about the Western countries telling them what to do. They know they have a problem, but they want to be involved in the research going on. Therefore, the Indian Council for Medical Research, by law, needs to supervise or be responsible for all clinical trials concerning contraception or family planning. Contraception is probably the most politically sensitive area, along with the related use of abortifacients. There are many countries in the world, particularly in Latin America, where in the foreseeable future, an abortifacient drug approval will not be obtained.

There are economic factors to be faced. The nature of pharmaceutical products is such that the most efficient way to operate is to manufacture in a large efficient complex and export all over the world. The reasons for not doing this are legal and political, not technological or scientific. There is a hierarchy of legal barriers to doing business in this manner — import restrictions, import duties, regulations that require manufacturing in-country, and prohibition of the import of finished pharmaceuticals. This can have an impact on dosage form design as well due to restrictions placed on the importation of excipients.

Regional preferences for dosage forms are evident by the use of suppositories in France, unreconstituted powders/granules in Japan, and surveys taken by marketing people to determine where prefilled disposable syringes, ampules, vials, etc., are most widely accepted. Included in these surveys are the flavor and color preferences expressed by different countries. These preferences must be considered by product development groups. Japan, for instance, prefers white solid dosage forms, which may necessitate a separate production procedure if colored tablets are marketed elsewhere.

During product development, it is essential that formulators request their international regulatory people to determine whether or not all the ingredients in a formulation are acceptable in countries targeted for marketing. Japan prefers white tablets. In addition, there is a very strong culture-driven need for small, defect-free solid dosage forms. The tablet size issue in Japan has significant implications for dosage form design. Acceptable ranges of commonly used excipients, and their approval status in Japan, need to be addressed early in product planning. As in the case of Japan's preference for absence of colors in tablets, Scandinavian countries are now prohibiting the use of yellow #6. In Latin America, there are import restrictions on compound excipients such as wetting agents and lecithin-coated penicillins. Japan, again, has a preference for parabens in place of benzyl alcohol, and the use of EDTA is frowned upon. These are but a few examples of excipient problems facing formulators. These problems can largely be avoided if key people are involved in the product development program at its inception. The time required for product development is critical, and clinical efficacy studies need to begin as early as possible. However, registration and data analysis problems can be greatly alleviated if the dosage form tested for efficacy qualitatively represents the product to be marketed.

D. PRODUCT REGISTRATION

Product registration is a complex, multidisciplinary operation. The pharmaceutical industry is a government-controlled business worldwide. Almost everything within research and marketing, including labeling and promotional materials, in some fashion or another goes through government regulatory authorities. When considering research activities, it is important for multinational companies to know what data will be required in order to accomplish government approval to market a product. This is best done by having company regulatory people involved throughout the entire product development process. Their involvement with new-product project teams will help assure that the studies being conducted will provide the appropriate data for product registration purposes. It is part of the responsibility of these regulatory people to know what the requirements are in each country. It is essential that, whenever a potential new product is developed by research, a copy of that formulation be sent to all the company affiliates to verify that all the ingredients are acceptable. If a government is not aware of a particular inactive or inert ingredient, the company may need to present to that government full data to verify that it is not a toxic substance. In some countries it is necessary to become familiar with advances in packaging material requirements, especially for plastic bottles. The identity of all of the components of plastic bottles that come into contact with the product must be indicated and verification made that each is safe with no toxicological effects. Processing requirements should be considered when gathering data for submission. In Nordic countries (Sweden, for example) topical ointments must be sterile. This is a requirement of the Nordic Pharmacopeia.

It becomes necessary to construct regulatory operations in such a manner as to be able to keep track of political, economic, and data requirement trends which impact on the ability to obtain and maintain product approval. This structure should allow a quick reaction to any changes in policy, not just in individual situations, and should serve as a comprehensive network of communication on a global basis. The world is shrinking in size as the communication gap narrows. There is not a regulatory agency in the world that does not know what another regulatory agency is doing, eventually. The networks between the governments are extremely active. There is, particularly within the EEC, for example, a "quest for the harmonization of the pharmaceutical product registration process". Common registration data and data presentation guidelines have been issued.[6] The nationalistic focus of each country, however, continues to be directed to local needs, including pricing and labeling concerns, and support of the economic infrastructure.

Any company deciding to go global is going to make a large investment in expertise and in dollars. This is one of the problems that local companies in many nations are facing. They do not have the economic resources and overall technical and scientific capabilities that the multinationals do. This is why some firms may be in just the chemical business, selling the drug. They do not try to set up a network of overseas affiliates to manufacture and sell products.

Governments are subject to many factors, all of which have a local, regional, and national flavor. Economic, political, social, and cultural factors all impinge upon the governments' consideration of what they will allow. Other factors which governments consider, of course, are the scientific, medical, and technical data which verify the safety and efficacy of the product. It is suggested, however, that even superseding these concerns which the industry is most able to meet are the complex economic, political, social, and cultural considerations taken into account by the governments. This may explain why many countries require local manufacture. Every nation is concerned with their balance of payments, development of technology, and the creation of jobs within their country. In many countries, the health authorities are political appointees, and therefore even more subject to internal pressure.

Many countries require the availability of local data. At least 12 countries now require local clinical studies. The drug action must be tested in patients in their country before the product is approved. This is not restricted to sophisticated countries. The reasons are for propagation of the local medical community and recognition of racial and physiological differences in people. Testing of a drug in the U.S. on an American caucasian with American eating habits may not reflect what will happen when the drug is used in Indonesia or Singapore or Japan. The absorption, distribution, metabolism, and excretion of the drug can potentially be different. Some countries may require that animal work be done locally. In this manner, as with clinical studies, governments are able to control foreign companies, can continue to protect the local industry, and can meet legitimate scientific objectives.

Following the actual registration process based on review of the scientific and medical data is approval of the price. Price approval is often handled by a separate governmental agency as is the case, for example, in France. The government may not want additional products on the market which they do not feel are totally new life-saving entities, because they do not want to have to reimburse.

Postmarketing data requirements and postmarketing surveillance are developing trends. They are coming on a worldwide basis and will probably be seen first on a firm basis in Europe. Very close monitoring of the use of drug products will be implemented with periodic issuance of reports to the government. This is now becoming a requirement in European countries. Every 6 months for the first 2 years, reports of adverse reactions are issued. Some countries are demanding, as a condition of approval, that the companies agree to carry out postmarketing surveillance.

V. MANUFACTURING AND QUALITY CONTROL TECHNOLOGY TO MEET THE NEEDS OF GLOBAL MARKETS

A. MANUFACTURING STRATEGIES AND TECHNOLOGY

A complex set of alternatives must be analyzed to determine the most appropriate product sourcing strategy for each country. The determining factors are economic and political risk assessment, volume and profit projections, local technical capability, plant capacity utilization and economy of scale, and most important, host country requirements and restrictions. Among the business structures which might be employed are importation, joint ventures with a local company, licensee manufacturing, local contract manufacturing, or a wholly owned manufacturing investment.

The economic priorities of many countries require local manufacturing rather than importation. This trend is likely to continue, as pressures continue for local technological development and for control of key industries.

The use of local contract manufacturers or licensees may be limited by GMP considerations. For the developing countries, it is often difficult to find a local company meeting the minimum GMP standards used by most multinational companies. It is essential that candidates for local manufacturing be carefully screened for GMP compliance: physical facilities; equipment;

systems and procedures; personnel qualifications and attitudes. Routine GMP compliance audits must also be performed subsequent to employing a contract manufacture or licensee.

Typically, companies operating globally must invest in manufacturing facilities in a number of countries. These plants must produce products of identical quality worldwide. However, overseas production facilities will vary considerably to meet the needs of each market. The product mix, volume, and growth rate are the principal factors affecting plant size, layout, and equipment selection. Additional factors which must be considered include the local level of technology, the availability of skilled people, and the relative costs of labor and equipment.

Manufacturing procedures must be modified and validated as lot sizes, equipment selection, and packaging are determined for each facility. Any modification to original or primary packaging must be thoroughly investigated and confirmed by stability data. This is essential in order to assure bioavailability and efficacy. The original product formulators must be aware of the worldwide capabilities of their plants, climatic conditions in the planned markets, the processing equipment to be used, and the packaging required in order to effectively design dosage forms for global markets.

When selecting pharmaceutical processing equipment, many factors must be considered. Every effort should be made to standardize critical equipment such as freeze-dryers, autoclaves, tablet presses, and coating systems. Selection factors include cost, availability of local servicing, level of automation needed, and user experience. Processability of local packaging components is a key factor in determining line speed and type of equipment.

In spite of the problems inherent in producing pharmaceuticals on a world-wide basis, there is a growing need to utilize complex and sophisticated equipment and elaborate environmental controls, and to restrict the extent of equipment or processing variation allowed.

Some technological considerations which must be included in overseas plant design and operation are listed below.

1. More complex and costly utility systems to provide increased product protection and operation protection, which results from increasing concern over drug cross contamination during processing and for operator protection from hazardous substances, with great emphasis being placed on water systems design and quality control, especially in parenteral products production
2. Plant layouts which provide effective isolation of unit processes, and the use of "black", "grey", and "white" zoning concepts, including strict personnel access control
3. The imposition of strict microbial contamination limits for nonsterile dosage forms
4. More stringent potency variation limits, requiring improved process controls
5. A strong and growing requirement for process validation data to substantiate all processing operations or changes
6. Changes in sterilization requirements, including aseptic compounding prior to terminal sterilization, use of cold sterilization by filtration only as a method of last resort, and discontinuing the use of ethylene oxide sterilization because of environmental concerns and toxic hazards due to residues
7. The use of more complex, automated tablet mixing, drying, compression, and coating systems for improved process control
8. Automatic, electronic sterile products inspection equipment to minimize the variation inherent in the present visual methods
9. Automated weighing and recording systems for raw materials
10. On-line automatic check-weighing and label code identification
11. Electropolished stainless steel vessels for parenteral products processing
12. Continuous "tunnel" systems for parenteral container washing, sterilizing, filling, and sealing

13. Increasing worldwide concern over environmental hazards and waste disposal, and the need for "environmental impact" data.

B. PLANT DESIGN REQUIREMENTS AND RESTRICTIONS

The construction of a high-technology facility such as a pharmaceutical plant in a foreign country involves many complexities unique to each country. The government may require or encourage site selection in undeveloped areas remote from population centers, transportation, labor, and other vital services. Securing the necessary approvals for investment and construction can be a time-consuming and costly process.

Some countries impose requirements that are difficult to reconcile with rational facility design. Korea, for example, arbitrarily designates the minimum space which must be provided for the production of each dosage form. Korea also requires separate plant areas and equipment for antibiotic and nonantibiotic products, regardless of cross-contamination potential. Some countries require separate facilities for the production of veterinary pharmaceuticals, even if these products are identical to those for human use.

Plant and utilities design must provide for adverse environmental conditions such as tropical humidity, impure water, or insects.

The exacting requirements of pharmaceutical plant design are unfamiliar to contractors in many countries. The use of an experienced local architect and screening of contractors are mandatory.

C. TECHNOLOGY TRANSFER

Much has been written concerning the complexities of transferring technology between one culture and another. An understanding of, and adherence to, the principles of international technology transfer is of critical importance in designing, building, validating, starting up, and providing continuing technical support to an overseas pharmaceutical facility.

Technology transfer at professional and technical levels is the most complex challenge. A common understanding of design criteria, equipment selection, and operating procedures must be achieved, with as much participation by the local people as the situation permits. Areas of authority must be clearly defined. The U.S. or other groups in charge of a foreign pharmaceutical project must do everything possible to understand the culture and attitudes of the country involved. This is particularly true in the Orient, and in developing countries whose people may resent U.S. technical and economic dominance.

Expatriate managers or technicians must be carefully selected for those personality characteristics essential to success in a foreign environment. They, and their families, must be thoroughly indoctrinated before moving to the host country.

The training of nonprofessionals presents different problems, and is best conducted by professionals and managers of the same nationality. Audio-visual training aids are very valuable in teaching basic concepts such as GMPs, asepic techniques, and in demonstrating manual operations such as in packaging or sterile products inspection. Several commercial films are available. Slide presentations prepared in an operating plant can be used in training personnel in a new facility, with the local supervisor translating a script into the appropriate idiom.

D. PACKAGING DEVELOPMENT

New products will often be introduced internationally before they are marketed in the U.S., yet there is still a tendency by some U.S. companies to impose U.S. packaging standards on overseas markets. For example, continuous-thread closures with screw caps on standard glass and plastic bottles are used in the U.S., but are less common overseas. Unit-of-use dispensing is much more common in Europe than in the U.S. In Belgium, Holland, Germany, and France, for instance, simple plugs or snap-caps are commonly used. Push-through blister presentations are widely accepted, but peel-off blisters are generally unacceptable in Europe, especially in

France, for pharmaceutical products. Although not a common practice, outside consulting firms may need to be brought in for assessing the acceptability of a new package or device in a foreign market. This approach may avoid generating stability data in a package that cannot be successfully marketed. The preference for smaller packages (ie., unit-of-use) creates a larger surface-to-volume ratio. Consequently, more product to primary container contact places greater demands on packaging material compatibility. It becomes evident that multinationals should determine where the product is going to be initially introduced and what the package preferences and regulations will be for that market before product stability is started. The affiliate should be told exactly what the dosage form will be — capsule, compressed tablet, coated tablet — and the affiliate should be asked for exactly what they want for a package presentation — push-through blister package, snap-cap vial, etc. In this manner the market package for international can be identified and placed on stability along with the desired U.S. packages.

Stability studies should be structured to reflect the environmental conditions for the market. One approach may be to package a product in push-through blisters, for example, and send these blisters to several different countries. These packages may be stored for up to 2 years, with samples being tested periodically for evaluation of package performance. This method may not follow routine stability guidelines, but may be a more realistic approach for evaluating packaging under actual conditions of use. Some countries, particularly those in the Middle East and North Africa, have unusual accelerated stability testing requirements. Multinationals must be aware of these requirements when planning registration strategies. Vinyl blisters would not pass high-humidity, high-temperature conditions, but they are being used in countries that do not need that type of protection for economic and marketing reasons. In the development of a product for international markets, a set of complex parameters should be considered very early, not only for the formulation ingredients, but for the packaging area and acceptability by the countries involved.

In many countries, pharmacists dispense much differently than they do in the U.S. In most of Europe and in other countries, original package dispensing is mandatory, and the pharmacist is not permitted to partially dispense from bulk containers. Yet in some of the poorer countries it is not uncommon for someone to stop at the local pharmacy every night on the way home from work to get a few antibiotic tablets for the next day. These will be dispensed in a blister, not as a prescription for a course of treatment all at once. When the economies of various countries are examined, an indication of the buying power of the people is revealed. Many cannot afford to buy a prescription for 30 doses in some underdeveloped countries, but they can afford to buy one or two. Holland is an exception to original package dispensing. Their pharmacies are very similar to those in the U.S. England is closer to the U.S. than the rest of the continent, but is now changing to original package dispensing. Japan, and to a larger extent South and Central American countries, prefer foil-to-foil unit dose packages for product protection, while countries with more temperate climates may prefer transparent films.

Bid and tender business is usually conducted through a Ministry of Health. Countries in North Africa and the Middle East engage very heavily in this business. They may indicate they want to buy several million antibiotic tablets, and the pharmaceutical multinationals will submit a bid. This bid is usually based on delivery of bulk tablets packaged in bottles of 500 or 1000, although the trend may be to supply in larger containers. The bulk may then be repackaged in-country for unit dose dispensing. An alternative would be for the multinational to individually package in blisters and deliver blisters in bulk. The pharmaceutical company is told by the individual country governments exactly what should go on the label copy, including various symbols and characters that are unique to that country. The U.S. companies also need domestic approval through regulatory agencies to ship drugs. They cannot ship international products that are not approved in the U.S. except to designated countries with sophisticated regulatory systems. These products must be under active NDA study, and cannot be re-exported from the original destination country. Bid and tender business has historically provided the least expensive means that will deliver a product as well as maintain product and package integrity. The packaging involved frequently eliminates cartons and uses the least expensive closures without sacrificing quality. Child-resistant closures, for example, are not universally required. The need for child-resistant closures is changing and should be considered on a case by case basis.

Tamper proofing and counterfeiting are issues of concern for multinationals. They tend to be of greater concern internationally than in the U.S., where stringent efforts are not currently made to tamper proof prescription drug products. Internationally, however, some countries have a strong preference for tamper proofing all items.

The problem of counterfeiting is most severe in underdeveloped countries where the distribution infrastructure does not lend itself to regulation and monitoring. One approach being taken to minimize counterfeiting is to utilize characteristic and hard to duplicate packaging materials.

The availability of in-country packaging components should be determined before product stability studies are initiated. Some countries, such as Mexico, state that if the packaging material can be manufactured in Mexico, it cannot be imported. Data must be available to show that there is something unique about a packaging material. If it cannot be manufactured in Mexico, then agreement may be obtained from the glass, plastic, or rubber industry, along with authorization by the government to allow import. When selecting a closure, worldwide outlets, licensees, and rubber manufacturing facilities should be identified. Many countries, such as Brazil and Mexico, have import restrictions which prevent the use of certain closures. There are more tubing manufacturers for vials throughout the world than there are for molded containers, because the pharmaceutical industry is not a large user of glass containers compared to consumer products. The demand for tablet bottles is not as great as the demand for other types of bottles. A specification may be made that a product must be packaged in a 100-cc molded container of Type I glass, but it may not be available. In some countries, very few quality packaging materials are available, and the multinational may opt to export packaging material components to them even though large duties may be involved.

E. GOOD MANUFACTURING PRACTICES

Under the U.S. Federal Food, Drug and Cosmetic Act, a drug is deemed to be adulterated unless the methods used in its manufacture, processing, packing, and holding, and the facilities and controls used therefore, conform to current GMP so that the drug meets the safety requirements of the act and has the identity and strength and meets the quality and purity characteristics that it is represented to have. The regulations are being updated and made more explicit, and therefore less subject to varying interpretations, to assure that all members of the drug industry are made aware of the level of performance expected of them to be in compliance with the act.[7]

International Drug GMPs provides a summary of basic GMP requirements for pharmaceutical manufacturers worldwide and contains the original texts of all applicable national, regional, and international requirements.[8] Part I presents a tabulated summary that allows quick reference to the GMP requirements of 66 different countries. Those countries subscribing to the WHO or European Free Trade Association (EFTA) requirements can readily be identified as can those that have legislated their own national requirements governing drug manufacturing. Part II provides the full texts of all applicable national, regional, and international GMP requirements. Comparative entries are arranged in the textual sequence of the U.S. GMPs. Consequently, one can easily compare WHO and EFTA requirements with various national requirements. The editors point out special features of national requirements wherever they exist.

The introduction of *International Drug GMPs* makes the following observations.[2,9] The 1970s saw significant advances in the field of pharmaceutical manufacturing technology. These strides have necessitated national regulatory agencies implementing or modifying regulations concerning GMPs for drug products.

Concurrently, the increase in the number of drugs being manufactured in one country for ultimate use in another has given rise to a need for ways of evaluating whether or not those drugs exported meet the criteria of quality and purity expected by the importing country. While point of use sampling and testing is certainly applicable, the complexity of drug technology necessitates that the conditions under which a drug is designed and processed be validated to assure the drug user that the probability of the drug being adulterated is minimized. This assurance is best provided under conditions that meet current GMP guidelines. GMPs must be considered minimal rules for manufacturing to assure drug product quality, purity, potency, safety, and effectiveness.

Exporters need be cognizant that drug products must be manufactured and tested in a manner that meets the GMPs of the country of manufacture as well as the GMPs of the country of use.

With the exception of Japan, categorization of GMP requirements has proved to be a rapid and systematic method of comparing GMPs for all countries. The Japanese GMPs consist essentially of three overlapping parts — GMPs expressed in the form of job functions, GMPs expressed in the traditional facility processes format, and GMPs expressed in terms of dosage form.

Among the different approaches taken to outlining national GMPs, it may be of interest to note those of Canada and Japan. The Canadian GMPs, in addition to outlining the requirements necessary for compliance, have established a numerical grading system to help quantify the extent to which a manufacturer complies with the regulations. This approach is especially noteworthy insofar as many less developed countries look upon the Canadian GMPs as a role model for formulating their own requirements.

The Japanese GMPs are unique, as described above, in their approach to spelling out GMPs in terms of job functions for various tasks to be performed within the pharmaceutical manufacturing process. These functions include manufacturing control manager, manufacturing process supervisor, storage supervisor, and manufacturing hygiene supervisor. The Japanese GMPs are further unique in their elaboration of GMPs in terms of dosage forms and the GMPs that uniquely apply to the dosage form being processed. The dosage forms covered by these regulations include injectables, oral solids (powders, granules, capsules, tablets, and pills), ointments, oral liquids, ophthalmic liquids, and liquids for external application.

Much effort has been expended on the national and regional level to unify GMP requirements. Most notable in their efforts at standardization of GMPs have been the member states of the EFTA. Until GMPs worldwide are standardized, much confusion and contradiction will remain between existing regulations. It should be noted that national (local) requirements always take precedence over regional requirements and that these in turn take precedence over international requirements. Where no notation is made, that country has not issued its own GMPs nor officially subscribed to any regional or international requirements.

F. PROCESS VALIDATION

As noted in the above section, the complexity of drug technology necessitates that the condition under which a drug is designed and processed be validated to assure the drug user that the probability of the drug being adulterated is minimized, and that this assurance is best provided under conditions that meet GMP guidelines.

The FDA regulations for drug products assert that all processes and procedures required must be validated. The concept of validation is the cornerstone of the GMP rules. The first official FDA attempt at a formal definition for validation appeared in an FDA Compliance Program issued to field personnel in December 1978. It stated simply that a validated procedure is one which "has been proved to do what it purports or is represented to do". The former Bureau of Drugs Associate Director for Compliance, Theodore Byers, the lead agency official in the monitoring of GMP compliance, offered the following definition: "Process validation is the attaining and documenting of sufficient evidence to give reasonable assurance, given the current state of science, that the process under consideration does, and/or will, do what it purports to do."[10] Validation is the core of a quality control system integrated throughout the manufacturing system. Quality is built in, not tested in, by means of a systematic approach determining whether or not equipment and processes meet design specifications. Such a system of ongoing checks, indication that equipment is properly calibrated and operated, materials properly monitored and handled, and sterility seals properly installed and maintained, serves to assure manufacturers (as well as regulators) that a manufacturing operation works as it should, time and time again. Instead of judging product quality solely on the basis of finished-product testing — often inadequate or cumbersome — process validation collects data from raw materials to end product, following everything that happens in between. Its purpose is to demonstrate consistent performance of the manufacturing system. Validation calls for manufacturers to keep abreast of current technology and practice, using state-of-the-art monitoring devices, electronic control mechanisms, statistical analysis, and special tests designed to "challenge" the system as necessary to demonstrate the integrity of the system. Validation may be outlined as follows:

1. Choosing the desired attributes of the product
2. Determining specification for those attributes
3. Selecting appropriate processes and equipment
4. Monitoring and testing processes, equipment, and personnel while in operation
5. Examining test procedures themselves to ensure their accuracy and reliability

It becomes readily apparent that process validation encompasses many key or critical steps in the manufacturing process. The formal documentation of validation is relatively new and may be found in various stages of implementation by pharmaceutical manufacturers worldwide. The degree of sophistication of GMP for any particular country generally is a good indicator of the state of validation being implemented.

Whereas process validation is concerned with the manufacturing process and identification of critical steps, the basic objectives of a system suitability test (SST) is to manufacture, filter, and fill a growth medium into a final market package without introducing any microbial contaminants. Thus, an SST is in actuality a comprehensive validation study designed to evaluate the three major components of a sterile processing area: (1) the personnel who work in this environment, (2) the suitability of the equipment used for the tasks they perform, and (3) the general cleanliness of the sterile area itself. The formalization of this testing procedure is also relatively new, particularly in developing countries, and is extremely important. The successful completion and documentation of SSTs has become a prerequisite for the processing of sterile clinical goods and parenteral products in the U.S., and is now being implemented overseas with GMPs.

G. QUALITY CONTROL

Quality control is in different stages of development throughout the world. The U.S., Canada, Europe, and Japan are generally considered to be the leaders in terms of standards such as registration requirements and the enforcement of these requirements. U.S. multinationals have adopted the policy that they will accept anything that is stricter than what their standards are in the U.S. In Sweden, topical ointments must be sterile. In addition, the manufacturing of sterile products must start with a material that has a very low microcount, and Sweden specifically wants everything possible terminally sterilized. Therefore, there is a stricter requirement in Sweden in terms of microbial purity of a material that is going to be sterilized, as well as the requirement for topical products to be sterile. The European Pharmacopeia requires antimastitis products to be sterile, which is not the case yet in the U.S. There has been a movement to have WHO regulations take precedence over many local pharmacopeias, but this goal has not been achieved. The USP/NF continues to be a guiding standard for many countries, but the European Pharmacopeia has achieved parity in many parts of the world, especially Europe. The WHO has a quality control training program to improve quality control in developing countries. The pharmaceutical industry is actively supporting this undertaking.

Assay specificity and stability-indicating assays in Europe, Canada, and Japan are very similar to those in the U.S. Other countries are developing in these areas. The multinationals attempt to start with one control procedure. However, if an HPLC assay, for instance, is required, it will soon beçome evident that some countries not only do not have the equipment, they will not accept the procedure. An alternate assay method must be developed. Other countries without this instrumentation will allow the registration of a product with a high-performance liquid chromatography (HPLC) assay method as long as the company performs the assay. These restrictions vary from country to country. Japan insists on microbiological assays for antibiotics. They will not accept gas chromatography or HPLC assay methods. The availability of in-country equipment service and appropriate reagents must be considered when registering an assay to be run by HPLC. There may be no service available, or only one or two representatives in a large geographical area. Multinationals may want to provide the latest technology, but may be prevented from doing so for lack of instrument service or assay materials.

Environmental control programs are often difficult to implement. Validation and systems suitability testing programs are needed to regularly monitor conditions in sterile manufacturing areas. Difficulties arise when multinationals must work with contractors in countries where their own facilities do not exist, and where the technology does not exist to understand what is wanted. Biological control systems are also difficult to implement.

The administering of quality control programs internationally must cope with many problem areas such as communication, language, consistency, technical competency, problem solving, and organizational depth. These may best be addressed by careful selection of people for key positions in the affiliates, regularly scheduled plant audits, and the conducting of extensive training programs by the parent company.

ACKNOWLEDGMENTS

The authors thank the following people for their invaluable help in providing information in their areas of expertise: A. J. Aartila, G. K. Crankshaw, L. E. M. Hines, O. A. Kreuzer, W. A. Struck, and J. S. Turi, J. W. Munden, E. A. Hardwidge, and A. D. DeVisser. Special acknowledgment is extended to P. C. Carra for his editorial comments and encouragement.

APPENDIX

Additional Sources of Information

A. General Reference Sources

1. Pharmaceutical Manufacturer's Association, International Division, 1100 15th St. N.W., Washington, D.C. 20005.
2. Proceedings of the Conference on Pharmaceuticals for Developing Countries, National Academy of Sciences, 2101 Constitution Ave. N.W., Washington, D.C. 20418, January 29 to 31, 1979.
3. International Federation of Pharmaceutical Manufacturer's Associations, Nordstrasse 15, P.O. Box 328, CH-8035, Zurich, Switzerland.
4. World Health Organization, Director Division of Prophylactics, Diagnostic, and Therapeutic Substances, 1211 Geneva 27, Switzerland.
5. Pan-American Health Organization, 525 23rd St., Washington, D.C. 20037.
6. Vernon, R. and Wells, L. T., Jr., *Economic Environment of International Business*, 2nd ed., Prentice Hall, Englewood Cliffs, NJ.
7. Kapoor, A. and Grub, P. D., Eds., *The Multinational Enterprise in Transition*, The Darwin Press, Princeton, NJ.
8. The World Today Series, Skye Corporation/Stryker — Post Publications, Washington, D.C.

B. Technology Transfer — General

1. *Survival Kit for Overseas Living*, Intercultural Network/Systran Publications, Chicago, IL.

2. Samovav, L. and Porter, R., *Intercultural Communications: A Reader*, Wadsworth Publishing, Belmont, CA.
C. Pharmaceutical Training Films and Slides
    1. Good Manufacturing Practices training film series: *Growing for Aseptic Areas: Handling and Control of Materials*; and others. Parenteral Drug Association, 1206 Western Savings Bank Building, Broad and Chestnut Sts., Philadelphia, PA 19107. Distributor: Milner-Fenwick, 2125 Greenspring Drive, Timonium, MD 21093.
    2. Microbes, Sanitary Practices, and You, Cosmetic, Toiletry and Fragrance Association, 1625 Eye St. N.W., Washington, D.C. 20006.
    3. No Margin for Error, U.S. Food and Drug Administration. Distributor: Precision Film Laboratories, 639 9th Avenue, New York, NY 10036.

REFERENCES

1. *Health Horizons*, International Federation of Pharmaceutical Manufacturers Association, No. 5, September 1988.
2. **Anisfeld, M. H. and Anisfeld, E. R.,** *International Drug G.M.P.s,* Interpharm Press, Prairie View, IL, 1979.
3. *Script World Pharmaceutical News*, p. 10, July 28, 1980.
4. *The World Drug Situation*, V, World Health Organization, Geneva, 1988.
5. *Script World Pharmaceutical News*, p. 10, July 28, 1980.
6. **Kreuzer, O. A.,** International Drug Registration, *Food Drug Cosmet. Law J.*, 43 (3), 564, 1988.
7. *Fed. Regist.*, 43(190), 45014, 1978.
8. **Murty, R.,** International G.M.P. requirements, *Pharm. Technol.*, 4, 177, 1980.
9. **Anisfeld, M. H. and Anisfeld, E.R.,** *International Drug G.M.P.'s*, Interpharm Press, Prairie View, IL, 1979, 2.
10. Process validation in drug manufacture, *Drug Cosmet. Ind.*, 44, 1980.

INDEX

40 CFR 160, 103
40 CFR 792, 103
U.S. Code, Title 35
  Section 101, 232
  Section 102, 232—234
  Section 103, 234
  Section 112, 234—235
  Section 116, 235
U.S. Food and Drug Act, drug screening under, 52
Uric acid, metabolism analogy in drug design and, 46
Usage, drug, approved, 2

V

Validation procedures, for computer systems, 37
Validation studies, statistical support in development
  of, 97
Venture capital funding, start-up companies and, 60

W

Warnings, attached to product
  adequacy of, 224
  false assurances and, 225
  limitations on duty and, 224
  postmanufacture, 225
  reasonably foreseeable misuses and, 225
  scope of duty and, 224
  standard of liability and, 223—224
  unreasonably dangerous nature of product despite
    warning and, 225
Waxman-Hatch Act, generic versions of post-1962
  drug products and, 214
Western Europe, see also European Economic
  Community

multinational pharmaceutical companies based in,
  268
  pharmaceutical industry in, 279—280
WHO, see World Health Organization
Word processing, in administrative management, 33
Work-load measure, in program project plan, 8
World drug consumption, geographic distribution of,
  272, see also Drug consumption, per capita
World Health Organization (WHO)
  Essential Drug Programs of, 276
  Nairobi conference under auspices of, 283
  national expenditure on health assessed by, 271
  quality control regulations of, 294
  twenty largest drug markets assessed by, 278
  world consumption of pharmaceuticals by region
    assessed by, 278
  world drug consumption assessed by, 271
Wound healing, therapeutic innovations in biologics
  and, 64
Written description requirement, patentability and,
  235

X

Xanthine oxidase, metabolism analogy in drug design
  and, 46
X-ray crystallography, designer drug development
  and, 70
X-ray spectroscopy, biochemistry of disease assessed
  via, 46

Z

Zero defects approach, to pharmaceutical elegance,
  281